Committed to the Sane Asylum

Committed to the Sane Asylum
Narratives on Mental Wellness and Healing

Susan Schellenberg
Rosemary Barnes

Wilfrid Laurier University Press
[WLU]

We acknowledge the support of the Canada Council for the Arts for our publishing program. We acknowledge the financial support of the Government of Canada through the Book Publishing Industry Development Program for our publishing activities.

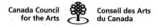   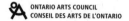

Library and Archives Canada Cataloguing in Publication

Schellenberg, Susan, 1934–
    Committed to the sane asylum : narratives on mental wellness and healing / Susan Schellenberg and Rosemary Barnes.

Includes bibliographical references.
ISBN 978-1-55458-034-7

    1. Schellenberg, Susan, 1934– —Mental health.   2. Barnes, Rosemary Ann.
3. Mental illness—Treatment.   4. Art therapy.   5. Narrative therapy.   6. Artists—Canada—Biography.   7. Mentally ill—Canada—Biography.   8. Psychologists—Canada—Biography.   I. Barnes, Rosemary Ann II. Title.

RC339.5.S33 2009   616.80092   C2008-901649-1

Portions of the Introduction and some of Susan Schellenberg's artworks were published previously in "The Pleasures of Healing, the Possibilities for Mental Health Care," by R.A. Barnes and S. Schellenberg, *Canadian Woman Studies/les cahiers de la femme* 24: 194–99.

The lines by Raymond Carver at the end of chapter 8 are used by permission of Grove/Atlantic Inc. Copyright © 1989 by the Estate of Raymond Carver.

Cover design by Chris Hoy and David Schellenberg. Interior design by Pam Woodland.

∞

This book is printed on Ancient Forest Friendly paper (100% post-consumer recycled). The paper used in the colour section is approved by the Forest Stewardship Council (FSC).

Printed in Canada

There is a crack in everything.
That's how the light gets in.

●

From "Anthem," *The Future* (1992),
written and sung by Leonard Cohen,
produced by Leonard Cohen and Rebecca DeMornay

Contents

Acknowledgements

WE THANK THE MANY PEOPLE who have encouraged and advised us. The medical record librarians at the former Queen Street Mental Health Centre and Kingston Psychiatric Hospital kindly assisted in locating the clinical records of Susan and her uncle, Leo Marrin Regan. David Guiffrida, Legal Counsel to the Psychiatric Patient Advocate Office, provided us with information about legal considerations in the use of clinical records. Dr. Mary Seeman, Dr. Brenda Toner, Dr. Margaret Malone, Paul Hogan, Helen Porter, Gail Regan, and Dr. Cheryl Rowe all generously donated their time not only for conversations but also to review background materials and to read and correct transcriptions of the conversations. Dr. Seeman has encouraged our work in important ways well beyond conversation with us. Gail Regan has been generously supportive of our creative efforts over many years. Helen Porter died in September 2007 as we were in the final stages of preparing this book; her life and stories were an enormous inspiration and we deeply miss her. Psychologists Dr. Patricia DeFeudis and Dr. Rickey Miller contributed much insight into hospital functioning. Heather Jacko and Gayla Aitkens completed initial transcriptions of our tape-recorded conversations. Psychiatrist Dr. Cheryl Rowe, psychologist Dr. Sarah Maddocks, Nancy Webb, and Maureen Edgar read and commented on earlier versions of the manuscript and provided much appreciated encouragement; Dr. Rowe repeatedly answered questions and shared her considerable knowledge about the concerns and psychiatric care of people with serious mental illness. Nancy Webb assisted greatly on a final edit of this text, particulary with names and references.

Jacqueline Larson provided gentle encouragement and incisive critique during the final stages of manuscript revision and steered us to Wilfrid Laurier University Press, where the guidance and enthusiasm of editorial, production, and marketing staff have sustained us to complete the final work associated with publication. Jacquelyn Waller-Vintar provided professional editing services for an earlier version of the entire manuscript. Family, friends, and the gang at Fraser Lake supported us in many ways including providing feedback on various title and book cover suggestions. James Madden read sections of the manuscript and pointed out the need for a glossary. Chris Hoy and David Schellenberg provided us with helpful technical support as well as a lovely cover design. Various individuals at the Centre for Addiction and Mental Health (CAMH) supported us—we would like to give particular thanks to Jean Simpson, former Chief Operating Officer at CAMH and Dr. Paul Garfinkel, former Chair, Department of Psychiatry, University of Toronto, and President and Chief Executive Officer of CAMH.

Susan Macphail, Louise Fagan, Elaine Pollett, and Sheila Simpson, who formed the Shedding Skins Committee of the London Women's Mental Health and Addiction Action and Research Coalition (WMHAARC), invited us to present a talk and slide presentation to a large London, Ontario, audience in April 2000. The standing ovation we received at the end of the evening encouraged us to believe that this book could offer hope to many people.

Introduction

Susan

"There will be a place for Susan after the war, Mrs. Regan," was the doctor's response when my mother asked if something could be done about my artistic nature. It was 1939. I was five years old and the Second World War had just begun. Armed with my father's promise that a day would come when pictures of war would no longer be on the front pages of newspapers, I settled into dreaming as I waited for war to end.

Close to VE day, I dreamed a marriage between two fish. The fish, dressed in traditional human wedding attire, sailed off to their honeymoon in a seahorse-drawn carriage. My grade five teacher and my mother, both disturbed by the excellence of my fish composition, jointly concluded that despite my effort, a grade of 60 rather than 100 percent would better serve the taming of my imagination and good of my soul.

There was no let-up in my Irish Catholic grooming. I was taught to pre-weigh each pleasure for its potential sinfulness, to confess my sins on Saturday, and to artfully express loveliness with practised white-gloved receiving-line entrances. While the seeds of the Vietnam war were being sown and the Korean and Cold wars were raging, I trained as a nurse, travelled the obligatory three months in Europe, then broke with the Regan tradition of marrying Irish by falling in love with a first-generation German Canadian. While my husband worked at excelling in business, I gave birth to the first four of our five children in four years, helped nurse a dying father and a mother who suffered a stroke shortly after his death, and gave my all to being a glamorous corporate wife. Though exhausted, I blossomed.

Then, in 1969, as an estimated 1 million Americans across the US participated in anti–Vietnam War demonstrations, protest rallies, and peace vigils, I too began to protest, but my demonstrations took the form of a psychosis.

I was treated solely with prescribed antipsychotic drugs during my three-week stay in Toronto's Lakeshore Psychiatric Hospital and for the ten years that followed. My former husband and I understood psychiatrists had explained that my illness was schizophrenia. My willingness to take the drugs was influenced by a nursing background that taught how schizophrenia was a chronic, irreversible, degenerative illness controlled solely by drugs; I was also compelled by my four small children's need of a well mother. I was additionally persuaded that drugs were a necessity by graphic and disturbing extremes in schizophrenic behaviours that I witnessed during my nursing career as well as during my stay at Lakeshore Psychiatric Hospital. The lack of any other explanation or meaning about my diagnosis given to me by my caregivers, and my willingness to place sole authority for my health in doctors' hands increased the effect of these motivating factors and contributed to my certainty that I suffered from a chronic illness with no hope for recovery.

Ten years later, while Quebec was considering a split from the rest of Canada, I too threatened to split apart. My suicidal urges triggered by antipsychotic drug side effects began to manifest and accelerate. On one of the darkest days in that period, the smallest of acts (my first ever in my own best interests), led me to find a psychiatrist willing to supervise my withdrawal from the drugs. Soon after my decision to withdraw from drugs, I made deep commitments to heal my mind from the causes of my psychosis, to heal my body from the drug side effects, and to paint a record of my dreams as my mind and body healed.

Reagan in the White House in the early 1980s mirrored my repressed maiden Regan parts. *My* "white house" was a construct of frozen feelings, knock-off Nancy suits, and patriarchal drives. But random dreams in this period echoed hints as well of Trudeau's attempt to repatriate Canada's constitution. The beginning of this coming home to myself was announced through a dream that voiced, "I feel as if I have been asleep for over a thousand years." The dream's "Sleeping Beauty" mysteries unfolded over time through the ordinary processes of my decaying suburban life and marriage.

I was forty-six. My once-auburn hair began to need hennas. A full year's tests and failures of available mascaras to correct my newly blurring vision prefaced my first pair of prescription glasses. I was patriarchal woman to the core. Yet, the extraordinary other occurrence of this time was the appearance in my life of mentors and helpers. The feminine principles that informed the mentors' art, dream, and story skills set the foundation for the change in my patriarchal codes of self-governance.

As the Cold War was coming to an end, the front lines of my war moved through our front door. Traditional marriage values clashed with my withdrawal from the antipsychotic drugs. The simultaneous loss of my religious beliefs stirred additional conflict. Whether driven by humour, compassion, or both, the energies or inner wisdom providing me with mentors and helpers made enormous allowances for my emerging, anxious/depressed, rage-filled, unlady-like self as well as for my increasing assumption that I was in league with the devil.

The more I dared to rebel and benefit from my mentors' diverse perspectives on story, myth, symbol, and dream, the more permission I found in the early Sleeping Beauty dream to wake from the life I was living. As I unlearned old myths that named women's growth suspect and wrongfully opposite to serving the Catholic patriarchal ideal, I came to see wellness and its pleasures as a good.

I met Rosemary Barnes in 1990, close to the time my dream art first went public. Although we have never shared a psychologist/client relationship, Rosemary is prime among my mentors. The steadfastness of her friendship, kindness, humour, and encouragement of my commitment to heal have been of invaluable support while I resolved the last issues at the core of my earlier psychosis and also came to peace. While writing this book, Rosemary organized a series of conversations on my illness and psychiatric records with leading people in the fields of psychiatry, psychology, sociology, art, healing, and business. The feeling of being safely contained in these conversations allowed me to bear the original feelings that accompanied the onset of my illness. It also helped me to make sense of and overcome the harms that were caused by the wrongfully explained diagnosis and treatment methods I experienced. The same series of conversations provided me with a more global view of women's mental health and how it has been traditionally perceived and treated. Seeing the treatment of my illness as one small piece of the twentieth century's mosaic of psychiatric care released the shame I'd felt about my own mental illness, so I could eventually replace my rage with justifiable anger before finally letting it go.

Before meeting Rosemary, no mental health practitioner I had encountered as a patient or during my training as a nurse encouraged or gave me hope that I could commit to healing and growth as I understand and live it today. Any antipsychiatric literature I read prior to writing this book echoed and validated my early rage and cry for help but failed to offer me ways to heal and move away from the rage.

As I uncovered and moved away from rage, new realizations emerged about events in my earlier life. My story describes these realizations and their occurrence within my chronological history. My goal in telling my story is to track a single commitment to heal and to illustrate how this long-ago and initially fragile expression continues to this day to sustain and nurture growing degrees of wellness in me. Because art was as unique to my talents and interests, it served as my important means of healing. I believe commitments to heal can be as varied in their processes as the people who make them.

In offering my psychiatric hospital records in Appendix II, I hope readers from the mental health professions will benefit from knowing the hospital's side of my story. My final intention is to illustrate as well as celebrate how healing occurs in relationship. Before and since I dared to know, speak, or write my story as I do now, my relationships with mentors, family, friends, as well as with adversaries and strangers mirrored my soul in ways that inspired, encouraged, empowered, or forced me to gain wellness through expressing my story.

My outer journey from despair to a meaningful life and my inner journey from unconscious knowing to conscious understanding of my psychosis core were marked by a light and dark that grew synchronously lighter and darker over time. The slow cyclic deaths of my false selves and tiny perfect births of my new self were informed by images found in dreams and the arts. The many wars that marked the historical eras in which my mental illness and healing occurred are briefly remembered at the beginning of each chapter. Where spindoctors sell war as a noble or even entertaining human endeavour, I hope our reminders of war will lend insight to the fact that my illness did not occur in a void nor can it be dismissed as a chemical imbalance. Within my psyche, the inner light and dark at war support my healing by forming a Zen-like koan, a spiritual exercise, an idea without apparent logic that, when resolved over time and through the imagination, arrives again and again at an increasingly peace-filled truth. At the point where I knew the truth of my psychosis story, the image of war and its by-then-outworn subjective and symbolic meaning dissolved into our book's metaphor for madness.

Rosemary

Healing was never mentioned when I began training as a clinical psychologist, about seven years after Susan was hospitalized with a psychotic break. Although my graduate studies in psychology had prepared me to become a university professor, scarce employment opportunities forced a career change. In September 1976, I began a postdoctoral fellowship in clinical psychology at the Clarke Institute psychiatric hospital, an apprenticeship of the kind undertaken by students in every health profession both then and now. Had any one mentioned healing, which few did in mental health settings, I would have considered the word flowery, quaint, or quirky with connotations of primitive or marginal beliefs and practices, as in "faith healing." Had I been challenged, I would have argued that patients improved, so clinical practices must be beneficial; a poetic word such as healing was simply inappropriate in a scientifically grounded professional setting. At the time, I would not have recognized that clinical constructs and terminology could be hiding some significant lacunae in theory and practice.

In 1969, as Susan protested through psychosis, I protested by falling in love with one woman, then another. Because I had grown up in a conservative religious American family, I understood these experiences to be equivalent to mental illness and deeply shameful. By 1976, I reluctantly reconciled myself to the conclusion that such feelings meant I was a lesbian. I met other lesbians and gay men in the 1970s ferment of the gay liberation and feminist movements. Lesbian-feminist groups, new friendships, and the electric creativity of the day allowed me for the first time to locate myself with confidence in the larger world. Feminist ideas infused my life with new meanings and possibilities. I learned feminist and antipsychiatry critiques of mental health care and resolved to be a better professional than those I read about.

For some years, I had a professional career that I understood and enjoyed. After postdoctoral training, I worked for nine years as a staff psychologist at Toronto General Hospital, a university-affiliated facility, and matured as a clinician and researcher. In 1986, I moved to the smaller Women's College Hospital as head of the psychology department and moved to address the split between my personal and professional lives by joining a small informal group of hospital professionals working to nurture feminist values in health care. I met Susan when she and I worked in the same political faction during the turbulence surrounding a proposed merger between Women's College and Toronto General Hospital.

Then I became lost. My ability to live with the split between feminist values and professional career commitments eroded as I became increasingly unconvinced that hospital mental health care gave paramount concern to human well-being. I felt cynical, exhausted, and angry about my apparently successful career.

Although we had met earlier, I learned of Susan's experiences with mental health care in 1992, when she exhibited her paintings at Women's College Hospital as part of a commemoration for women staff and engineering students who were murdered in Montreal on 6 December 1989. What Susan had to say exceeded the limits of the exhibit and reflected the dilemmas in mental health care that I found persistently troubling. Around the time we agreed to work together, I resigned my hospital position to begin an independent clinical practice. I was relieved to no longer have to support an institution that I found hostile to my own well-being and that of my patients, but I felt a failure for abandoning a career path associated with power and prestige.

I realized gradually that I was working with Susan with the hope of healing this wound within myself. My inability to reconcile my work as a hospital psychologist with my commitment to feminist values and process was a major reason that I left hospital practice. Though I never wished to reverse the decision, I wandered for years, troubled about the choice and what I might have done differently. Susan's taking responsibility rather than blaming, her introductions to artists and writing on art, and her insight into the connection between healing of the person and healing of the world all influenced me profoundly. Healing required collecting the disparate and conflicting fragments of my personal and professional experiences and fitting them together to form a new story of my life's work.

Susan and Rosemary

What goes wrong in conventional mental health care has been catalogued at length by feminist and antipsychiatry critics for over thirty years: Restrictive gender stereotypes, questionable diagnostic systems, patronizing or abusive professional practices, harmful psychoactive medications, and disregard for more humane and effective approaches to care.[1] We like a critique provided by Marilyn French, who argues that our choices about the world originate in our values.[2] In her critique of mental health care, French examines the valuing of power and transcendence that is enacted when doctors and patients engage in subduing passions, illness, frailty, and dissent for the sake of "normality" and "success." We travelled this road, we tried to transcend—Susan, for the sake of becoming a "normal" wife and mother, Rosemary, a "successful" professional. We tried, as French puts it, "to produce humans fit for this world rather than a world fit for humans."[3] Fortunately, we failed.

French's alternative is a new ordering of human values to give the highest priority, somewhat shockingly, to pleasure. French suggests turning within to identify what makes living desirable and satisfying, accepting our dependence on the earth and other people, and leading lives that give the greatest importance to the deep pleasures associated with the beauty of the earth, the company of others, and the freedom to choose our commitments and the means of self-expression.

When experiencing unbearable despair, each of us, first with wordless groping, later with increasing clarity, committed to live differently, to engage in a creative undertaking. We turned within and examined our lives to locate our deepest values, then worked to honour these values in our day-to-day thinking, relationships, and activities. We came to prize living "with an eye to delight."[4] We focused, to put it in health care lingo, on well-being and quality of life.

If the shift to valuing pleasure sounds oh-so-lovely (cue sunshine, birds chirping, soft music), please excuse us for being completely misleading. Read on and you will find that we both moved in desperation across dark and terrifying landscapes, certain only that we could not go on as we had before. We will tell of inching along shadowy precipices of fear and doubt, harrowing encounters with outer and inner critics, lonely nights in moonless landscapes, painful deaths of false selves, and other trials too terrible and numerous to mention just yet. We also mention diverse mentors who appear, unanticipated sunlit meadows of light and calm, and the springs of confidence and fruits of knowledge that became ever more abundant as we travelled. It is only looking back along the path that we appreciate the movement from inner realm to outer and outer realm to inner, one realm constantly informing the other; the encounters with the unexpected, painful, or delightful; and the reliable freshness, earthiness, colour, and creative possibilities. Along the way, Susan became an artist and Rosemary, a different kind of psychologist.

In the spirit of living with an eye to delight, even in the midst of war, we write to offer thoughts on a different vision for mental health care. We feel it is helpful to talk about healing. Healing is different from "conquering" disease, achieving a "cure," or "managing" a condition; indeed, such concepts and terminology reinforce the discourses of power and transcendence. We think of healing as growth in ability to love and forgive self and other, to cope, to feel pleasure, to engage in meaningful activity, and to follow the psyche's inner direction away from addiction and towards greater wholeness. Healing is a creative process relying on an inner capacity that is neither created nor destroyed by professional care, but amenable to nurturing.

We believe that healing is relational and tied to the earthy specifics of individual and community life. We tell our personal stories together in order to challenge the conventional doctor/patient relationship and to show how this crucial relationship can and should be reorganized. We mean *doctor* broadly to refer to any professional providing patient care, for example, physician, nurse, psychologist, social worker, physiotherapist, and *patient* to describe individuals seeking care from doctors. In the *realpolitik* of conventional mental health care, the doctor (or nurse, psychologist, social worker, occupational therapist) is seen as the confident, powerful, infallible expert responsible for maintaining order by making quick, accurate diagnoses and providing effective treatment. Patients are seen as weak, distressed, needy, foolish, and sometimes threatening dependents responsible for "getting well" by following the directions of the doctor. Such relationships form a command-and-control system of the type that is being abandoned as ineffective in many areas of commerce and business. Such relationships leave many patients and doctors as exhausted, harmed, and frustrated as it left each of us.

To be clearer about how her professional practice has evolved, Rosemary uses Susan's experiences to present a series of imaginary case studies. In each of these case studies, Susan's difficulties and life circumstances are assumed to be as they were at the time of her 1969 hospital admission and Rosemary role-plays the professional providing care to Susan. What changes over the series of case studies is Rosemary's approach and the setting as Rosemary moves from hospital to hospital and then to independent community practice. In contrast to the usual practice, the doctor rather than the patient is the focus of these case studies.

Other people have been profoundly important to our healing, and we will relate readings and conversations with scholars, mentors, and colleagues. We were particularly moved by a series of conversations that we had in 1996 as we began this book. In 1995, Susan pointed Rosemary to the work of art historian Suzi Gablik on the possibilities for a paradigm shift in art. In *Conversations Before the End of Time*, Gablik converses with individuals immersed in the world of art concerning whether the current approach to art is sustainable in a world facing unprecedented ecological and political crisis.[5] Rosemary admired Gablik's way of providing a respectful place for multiple perspectives and felt that she and Susan could honour the diverse interpretations of Susan's emotional crisis in the same imaginative way. So we sought out people with an interest in mental health and healing and arranged a series of conversations with six individuals who had backgrounds in mental health, the arts, and business. We quote from these conversations in some detail because they ultimately became important aspects of the healing that we both experienced. We keep in mind, and hope our readers will as well, that these individuals may think or talk about things differently now than they did at the time that we conversed with them.

We met in the context of local hospital politics (a kind of war zone), worked together as friends, and have never been in a doctor/patient relationship. However, our ability to learn from one another, to collaborate, to nurture each other, to appreciate strengths, and to balance weaknesses is an example of the honest, mutually respectful, interdependent relationship we see as essential to healing and well-being. We believe that such a healing relationship is possible in many contexts, including the doctor/patient relationship. We represent this in the writing ahead as we have so far, that is, by passages where we each tell our separate stories, as well as passages where we relate shared conclusions.

We hope that this book shows in practice what we deeply believe: that emotional disturbance—and who among us has not experienced this in some form?—can be best addressed by living with an eye to delight and commitment to the creative, relational, earthy process of healing.

Notes

1 See for example Persimmon Blackbridge and Sheila Gilhooly, *Still Sane* (Vancouver: Press Gang, 1985); Peter Roger Breggin, *Toxic Psychiatry* (New York: St. Martin's, 1991); Bonnie Burstow and Don Weitz, eds., *Shrink Resistant: The Struggle against Psychiatry in Canada* (Vancouver: New Star, 1988); Pat Capponi, *Upstairs in the Crazy House* (Toronto: Penguin, 1992); Phyllis Chesler, *Women and Madness* (New York: Avon, 1972); Barbara Everett, *The Fragile Revolution: Consumers and Psychiatric Survivors Confront the Power of the Mental Health System* (Waterloo, ON: Wilfrid Laurier University Press, 2000); Courtenay M. Harding, Joseph Zubin and John S. Strauss, "Chronicity in Schizophrenia: Revisited," *British Journal of Psychiatry* 161 (1992): S27–S37; Irit Shimrat, *Call Me Crazy: Stories from the Mad Movement* (Vancouver: Press Gang, 1997); Thomas Szasz, *The Myth of Mental Illness* (New York: Harper and Row, 1974); Thomas Szasz, *Schizophrenia: The Sacred Symbol of Psychiatry* (Syracuse, NY: Syracuse University Press, 1988); and Philip Thomas, *The Dialectics of Schizophrenia* (New York: Free Association, 1997).
2 Marilyn French, *Beyond Power: On Women, Men and Morals* (New York: Ballantine, 1985).
3 French, *Beyond Power*, 382.
4 French, *Beyond Power*, 542.
5 Suzi Gablik, *Conversations Before the End of Time* (New York: Thames and Hudson, 1995).

1 Normal Beginnings

> A shadow has fallen upon the scenes so lately lighted by Allied victory. Nobody knows what Soviet Russia and its Communist international organization intends to do in the immediate future, or what are the limits, if any, to their expansive and proselytizing tendencies.... From Stettin in the Baltic to Trieste in the Adriatic, an "iron curtain" has fallen across the Continent.... The Communist parties ... are seeking everywhere to obtain totalitarian control.
>
> —Winston Churchill, "The Sinews of Peace"[1]

SUSAN
A Daughter, a Wife, a Mother

I WAS BORN IN 1934, into a "power-over" struggle between my mother, her deceased victim mother, and their shared story that began to haunt my life as the rise of fascist governments seeking world domination were determining the 1939 outbreak of World War II. By the time I was a young adolescent, an iron curtain had been drawn through my inner geography that mirrored postwar Europe's geographical and adversarial split into two political systems. By the time I was a young adult, the wall of rigidity that defined my "sweetness/badness" split and its domino effect of other selves came to be as rigorously guarded, as systematically toxic, and nearly impossible to breach as the Cold War's Berlin Wall.

I don't mean to mistake my own experience with the real war experiences of real peoples. I instead use the idea of war partly within an art history context that reminds us how evolving outer world events are echoed in the arts as well as in the diverse forms of thought, science, and mechanical invention that influence life in each era. War as an image serves as the toughest and oldest of realities to push against, especially when my personal life choices at the time were narrowed to making war or making peace. The twentieth century's story and mine mesh at certain points—making peace with self holds the much-needed possibility of benefiting our children and their future generations and the potential as well to widen acts of conscious care of self into care of each other, the environment, and planet.

Daughter

I was the second of four children born to a third-generation Irish, middle-class family. My mother, Ann Catherine (née Ronan) Regan, and father, Joseph Patrick Regan, provided my siblings and me with an education, social life, and spirituality based on the ideals and ancient rituals of their rigidly upheld Roman Catholic faith. My secondary convent schooling, post-secondary training as a registered nurse at St. Michael's Hospital, and public health studies at the University of Toronto represented an advanced education compared with what my parents received from their parents.

Appearances were important to my parents. My mother possessed a unique sense of style. Prior to her marriage at age twenty-two, my mother had modelled and sold a line of women's clothing right across Canada. My father's father was a tailor, so dress was integral to his expression of self as well. My parents adhered to a religious philosophy that placed a high value on Catholics converting non-believers by presenting an appearance of goodness, happiness, and success. Conditioned to believe that money was the "root of all evil," my parents measured acceptable material success by what they achieved—to the penny—and regarded anything beyond what they had earned as a potential danger to the soul. They were critical of people who were more financially comfortable. Those with greater wealth who happened to disclose their humanity and good works before the fact of their wealth were automatically exempt from this judgment and treated as family. But, where status was concerned, it was the friendship of the parish priests who frequently visited our home that was my parents' most sought-after and revered social contact. While the morals of the larger culture were held in question, family appearances were still influenced by idealized images of family, as depicted in artist Norman Rockwell's *Collier's* magazine covers of the 1930s and '40s and reinforced in radio and later television programs of the *Father Knows Best* genre.

A complex story cooked below our happy family surface. My mother was hard on the outside, fragile within. Traumatized in childhood by her own father's abandonment of his family, she was further hurt by her Catholic community's marginalizing of the fatherless family and by the resulting poverty and added hardship of the Great Depression. She worked ceaselessly throughout her life at being first in my father's and her Heavenly Father's affections. The religious goal caused her to be rigorous about organizing her children's salvation. My mother also determined to make me tough, so I would survive and escape her own victim mother's fate.

My mother remained at home after her marriage, keeping abreast of the world and informing the integrity of her homemaking skills with popular women's journals. She gained energy through daily phone calls with a life-long friend from her modelling days and both women shared close friendships and monthly bridge games with six other women. My mother provided us children with superb physical care and created nurturing social rituals with extended Catholic family and friends.

Despite these social relations, my mother believed that "he travels fastest who travels alone" and "you do not want to be like the pack"—these oft-repeated expressions encapsulated her ways of coping. Equating survival and success with isolation caused her to dress in a more stylish manner than her friends and to direct us to stand out rather than to blend comfortably with our friends. I sensed deep scorn for my friends in her use of these sayings.

Shortly after I entered nursing in 1953, my parents moved to Thornhill, which was then a small village north of Toronto. My father's postwar business success, reflected in the home they bought, gave my mother the sense of security she lacked from childhood and through the war years. My mother joined her new parish's Catholic Women's League (CWL). Although she saw herself as unlike the pack in the CWL setting and was constantly annoyed by the group, she moved up quickly to become vice-president of the Toronto Archdiocese CWL and was asked to also join the board of the Toronto Catholic Children's Aid Society. In these positions, she admired the organization heads but mainly scorned her peers.

Her sophisticated European style of dress fuelled her bravery and sense of self. It was apparent to me that she also grew spiritually through dress and used fashion in the best sense of theatre to bring life to my father. In the world beyond our home and while she held executive positions in Catholic agencies, I sensed that clothes were my mother's protective armour.

Her managerial skills were best shown shortly after I married when she helped spearhead a Thornhill community effort to bring a middle-European refugee family of seven to Canada. My mother befriended the family long after the committee that brought the family to Canada disbanded. In addition to arranging a rent-to-own home agreement between the bank, the family, and railway—on whose land stood the original shell of the home the town had renovated by hand and made livable for the family—she made certain the father always had work until he found a well-paying lifetime position with benefits and pension.

I was deeply touched the several times I accompanied my mother on afternoon visits to the mother of this family. For those visits my mother, dressed simply and without any of her usual "one up/one down" dynamic, would sit and share mutually with the woman under a tree in her garden. I recall my mother being more relaxed and at home in the refugee woman's garden than in her own home.

Throughout my childhood, my mother's disapproval of me was often expressed with the reminder "I have never been able to stand the sight of your face, not since the day you were born." She followed this remark by ordering me to confess to the priest how I had been the cause of her anger. When I was sixteen, my mother's oldest and most toxic sister informed me that my mother was furious when she discovered she was pregnant with me.

My mother disciplined me severely with frequent spankings and enemas and forced me to repeat a hundred times into a mirror that I was a liar or bad. My bowel training began when I was old enough to sit upright on a pot and persisted until my pre-nursing physical at age nineteen. At that time, when the family doctor asked me, "How are your bowels, Susan?" my mother answered, "Bill, I still cannot get her to have her movement first thing in the morning." The doctor's "Oh, for Christ's sake, Ann!" brought my bowel training to an end.

At the beginning of each school year, my mother made a point of informing my teachers that I was deviant and encouraged them to strap me when needed. Following these visits, she relayed her school visits to the family in a way that implied "Susan won't be pulling the wool over the teacher's eyes this year." Shortly after one school visit, the teacher, without mentioning my mother by name, locked me in her stare while explaining my mother's directive to the class and asking them to consider the mother's sorrow at being driven to these lengths.

At age eleven, I openly felt hate for my mother after she struck me forcefully on the side of the face with a steel hairbrush. I withdrew in silence for several days until I could no longer bear my separateness or her rejection—I reluctantly broke our separation by creating cards and poetry that expressed my apologies and intentions to never cause her to be angry again. Art from early on proved a successful tool whenever I needed to atone, to pacify, or regain my mother's forgiveness and approval.

My mother's inability to nurture psychologically caused me to embrace the Catholic god and my father as the major love figures in my life. Having to choose between God and my father, I chose God who seemed the safer bet (except for His aversion to sin, which I became over-scrupulous in guarding against). The close bond between my mother and my father dictated his standing behind her every decision whether or not it was fair. My constant childhood need to keep my mother and God appeased was so evident that a parish curate confessor encouraged me to begin spiritual training to become a nun.

My siblings and I were expected to demonstrate pathological levels of obedience and were forbidden to speak up, or out, or back—a conditioning that shaped my later habit of seeing other people as being in authority, and repeatedly pleasing others whether it was warranted or deserved. After I'd worked a year as a nurse in St. Michael's emergency department, my mother, fearing that hospital shift work would lessen my chances of finding a husband, forced me to take a Bermuda vacation on my own. During my Bermuda absence, my mother arranged with the Victorian Order of Nurses for me to receive a bursary to study public health at the University of Toronto and agreed on my behalf that I would work for that organization for a year. By the time I married at age twenty-six, I was submissive to the degree that I acquiesced to my mother's purchase of my wedding gown without me, and accepted that I could not see the dress until the night before the wedding.

My first awareness of the pain in my mother's extreme self-loathing came in the last hours of her life. Her final words, "I don't know how anyone like me could have had a daughter as lovely as you," shocked as well as freed me to later explore her effect on my life. My mother's words and the freedom I felt when our years of ritual mid-week lunches, Sunday dinners, and her daily phone calls ended were such a contrast to the way her grandchildren saw her and how much they missed her and the approval she had showered on them. In her later years, both the parish priest and family doctor suggested that she might be mentally ill; this allowed me to persevere through art and therapy processes until I found and accepted her full humanity.

My father was thirty-three, eleven years my mother's senior when they met during the Great Depression. He was a master salesman and owned several homes. But he was also a party boy and in debt. My mother assumed and maintained control of their finances which helped him clear his debt, change his friends, and give up drinking for life in the first two years of their marriage. He experienced financial setbacks during the war years, but prospered in the post-war years. My father was elegant in his dress, wearing clothes like a second skin. He blended in anywhere because he cared deeply about people. Growing up in Toronto when Bloor Street was the city's northern limit and signs reading "CATHOLICS NEED NOT APPLY" closed doors to employment and large segments of the community, my father learned charity in a church that took care of its own through building hospitals, schools, and varied facilities for Catholics in need.

I cannot recall walking in the downtown area with my father without his meeting a boyhood friend. Many of these men were in dire straits and my father would pass them a ten- or twenty-dollar bill hidden in his handshake. His greeting always suggested true friendship and delight in the meeting. As if to name his kindness and charity, he sometimes said, "The only thing you can take with you is what you give away." My father was a mentor to a number of young men. He was humorous, and loved and respected by many. His doting on me was a great buffer against my mother's harshness. My mother's behaviour toward my father was that of a bossy, loving courtesan. My father adored her and assumed a nice-guy role with us children. Whenever the affection or gifts that my father gave to us seemed excessive to my mother, she would react negatively towards us rather than confront him. Although he failed to protect us from my mother's abuse and was uninvolved in our disciplining, I equated my father's passivity with gentleness and favoured him more than my mother. My father died in 1962 at age sixty-four, three months after my first child was born. Two years after my father's death, my mother suffered a massive stroke. She struggled to regain a restricted but independent life until 1974 when at age sixty-six she died of another stroke. My fifth child was two years old at the time of her death.

My parents achieved a close, loving relationship though they held many opposite views, particularly concerning finances and how children should be taught to regard money. When I began to babysit in my teens, my mother told me to refuse payment for my services. When I received my first paycheque after graduation from nursing, my mother demanded the return of the entire weekly allowance she had given me over the course of my three-year nursing training. Two dollars weekly allowance in the first two years and three dollars in the last year was large in terms of my twenty-six-hundred-dollar yearly salary. In that instance, my father, rather than confront her over this lack of fairness, gave me operating money for my second month of work and never asked to be—nor was he—reimbursed. Similarly, despite the fact that I was given no say in the planning or budgeting for my wedding and I was allowed only two friends as guests, my mother expected me to cover a substantial part of its cost. My father rescued me on that occasion as well and suggested we not tell my mother.

Wife

At age twenty-six, I initiated an enormous break from my parents' Irish traditions when I met and married a first-generation German Canadian. My husband, a highly intuitive, hard-working, and ambitious engineer, excelled in marketing and business management.

His childhood during the Second World War was made difficult by the fact that his family were the sole Germans in a rural Ontario community of mixed middle Europeans. During his junior school's war effort, he was forced to do math on the blackboard for refusing to help with any project that might harm his parents' German relatives. "That is why I now excel in math!" was his response. Rather than being crushed, he also turned classroom humiliations, name-calling (he was called a Nazi), beatings, and bullying experiences into positives.

Although his family lacked the means to give him music lessons, they required him and his sister to listen every weekend to broadcasts of the New York Metropolitan Opera and New York Philharmonic Orchestra.

After winning a General Motors scholarship to train in auto mechanics in Michigan, he was persuaded by a teacher that he was capable of going on to university. One year later he enrolled, then excelled, in civil engineering at Queen's University. He was hired and trained by a large American company and eventually headed their Canadian manufacturing and sales subsidiary operations.

My mother made numerous attempts to derail our courtship. She projected of her own victim mother onto me: "You're a gentle soul like my mother, Susan. You will never be able to stand up to him." As I left for my honeymoon, her parting comment was, "He will be lots of fun, but he will never be faithful."

My fiancé and mother locked horns over issues of control. While they battled, I took on a peacekeeping role and developed short-term ulcer-like symptoms. My mother wanted a long engagement that would buy time for me to change my mind. My husband wanted a brief courtship and a Boxing Day wedding that would allow us to take a ski honeymoon and for me to be a tax deduction. My husband won Boxing Day at the pain-filled cost of acquiescing to my mother's demand that he replace his chosen best man with his sports celebrity brother-in-law.

In spite of their power struggles, my mother was charmed by the attention my fiancé paid her, and he admired and respected her courage. My husband reflected many of the brash, self-made qualities that my mother most admired in men. I now see that part of my attraction to my husband was a hope that he would gain me my mother's approval. His ritual gift to her—a bottle of champagne, which they'd drink together before our Friday-night dates—brought out her coquettish side and gave her enormous pleasure. I later saw how his belief that he had to win my mother to win me was linked to his self-assigned boyhood role of keeping his own victim mother happy. "It was my job to make my mother laugh." My mother and husband's honeymoon/fight relationship foreshadowed the cycles he and I would later enact as a couple. But, prior to marriage, both my mother and fiancé treated me as too gentle or naïve to keep up with their games.

My father was fond of my husband, enjoyed sharing time with him, and gladly mentored him in business whenever my fiancé sought his advice. Unlike my mother, my father encouraged me to marry my husband if I loved him. However, as my father's health worsened over the course of our courtship, we kept my parents company over numerous games of bridge. Though our bridge fights did not prompt my father to discourage us from marrying, he did suggest that since we planned to marry, we should buy a set of pistols. When my father died, shortly after the birth of our first child, my husband expressed his loss by saying, "He was more of a father to me than my own father."

German Husband

My husband's German immigrant background was an issue for my parents as well as for me. My mother's struggle for community approval from childhood onward was threatened by the fact her chosen community, in the postwar era, followed the larger culture's practice of conferring an inferior status on new Canadians by calling them DPs (displaced persons).

When my mother's efforts to break our engagement failed, she encouraged me to charm and persuade my fiancé to change his name to an Anglo-Saxon one. Timid as I was about taking on a German name so close to the war, I admired and found strength in my husband's pride of name and still hold to that pride when I sign myself Schellenberg.

My father placed an uncharacteristically harsh judgment on my husband's parents that implied they were Hitler sympathizers. More than once I heard him say, "The only thing they are sorry for is that Hitler lost the war." Considering that Mr. Schellenberg senior had often told me that he'd come to Canada in 1929 to avoid Hitler, I sense my father's failure in kindness and judgment was triggered when his feelings towards me and towards his many close Jewish friends became severely conflicted by my marrying a German Canadian in the acutely painful post-Holocaust period.

Being German through marriage brought unaccustomed social rejection after I married. My father's Jewish friends continued to call me "Miss Regan." Friendly Jewish merchants often turned hostile after I stated my married name for an invoice. In hospital, after the birth of our first child in 1962, a European nurse came to my room to give me perineal care, a procedure administered then with warm saline solution, gauze wipes, and metal forceps. As the nurse proceeded, I noticed her arm bore a Nazi brand of concentration camp numbers. Overwhelmed with guilt, I reached out, touched her arm, and said, "I am so sorry." As I did this her forceps pressed into and cut my perineum.

The Schellenberg seniors who had worked, sacrificed, and often insisted, "We don't matter as long as our son and daughter have everything," had, according to my husband, fought viciously throughout his childhood. These fights were distressing enough that my husband on one occasion drove his fist through a door in response. My husband would often invite his parents to visit us but soon after they arrived, he would drive to his office, leaving me to spend entire days with them. My mother-in-law, bringing her own pots, pans, and food, would announce, "I can't eat her food" (meaning *my* food), and tell the children they would eat and be properly looked after now that she had arrived. "I pity you children," she said.

On one of the Schellenberg seniors' early visits, their fighting caused me to scream hysterically at them, "You are not to fight in my home." My mother-in-law's response, "It's my son's home, not yours," added to the awfulness of their fight. To get distance from my in-laws on that occasion, I broke my own mother's rule that I was never to come home to her with marriage problems. I took the children to her home for a brief visit and tea, but felt too shamed to tell her about my in-laws' fight and insult.

My father-in-law, who held an idealized view of women and was far kinder to me than to his wife, expressed as the highest form of compliment that I was like his, "saintly victim mother." Mr. Schellenberg senior described his own father to me several times as a cruel, oppressive man. If Mr. Schellenberg senior was a loner by nature, he was isolated further by being German in a time of war and by his diverse intellectual capabilities. A master tool-and-dye maker by trade and a self-educated student of classical music and the humanities, he had a command of English that was uncommon among his co-workers. He and his wife built their own and two other homes in an isolated Ontario lakeside community. But he was Spartan to the point of never letting Mrs. Schellenberg decorate their home and he made a point of defining her work as solely a duty before their children.

Rather than Mrs. Schellenberg's own marriage experience encouraging kindness toward me, my husband's mother told me bluntly at our first meeting that her son deserved a wife with better social connections and a sturdier work physique. Her ritual welcomes to us as a couple over the years involved long adoring glances at her son accompanied by her saying, "Ach! Schelly, you are so beautiful!" Then shaking her finger at me she would say, "You are one damn lucky girl!"

Hardened by her husband's put-downs of her intelligence and his denigration of her importance to his and their children's lives, I believe that it was her grandchildren's love that eventually softened Mrs. Schellenberg. In time, Anna also came to show me the beautiful unused linens she had brought to her marriage from Germany. My mother-in-law never changed her wording, but the sting disappeared from her welcomes when our children began to show signs of becoming fine adults. From that time, she began to credit my contribution to their development.

My husband's and my Irish and German backgrounds found common ground where our shared traditional views on marriage were concerned. We agreed that he was to be the breadwinning head of the house, while I was to assume the role of a glamorous, obedient helpmate who provided children, along with sexual, domestic, and emotional support. In the early years, we mainly regarded our eccentric mothers as courageous warhorses and tried for each other's sake to be respectful and caring towards each of them. But our psychological naïveté and inability to individually, let alone mutually, resolve our childhood wounds fuelled many quarrels.

Mother

Our first four children were born between 1962 and 1966. At my mother's prompting my husband began a tradition of buying me couturier outfits after each of the baby's births. When our daughter was close to four months old, my husband, who was rarely home because of his work, witnessed me changing her diaper. He was so shocked at seeing her bowel movement he exclaimed, "My god! How often has that happened?" before rushing out to buy me roses. After the birth of our second child and my bout of infectious mononucleosis, my husband began helping me with diapering the children at night. I cannot remember him as being anything but caring and loving toward the babies when he was at home. He was also fully engaged later with my seeking and following the advice of the Institute of Child Studies, at the University of Toronto. We fitted a playroom with art materials and creative toys they'd recommended and over the years made a habit of buying only those toys that allowed the children to construct from their imaginations.

Our neighbours were cordial but distant, so I remained fairly isolated in our suburban home over the next twenty years. My nursing background was an asset to my care of the children, but rapid multiple pregnancies and my husband's extensive business travel and long hours at work led to my having near sole care of the children and being in a constant state of exhaustion. Our shared expectations for me to be glamorous and ready at a minute's notice for business events stayed in place when the children were little and later when I was drugged and they were in their teens.

Though we appeared to be and believed we were an ideal couple, our early happiness and passionate sense of adventure was very real only when I was pregnant. When I was not pregnant, my husband increasingly denigrated my appearance, sexuality, and interest in or practice of art. Even if I was told at the last minute to settle the children's needs and get myself ready to go to dinner with a customer, my husband would react to my hair or some part of my outfit being less than perfect by saying, "I am disappointed, Susan—I expect you to look perfect. You have a responsibility to the company and looking after the children is no excuse." Raised on criticism and accustomed to handing authority to others, I absorbed his comments as if I deserved them.

Economics played a significant role in our taking one-up/one-down positions in the marriage. Once married, I gave my entire paycheque to my husband. On becoming pregnant, I gave up my job and allowed him to sell my car and keep the sale monies. Without access to a bank account, without easy means to travel from our lakeside apartment in the suburb of Mimico, I was completely financially dependent on my husband. He gave me money daily as each grocery and household need arose. Weekly grocery shopping checkouts were anxiety filled because I was given only the amount of money I estimated our groceries would cost. I did not receive a household allowance for the first twenty years of the marriage and learned to get what I needed either by pleasing, being seductive, and/or being submissive. I was given beautiful clothes if my husband chose to give them to me, but his whim determined what I would wear and how my clothing and household needs got met. We were also conditioned to devalue my work of raising children and running a home because it lacked monetary value. When people asked, "Do you work?" I responded, "No, I am a mother."

ROSEMARY
Becoming a Doctor

In the 1970s, some years after Susan became a wife and mother, I learned to become a doctor, more specifically, a clinical psychologist. For six years, I had studied in a psychology graduate program at McMaster University where I trained in experimental psychology research. My specialty involved studying learning in simple animals as a means to understand human learning; for several years, I conducted scientific experiments on how motivated (that is, hungry) pigeons learned to identify a conditioned stimulus (in this case, the illumination of a plastic disc) as a signal for an unconditioned stimulus, that is, food. In June 1976, I completed the final academic test of my abilities by explaining and defending my research studies before a committee of university professors. My doctoral thesis was entitled, "The Effect of Temporal Spacing on the Development of Autoshaped Key Pecking in the Pigeon."

These graduate studies prepared me to conduct experimental psychology research as a university professor, but in 1976, thousands of young people were completing graduate training, and universities received hundreds of applications for every faculty position. For a year, I collected advertisements and mailed my resumé to psychology departments across North America. Mount Holyoke College, a small women's liberal arts college in Massachusetts, flew me in for an interview. I bought a blouse with a large bow at the neck, a pair of dressy pants, and a blazer to wear for the interview. I spent hours preparing a presentation about what influenced my pigeons' learning. However, when not offered a position, I was secretly relieved because I had not enjoyed research on animal learning and dreaded being pledged to teach and conduct research in experimental psychology. I had chosen to study psychology because I liked people. Intellectually exciting mentors had persuaded me to pursue research, but my heart lay elsewhere.

I applied for positions in clinical psychology, hoping that I could learn on the job. In the spring 1976, I had an interview at an Ontario residential institution providing services to people described at that time as mentally retarded. The older psychologist who interviewed me explained gently that he could not hire me because the colour of my hair was wrong. "If you had white hair, I might be able to hire you because, though you do not know anything about clinical practice, patients and their families would see your hair and think that you are old and wise. But you are young, you look young, and you are not qualified to do this work. Sorry."

I then looked for training and in September 1976 was accepted for a postdoctoral fellowship at the Clarke Institute (now part of the Centre for Addiction and Mental Health), a prestigious, university-affiliated psychiatric hospital in downtown Toronto. The postdoctoral position involved a clinical apprenticeship of the kind undertaken by students in every health profession both then and now. I was assigned to work with a staff psychologist and, under her direction, was responsible for conducting clinical assessments for the in-patient Mood Disorder Unit. As I became more knowledgeable, I was given opportunities to see patients for psychotherapy.

On the advice of Dr. Harvey Brooker, the senior psychologist who mentored me, I applied for a provincial licence to practise clinical psychology, which required my becoming a member of the Ontario Board of Examiners in Psychology (now the College of Psychologists of Ontario). To become a member, the aspiring professional must have a certain level of education, complete a period of professional practice under the supervision of a senior practitioner, pass written and oral examinations, and agree to work in accordance with ethical and professional standards. Any person who wishes to do so can provide counselling or administer psychological tests without the licence provided by membership in a professional college. However, because reputable institutions and businesses hire only licensed professionals, being a member in good standing has powerful benefits. Learning to work in a manner satisfactory to my psychologist supervisors at the Clarke Institute was essential to become a member in the Ontario Board of Examiners in Psychology. I bought new skirts, more bowed blouses, lined wool pants, and another blazer as well as dress shoes and nylon hose to wear on days when I put on a skirt.

Note

1 Speech given at Westminster College, Fulton, MO, 5 March 1946. Available at http://www.hpol.org/churchill.

2 Protests

"One, two, three, four! We don't want your fucking war!"
"Hell no, we won't go!"
"Make love, not war!"

—Slogans used by Vietnam War protesters
in the 1960s and 1970s

SUSAN
Patient

ON 2 SEPTEMBER 1969, as young Americans and students slated for draft into
the United States armed forces were questioning authority and protesting the
Vietnam war, the real me who had remained divided by an inner iron curtain
since childhood erupted in protest as well. My protest probably originated in
the legacy of repressed 1840s Irish Potato Famine rage that had gone unchecked
through generations of my maternal and paternal lines. My own outcry gained
my attention in the form of a psychotic break three years after the birth of my
fourth child in four years.

Like citizens who are given the facts of wars that are controlled, manipu-
lated, and interpreted by political, industrial, and media powers, I spent years
accepting the officially provided interpretations of my 1960s and 1970s experiences, for lack of other sources of information.

However, when the courage emerged to commit to changing my story and
the wisdom grew to see how psychic wars are solely lost or won on truth, I
embraced a thirty-year war between my "good" patriarchal woman self and

the real me she silenced. The spoils of that war were the awakening of a new feminine consciousness and abilities to feel, to nurture, and to create from the core of my being. As the conscious understanding of my story grew, I began seeing my hospital experiences through different eyes.

What follows is an account of the events and official interpretations as they unfolded in the era of protests. I was thirty-five years old at the time of the break and for the prior eight years had been isolated in Etobicoke, a Toronto suburb, while discovering my sexuality, raising children, and lending support to my husband's career.

Birth Control Issue

My first brief and guilt-ridden attempt at taking the religiously forbidden birth control pill lasted several months following the birth of my third child. After my fourth child was born, I stayed on the pill for three years. By the fourth pregnancy, our ability to afford live-in help allowed us to begin taking evening walks together. The added freedom and routine physical exercise allowed me to feel better at the end of the fourth pregnancy than I did at its beginning. Live-in help also enabled me to begin the study of art one day a week as soon as our fourth child was off his night feedings. Although I was free to garden and I enjoyed doing so, my husband, like his father with his mother, forbade home decoration as a needless frill. My husband's attitude so thwarted my need to create beauty that his control forced my buried artistic spirit to the surface.

The Three Schools of Art, where I studied, was on Markham Street, a trendy, boutique-filled street in Toronto's Annex. My one day a week at art school filled me with energy and contentment. At home, one side of the kitchen counter began to hold baby foods and the other my paints and brushes. I expressed with growing skill and abandon and enjoyed the company of artists for the next the three years.

By my third year on the pill, the freedom to enjoy my children, to study art, as well as to cook and to meet new artist friends could no longer mask the lessening of my husband's affections when I was not pregnant. I wanted to please him, missed his affection, and felt guilty about being on the pill. However, because I was too Catholic to consider therapy to help me deal with these difficulties and too exhausted to face another pregnancy, I shrunk my unconscious dilemma to an action I could cope with at the time. I went to a Catholic retreat to look for a loophole that would allow me to continue using the birth control pill.

I held the considerable inner conflict I brought to the retreat in a slender coltish body. I was slim, but heavy with fatigue from a bout of infectious mononucleosis I'd contacted in July 1963 between the second and third child, and from an exhaustion that built between the births of my third and fourth children when I helped nurse my mother over a six-month period following her 1964 stroke. Weeks prior to the retreat and my breakdown, I was weakened further by a pericardial infection.

The Retreat and Onset of Psychosis

My husband, with our four children in the back of the car, drove me to the retreat. He was cross during the drive saying, "I don't like your doing this" and "I don't know why you need anyone's permission to use birth control." I felt the loss of his love, a loss of the kids, and alone. As I entered the retreat space, I was isolated further by the fact that 90 percent of the retreatants were nuns and priests. Many of the clergy appeared to know each other well. If I took an empty chair at one of the dining tables, the clergy would politely ask my name, give their "How lovely" approval when satisfied that my four children under six years of age signalled adherence to my Catholic duty, then resume their private conversations without me.

At one of these lunches a priest repeatedly pushed a dessert at me and ordered me to eat it. Though I was trained in pathological obedience to the church, priests, and my mother, an acute loss of appetite caused me to politely but repeatedly refuse the dessert to the point that another priest beside me yelled at the bully priest, "For God's sake, leave her alone."

Another retreat memory that stays with me involved the time I happened on a group of nuns delighting at how one of their sisters had dared in chapel to answer a priest who collectively asked the nuns, "What is it you nuns expect from us priests?" Pathological as the nun's celebrated response, "We expect you to be holy," later showed priest–nun dynamics to be, I interpreted the story as proof of the nuns' greater authority at the time. My birth control concerns paled in the shadow of the nuns' idealic expectations for men to be holy rather than human.

The clergy's celibate and pure status at that time in history carried the powerful energy of a "higher calling," which implied a superior status for clergy over that of lay people. My identity never being strong in the first place, I absorbed this devaluation of my gender and sexuality as an absolute in the retreat setting.

Although I had come looking for support of some kind for birth control, the retreat focused solely on social ministry as exemplified in the work of Mother Teresa. The steady rhythm of back-to-back sermons was presented without the aid of body work to assist the retreatants with their grounding of the spiritual information or their guarding against overload. After six days and nights of continuous sermons and sleeplessness, I began to manifest confused thinking outwardly and was in worse shape than when I arrived. At that point, the retreat director called my husband to come and take me to a doctor. I left the retreat convinced that I had failed and that my work at home was insignificant compared to that of Mother Teresa's.

The five days I spent at home following the retreat and prior to being hospitalized are difficult to recall or put into sequence. We were fortunate that we had a kind and excellent live-in *au pair* who remained supportive to the children and us even in the face of my building psychosis.

My husband's first response when I returned home was to ridicule the retreat. This put-down terrified me to the point I gathered all the children and *au pair* into the car and drove them back to the retreat, which was still in progress. I brought the children and *au pair* into the chapel just as a sermon was about to begin. Afterwards and without being invited, I took them into the dining area to join the other retreatants at lunch. We left for home after lunch. My sense now is that I was perceived as being mentally ill and was mainly left on my own during this visit.

My husband, the children, and I kept a family dinner invitation at the home of friends during my pre-admission time. Years later, the friend told me how bizarre their evening with us was. She mentioned that she and her husband realized I was mentally ill but because my husband kept joking and saying how great things were going for us, they felt helpless to help me. What I mainly recall of that evening was how my friend's exceptionally beautiful eyes filled me with terror whenever she looked at me.

I also managed in the pre-hospital days to paint a portrait of my second son that was favourably critiqued later, but my attempts to follow a daily routine were increasingly interrupted with delusions.

Psychotic Thinking

My psychotic types of thinking included thoughts that germinated from the retreat master's discussions on suffering and how each person was in some way wounded and in need of compassion. To illustrate his theme, the retreat master offered an image of the "other" as the "Suffering Christ" as a method of tapping into compassion for others. After my husband brought me home from the retreat, I tried to adopt this way of seeing him in the hope it would help our relationship. It was not hard to envision my husband as wounded because he had often shared information about painful events in his childhood. However, as my mind's "computer" broke, I could not keep metaphor and reality straight.

The more ill I became, the more I determined to fix our relationship by relating to his wounded side with the "Suffering Christ" image. As realities of the relationship that were too difficult to associate with the Christ figure came up, I reacted oppositely and confused my husband with the devil. My Christ/devil swings became more rapid and intense. Without treatment, I also spun out of control with fear, feelings of worthlessness, and with erratic, God-pleasing plans to correct my ways.

My God-pleasing peaked in a devastating manner. My medical records quote my husband as saying we attended Sunday mass, but over the years the memory of the second mass I attended that Sunday overshadowed my memory of the first. I recall how prior to leaving the house for the second mass, my eye caught sight of a painting I had done the prior Christmas. (The painting was a work I had created by drilling a gessoed board full of holes, threading wire through the holes, and then shaping and painting the wire into the three magi figures.) I grabbed the painting and car keys and when my husband rushed after and tried to stop me, I nearly drove him down as I backed out our drive. I drove to a church where I knew a late mass would be starting. By now I'd forgotten about the painting, and I entered and stood at the back of the church. Several priests and altar boys were walking in procession from the back of the church to the altar. The congregation was standing. I waited, staring into the church rather than taking a seat. The next thing I recall was the pull of a vacuum-like force propelling me towards the altar. When I arrived at the altar, the pulling sensation disappeared.

I became filled with the humiliation, knowing how fanatic and foolish my holding on to the main altar crucifix would seem to the congregation. Though I wore an appropriate cream-coloured dress and had continued, despite my emotional state, to exhibit habits of good personal care, I grew doubly distressed and convinced that the congregation was witnessing a menstrual stain on the back of my dress. One of the priests muttered, "Get her off the altar," and the next thing I felt I was being coldly (or more likely fearfully), off-loaded into a car and driven to Queensway Hospital Emergency. My husband, notified by the church, arrived in the emergency department sometime later. His first words were, "Get dressed; we are getting out of here." The nurse urged us to stay, saying I was schizophrenic and the psychiatrist had been called, but my husband's only goal was to get me out of there. When we arrived home, I would not go into the house and was forcibly dragged in by my husband.

I believe now that my husband's initial refusal to get psychiatric treatment for me resulted in part from his being conditioned by his father to believe that illness was something one should not display; his mother viewed hospitals as "death houses." His mother's death house concept appeared to be a passed-down European notion from the pre-germ-theory era when hospital childbirths routinely ended in childbed fever deaths due to a lack of doctor cleanliness. Though my father-in-law never lacked a good job and never missed a day's work after immigrating to Canada, I imagine his attitude towards illness was reinforced by the bleak economic circumstances he faced in Germany between the great wars and the fact that as an English-speaking German immigrant he was the only ship passenger to obtain work when he landed in Canada near the end of the Depression. In any event, my husband's unwillingness to seek treatment for me was not out of character. He himself sometimes endured severe bouts of pain for two weeks or more without seeking medical attention or even simple relief like aspirin.

For the two days following my being taken from the Queensway Emergency, my husband remained home from work and devoted his time to straightening my thinking. "Okay, Susan, now I know you can do it. Can you tell me who I am?" If I said, "Yes, you are Schell," he would say, "Good girl. Now are you sure of that? Shall we try one more time just to make certain? Take your time, Susan, and when you are ready, tell me who I am. Just remember, you are doing great. Who am I, Susan?"

As my tendency to swing increased, I probably responded next with "You are Christ" or "You are the devil," to which he would patiently reply, "No, no, no, Susan, you have to try harder, I know you can. Now I am going to give you a big hug and we will try once more." If he tried to hug me when I was in my devil thinking, I would shrink from him: "Get away from me, I know who you are—you're the devil."

Hospital Admission

The more my thinking deteriorated, the more my husband tried to make me well but eventually he was forced to ask for help. Our family doctor instructed my husband to bring me to the Emergency department at St. Joseph's Hospital where the doctor arranged my admission to Lakeshore Psychiatric Hospital (LPH). I was admitted to LPH on the evening of Tuesday, 2 September 1969.[1]

Despite having worked for a year as an emergency staff nurse following nursing graduation, I failed to connect to my reality in the hospital's emergency department. But as soon as our car pulled onto the LPH grounds, I realized it was a psychiatric hospital and that I was mentally ill. Although I did not want to be mentally ill or in hospital, I recall being relieved to know what was happening to me. Before leaving the car, to enter LPH's Cottage number three, my husband asked me to promise that I would get well and come back to him and the children. I was clear in my promise and determinations to get well from that moment onward.

Cottage Three's non-cottage-like mass was anchored between Cottages Two and Four. Years later, I recognized something of the essence of LPH's Cottage Three when photos I took of it in its 1996 barbed-wired and boarded-up state due to architectural similarities accidentally became mixed in with other recent photos I had taken of Auschwitz in Poland. In 1969, LPH cottages faced through barred windows onto short cottage lawns and a hospital service road before opening onto spacious tree-covered grounds that ended at the lake. Numerous similar cottages extended behind Cottage Three towards another open space that led back to the hospital's gated entrance. Beyond the hospital gates, Lakeshore Boulevard, dotted with used-car dealers, small diners, laundromats, drab box apartments, and broken-down shops established the sadness hidden behind the hospital's lush grounds and trees.

After completing my admission, my husband kissed me goodbye and a nurse took me to a bed in a sub-basement ward. With the exception of an older toothless patient who shuffled to my bedside to mumble a strange coded welcome, the other patients stared at or beyond me. As the nurse injected drugs into my hip, my body's chemistry changed instantaneously from one way of being into another and my mouth completely dried up. For the rest of my first night, I lay with terrible hallucinatory thoughts, experienced myself as being punished for being bad, and listened to other patients' horrific cries. I repeatedly prayed, "God, I promise never to be bad again if you'll just make this go away."

The drugs brought a quick end to my Christ/Devil thinking. My other types of psychotic thinking at the time of admission ended more gradually. Included in these was my speculation that I might be the Blessed Virgin Mary (BVM). My BVM notions grew from questions such as, "Well, who am I, if my husband is Christ?" Because my husband and I were so enmeshed in our everyday reality it seems reasonable to assume that I tried to construct a relationship of similar proportions during the psychotic period. My BVM thoughts warred with entirely opposite ones that argued I was delusional, a heretic, evil and grandiose for thinking of my husband and myself in these terms. It was humiliating to have to admit to doctors that I was thinking these thoughts, but I was also afraid I would not get well if I did not own up to them. My thoughts about being the Blessed Virgin did not originate in cockiness about having arrived on top of some cosmic heap—they terrified me.

My BVM struggles were further aggravated by the attending psychiatrist who, during my admissions physical examination, remained staring at my belly for a disconcerting length of time. While he looked and looked at my belly, I was still spinning with the notion that I might possibly be the Blessed Virgin, so I intuited that he was overly fascinated by my lack of stretch marks.[2] Having been told from childhood that Mary remained a physical virgin even after Christ's birth, I began wondering if the psychiatrist was as hooked on this Blessed Virgin business as I was. When he announced, "No stretch marks!" as if that was the main conclusion of his examination, I began to wonder if he might actually be St. Joseph. Curious to see if I was right but not wanting to look even more insane if I wasn't, I asked the psychiatrist, "Have we ever met before?" When he said we hadn't, I returned to accepting him solely as a doctor, but his "No stretch marks" comment contributed to my Blessed Virgin delusions lingering a while longer.

Bizarre and ill as my Christ/Devil and BVM symptoms were, I continue to see them as mirroring a pattern in my reality, given that I was prone to extremes in black and white thinking and that my husband and I increasingly related with enormous swings on issues of acceptance/rejection, closeness/distance, and tyrant/victim behaviours.

My efforts to be a model patient were aimed at obtaining a quick discharge. Each bed move that I made to an upper level of Cottage Three was the hospital's way of signalling my gain in stability. "Good," as in "compliant," patients slept on the top floor, the less good slept on lower floors. My move to the third floor meant my discharge was imminent if my progress held.

My sole rebellious act during my hospitalization came when I was taken to a room to package party balloons and whistles for outside manufacturers. I was instructed that yellow balloons were to be attached to the red whistles and red balloons to the yellow whistles, but the garish colours together were so offensive to me that I spent an entire morning attaching red with red and yellow with yellow. Scolded and ordered to go to the art room instead, I was happy that I never was sent back to the whistle factory.

My memory of being ordered to the hospital grounds for what proved to be a surreal game of dodge ball disturbs me to this day. To watch psychologically fragile people being hit with a ball was bad enough, but then their lack of coordination caused by drugs made them topple. Seeing them fall on the ground only to be told they had disqualified themselves from the game would no doubt have set me in a rage if I hadn't been as drugged or determined to be discharged.

The privacy I lost by being in a ward felt minor compared to certain shames I experienced, like being forced while in the visitor room with my husband to expose my hip for an injection in front of other patients and their visitors. It was also crushing to witness appalling patient behaviours and experience the sense of hopelessness that followed when nurses brutalized the patients who acted this way. Cottage Three held several patient cliques but the relating within these groups could turn on a dime from enmeshed to hostile so I was content to remain pretty much on my own.

Being on my own was also made easy by my husband who, because his office was not far away, would visit and walk with me once or twice a day on the hospital's beautiful Lake Ontario grounds. My husband's care and love for me at that time and in that psychotic state was a gift that painful later events dimmed for a number of years but did not and never will erase. A number of the women patients would routinely wait by the window for my husband to appear so his tenderness towards me brought hope to others as well.

The fact the children needed school clothes, and that I asked and received permission to go clothes shopping with my husband early in the second week, confirms my sense and what the records show—that I stabilized fairly rapidly in the first week.

The doctors' "happy ever after" message at the time of my hospital discharge implied that I was being officially returned to my former "normal" life and would fit perfectly into that life as long as I took drugs.

Who We Became after the Breakdown

The benefit of having domestic help and a busy routine after hospital discharge was that, unlike mentally ill persons who are placed in boarding homes and left to idly roam the streets during the day, my mind and body had a steady, easy-to-follow daily structure that allowed me to become naturally tired, to take charge of nurturing and relating to others, and to experience and encourage the life energy and play in my children's lives. With the avoidance of stimuli such as television and movies and the resumption of our evening walks, I made steady progress at becoming well.

As a couple we shared a deep appreciation for what we considered a second chance. The beginnings of our ability to laugh again came one night in the guise of a symptom that caused me to check with my husband if he too had just heard a neighbour's dog bark. The timing of his jest that he hadn't heard a sound, then seconds later assuring me not to worry and that it was a real dog, provided much-needed laughter and shared pride in our ability to survive a difficult time.

Normality, in terms of our traditional marriage, was achieved on many levels fairly soon after I returned home. Though it was a standard appliance to most of our friends, my husband's gift of a dishwasher left me feeling thoroughly spoiled. With my desire to do art nullified by drugs and the dishwasher leaving me more free time, I returned to my pre-psychosis "I-am-not-doing-enough-compared-to-the-work-of-Mother-Teresa" thinking. As a result, in the first year after leaving the psychiatric hospital, I began to voluntarily care for two intellectually disabled children one day a week. The children's parents were grateful for the relief this help brought them and I found relief in feeling useful.

In the context of my actual experience—I was giving care to my four small children, my mentally ill aunt (more on her later; see chapter 5), my mother, and the handicapped children—my exaggerated "I am not doing enough" might have been more appropriately viewed as low self-worth, guilt, and an agenda for discussion in psychotherapy.

But psychotherapy was never once recommended or prescribed. Month after month, year after year, I visited Lakeshore Psychiatric Hospital's outpatient department (OPD). For these visits I dressed my best and presented the perkiest face to ensure I would not be readmitted. My husband often accom-

planied me on the OPD visits in the early years. The psychiatrist would simultaneously write and query my husband if he were in attendance and me if I
were alone. After one or two questions the psychiatrist closed the visit by handing me a new prescription and saying, "I will see you again next month."

In the mid-1970s, my OPD care was transferred to our family doctor. The
doctor barely disguised his fear of me, barely disguised his annoyance that a
mentally ill woman had been thrown among his grander class of clients. My
psychiatric treatment from 1969 to 1980 never varied from this sole prescrib-
ing of antipsychotic drugs, together with a medical judgment that I later came
to view as steeped in gender bias.

One year after my hospital admission, I became pregnant with our fifth
child. More tired with the fifth than with my other pregnancies, I gave up my
care of the disabled children but continued with our evening walks. We originally wanted five children and my husband, though still very much wanting
a fifth, was afraid to have another child because the doctors told him I should
not get pregnant. My husband's "I would love to have a fifth, but am afraid of
getting you pregnant" became a terrible Catch-22 for my mind to hold at that
time. The pressure of wanting to please my husband while also obeying doctors led me to reduce the issue to a question of "fear" or "love" and to decide
for the pregnancy. However bizarre my decision may appear now, our fifth
child, born in June 1971, was, like all his siblings, a love child and continues,
as they all do, to be a joy to each of us still. My obstetrician, who later told of
the fears he had for me during the pregnancy, spoke of his amazement at my
becoming increasingly well as my term progressed.

The fact that the pregnancy anchored me so deeply in my body at a time
of mind/body splitting seems to have made an enormous contribution to my
recovery. Following the birth of my fifth child, and on the condition of my
husband and a St. Michael's Hospital committee giving their consent, I obtained
a tubal ligation. As a couple we had discussed the possibility of my husband
having a vasectomy at that time, but the procedure was too tied to loss of man-
hood for him and the peace of mind that I felt was necessary to my sanity could
be secured only with my having a tubal ligation. Rather than causing religious
torment, the surgery empowered my psychic health and provided a vital
demythologizing of my outworn beliefs about birth control. The surgery's
combined effects of relief and interruption to my daily routine caused my
mind to become slightly overactive short-term. But as I had taken the precau-
tion to ask for an increase in my drug dosage to tide me over the operation, I
stabilized and returned to a smaller drug amount quickly.

Even though I was still heavily medicated with antipsychotic drugs, by ending my need to seek the approval of a church that demanded more than I could

deliver and the social forces that named my reproduction choices pathological, I was more opened by the tubal ligation for the process of becoming me.

After the birth of our fifth child when life began settling into a more normal routine and the older children were at school full time, I made a decision
to go without the help of *au pairs*. Inspired by my husband's employer philosophy, "Pay well and expect hard work," I began tying the children's weekly
allowance to their helping me to clean the upstairs one week and the down-
stairs the next; they measured up magnificently. However, with my recovery,
my husband gradually returned to his habit of criticizing, silencing, and putting me down. To maintain my sense of reality when put-downs occurred was
even more difficult than before. His negative comments would take me into
my head where I would spin word scenarios hoping to come up with a cute,
endearing response that might appease him and prevent his becoming angry.
After the breakdown, I was less capable of not splitting during this mental
reaction. To prevent getting emotionally worn down again, I made a decision
to never communicate with my husband unless he spoke to me first.

My decision to not speak to my husband unless I was spoken to brought a
quick end to his put-downs and mental relief for me. But a September 1972
event involving his health suggests that my changed way of relating was deeply
stressful to him. My husband woke one night with an unusual request for a glass
of water. I was startled by the way something in his voice recalled similar requests
that dying patients had sometimes made when I nursed. Frightened, I turned
on the light to find him ashen, short of breath, and covered in sweat. I called the
fire department and ambulance and took him to a hospital where, through family, I had a connection to a heart specialist. My husband remained in hospital
and received extensive heart testing for the next ten days. On the second day of
his admission, I asked the heart specialist if my husband's problem could be anxiety rather than heart related. The doctor stated that, while he was quite certain
that my husband's problem was anxiety, he did not think it would be helpful to
burden my husband with a psychological diagnosis. The doctors never discussed
anxiety with my husband. They instead prescribed Librium for five years and
gave him a printout of his cardiogram to carry whenever he travelled.

My husband's health scare allowed the glue of our original contract to be
temporarily replaced with the glue of our shared loss-of-health experiences.
The next five years were a time set apart and our best as far as our being able
to work as a team, enjoy a peaceful home life, and give quality time to our children. The sweetness we held for each other during those few short years, and
the potential we demonstrated to form an alternate contract, made our inability to do couple therapy and to achieve the same quality of relationship without drugs all the more heartbreaking.

In the case of my husband's health, as in mine, our family, rather than being treated for its psychological health needs in the context of our actual dynamic, was once again affected by medical gender bias and wrongful diagnosis. The doctor's decision to mask my husband's anxiety as a heart problem compounded our inability to relate. I believe my husband was doubly convinced he had no part in the marriage breakdown by the heart specialists who told him that heart disease was the only thing wrong with his life. Placed in another double bind, my support of the doctor's fiction reinforced my role as the "mentally ill, silent partner" and my husband's as the heroic rescuer.

Not even in our worst fights towards the end of the marriage, when I was as mean as I have ever been, did I feel free to use the lie of his heart diagnosis as a weapon. The couples therapist who later helped us separate said, "Susan, your husband made a conscious decision not to do the work of looking into his past, and I think he made the right decision because looking into his past might have caused him to enter a black hole of depression he might never escape from." The scarcity of doctors who know the story in their own bodies and are able to truly recognize and help heal the stories in other persons' bodies makes my husband's decision to avoid an exploration of his own painful story more understandable. As for the health of his heart, when illness struck my ex-husband in his seventies, his doctor assured him that his heart, strong as a horse's, supported a favourable prognosis.

During my ten years on antipsychotic drugs, I developed a near-impossible-to-dissolve belief that I was chronically ill. My conviction was reinforced by symptoms of impaired speech, loss of physical coordination, and loss of memory. I was ignorant at the time that all the above were symptoms of a condition called *tardive dyskinesia*, which involved a set of problematic, sometimes permanent physical effects associated with long-term use of the type of medication I was prescribed. My sluggish thought processes and slowness of mind additionally affected our existing marital and communication difficulties. If I reacted forty-eight hours after a fact rather than immediately, my husband would respond with, "We had that discussion, it's over."

My husband's ritual offerings of flowers and gifts remained as constant over the years as his put-downs. As the intensity of our love/rejection relating patterns increased, the time between when I would be complimented and given a gift and when I would be told I was nothing and he was sorry he'd given me the gift narrowed from a span of several months at the beginning of the marriage to a matter of hours by the time we separated. My guilt that I was the sole cause of our problem was addictive in the sense that it prevented my taking action on my half of our joint problem and allowed me to continue responding to rejection with paralysis, self-blame, and efforts to be a "better" wife.

We had a range of opportunities to explore our backgrounds. My younger brother and his wife openly shared ideas from their T Group sensitivity courses at the National Training Labs in the US. Popular films of the time such as *Bob and Carol and Ted and Alice* also reinforced permission to explore relationship work. But though all our children, at one time or another, were called Nazi at school just as their father had been during his schooling, we never went near our pasts. When our daughter was ten, she came home angry from school saying that she wasn't Nazi, that she didn't do anything to and didn't care what had happened to the Jewish people. I did not possess enough self-worth myself to be able to convey to her that she did not deserve to be called Nazi under any circumstance. In her late teens my daughter sided angrily with her father against me on the Nazi issue when Mrs. Schellenberg senior told the family at dinner that there was no truth to the Holocaust story. I waited for my husband to respond to and correct his mother. When he did not, I took him aside and asked him to do so. When he said that his mother was an old woman and that I was to let her be, I returned to the table and told Mrs. Schellenberg and the children that the Holocaust did happen, was well documented, and that she was never to tell my family that it was otherwise ever again.

My husband never spoke of this to me afterwards. When my daughter told me I was needlessly harsh on her grandmother, I asked her to reserve judgment and to come with me to the film *Sophie's Choice*. The post-film image of my daughter's tears, look of lost innocence, and words "I never knew Mom" remain with me still.

I did not confront Mrs. Schellenberg often, but once I began to do so later in the marriage, she came to respect me and though we were never close, our relationship softened. As I became more aware of story's potential to heal, I encouraged Anna to tell me her story. I believe we both benefited from her sharing details of her hard life and accomplishments as an immigrant wife and mother.

ROSEMARY
Psychologist

Training Continues

I sat in a lecture theatre at the Clarke Institute of Psychiatry. The senior psychologist, Dr. Brooker, explained that assessment is one of the most critical and demanding aspects of our work. "The patient is distressed or facing problems in his or her life and looking to you, the doctor, for help. As a psychologist, you have two to five hours to interview the patient and to administer psychological tests. During these few hours, you are responsible for helping the person to feel comfortable with the interview process, obtaining information about every aspect of the person's life, and administering tests. At the end of the assessment, you are responsible for explaining your understanding of who he or she is as a person, how this problem has developed, and what can be done to help. Because the patient is apt to be at a personal crossroads in life and you are the doctor, your understanding and recommendations are likely to be very influential."

To assist students, a standardized questionnaire provided an interview guide. I learned to ask about the patient's presenting complaint, symptoms, and history (i.e., personal background). There was a place on the questionnaire for observations of the patient's appearance and behaviour such as personal grooming, speed of talking, degree of eye contact, and emotional expression. Psychologists in training were also given psychological test materials—we were to read the instruction manuals and practise with the materials in order to learn how to test patients. I took the tests myself and was anxious that my IQ score was not as high as I had expected; I wondered if I was smart enough to master this new line of work.

Case Study: Dr. Barnes 1976

I did not actually meet Susan for another fourteen years, but let's suppose that she had been hospitalized at the Clarke Institute and that I had been assigned to assess her in the fall of 1976.[3] I read over her medical chart on the hospital ward, then introduce myself to Mrs. Schellenberg as the clinician who will conduct the psychological assessment ordered by her psychiatrist. I arrange a time to meet with her in one of the bare, windowless, utilitarian student offices with grey linoleum floors. I focus carefully on the steps that I have learned. I explain that the purpose of the assessment is to understand Mrs. Schellenberg and her difficulties more thoroughly so that the staff can be more helpful. I interview her using the standardized questionnaire and administer the psychological tests.

At the end of the assessment, Mrs. Schellenberg's husband comes to meet her for their daily walk. He pulls me aside, asks what his wife's problem is and whether she is going to get better. My stomach churns and my head swims with information; I have little ability to judge the significance of what I have heard and no idea how to answer Mr. Schellenberg's questions. As the Schellenbergs are probably feeling the same way, sharing my confusion is hardly likely to be helpful. I say politely that I will have to score the tests and talk over Mrs. Schellenberg's case with my supervisor and that I will write a report to be placed in the medical chart and reviewed by the staff psychiatrist. Mr. Schellenberg looks disappointed and frustrated, but thanks me; he and his wife leave.

I spend the next week or so poring over books and articles about psychopathology, searching for descriptions that match what Mrs. Schellenberg reported and trying to understand the significance of her experiences. Is her account of being the Blessed Virgin Mary a neurotic symptom, a delusion, or a hallucination? I read carefully through the glossaries of medical texts. When I have learned what I can in the short time available, I write a report using the designated headings, Presenting Complaint, History, Presentation (those observations I made in the interview), Test Results, Summary, and Opinion. I meet with my supervisor, who explains that Mrs. Schellenberg's experience of herself as the Blessed Virgin Mary is a delusion. Her behaviour in taking the children to the religious retreat is evidence of poor judgment. Her belief that she does not do enough for others indicates poor reality testing. Because of these symptoms, and test results indicating similar difficulties, her diagnosis is Acute Schizophrenic Reaction. If she experiences such symptoms over a longer period of time, the diagnosis may change to some form of schizophrenia.

I attend ward rounds, the twice-weekly meetings of the professionals working on the Mood Disorders Unit. Such multidisciplinary mental health teams are always headed by a psychiatrist. At these meetings, each patient's status, diagnosis, and treatment are reviewed. Ordinarily such meetings are attended by the staff psychiatrist in charge of the unit, a consulting psychiatrist, a psychiatrist holding a research fellowship, two resident physicians who are training to become psychiatrists, a medical student who is being introduced to psychiatric services, two social workers, a social work student, the unit head nurse, a staff nurse, a public health nurse, a student nurse, an occupational therapist, the psychologist, and myself. Often, fifteen or more professionals and students are present. Usually during ward rounds, the staff psychiatrist briefly interviews a patient in order to address an issue of concern that has emerged from discussion of the patient's status. Such interviews are conducted in the presence of the mental health team. Because rounds are considered important to student training, psychiatric staff sometimes administer minioral examinations to residents or medical students during rounds and make a point of discussing a clinical issue or recent research finding. I strain to follow the discussions without drawing attention to myself.

My supervisor encourages me to report on Ms. Schellenberg's psychological assessment results at ward rounds. She wants me to be sure to mention that Mrs. Schellenberg wrote on one of the tests that her greatest fear was that the children would be hurt. I am unsure of the significance of this response, and nothing related to this possibility had come up in my interview with Mrs. Schellenberg. However, my supervisor feels that the response should be highlighted as the issue of the children's safety has not been raised by any other professional and it is important to demonstrate that psychological assessments can provide valuable information about patients that would not be otherwise known.

Aware of the professional eyes focused on me and the black, typed words on the yellow report form that I clutch, I try to summarize without appearing to be reading word for word, something that would make my report inappropriately long and unprofessional. Mercifully, the staff psychiatrist does not interrogate me. The psychiatrist is, however, interested in Mrs. Schellenberg's test response about her children and a discussion ensues concerning this matter. My supervisor is pleased. Because her diagnosis does not involve a mood disorder (i.e., depression or mania), Mrs. Schellenberg is transferred from the Mood Disorders Unit to an in-patient unit specializing in schizophrenia and I do not see her again. As I conduct more assessments, I carry out this process over and over, interviewing and administering tests, then studying and talking with my supervisor. Gradually, I become more fluent in professional language and practices.

The "Day Job" as Staff Psychologist

After postdoctoral training, I passed the exams and was accepted as a member of the Ontario Board of Examiners in Psychology. I was hired as Staff Psychologist at Toronto General Hospital, a university-affiliated general hospital where I worked with the SHARE (Self-Harm Assessment Research and Education) program. This program was devoted to clinical service, research, and education in the area of suicide and attempted suicide. The SHARE clinical team evaluated problems and suggested treatment for people hospitalized after coming to the emergency department thinking of suicide or having done something to injure themselves.

The SHARE team was headed by Dr. Analytic, a man about my age who accepted this position as his first job after completing training as a psychiatrist. Dr. Analytic took pride in his work and was deeply respectful of the patients; his attitude set the tone for the team and was somewhat remarkable, because emergency and other hospital professionals often disliked our patients, as did we ourselves on occasion. Dr. Analytic was interested in psychoanalytic theory and practice, so he was interested in the meanings of people's experiences and sophisticated in thinking about the patient-professional relationship. This perspective helped me to understand that hospital staff dedicated to saving lives felt confused, scared, helpless, sad, and finally angry when faced with caring for a person who had deliberately tried to die. Such feelings underlay the dislike for suicidal patients seen by the SHARE team.

Dr. Analytic's outlook influenced my thinking considerably. As I worked with the SHARE team, I learned that many individuals whom we saw during a suicidal crisis had experienced great hardship, often beginning in childhood.

One young woman whom I saw in psychotherapy for several years had been sexually abused by her father, mother, and several other men since she was very young, physically abused (e.g., punished for misbehaviour by having her fingers placed on a hot stove burner), and placed in foster care for a year or so as a young child. What was puzzling was not her despair, but rather her will to live in the face of profound emotional pain. The damage wrought by her severe maltreatment was apparent by her late adolescence and early adult life, a time when she had several admissions to the SHARE program. When some relatively minor thing went wrong such as a fight with a boyfriend, she lacked confidence in her value as a person, the skills to comfort herself or resolve problems, and the supportive relationships that might help her to put the matter into perspective. In despair, she impulsively cut herself or overdosed on medication.

In time, I came to realize that hospitals, like prisons, are caring for many such adults. Although mental illnesses can and do develop in other circumstances, a significant proportion of those hospitalized for mental health problems have been maltreated as children and thus had limited opportunities to mature psychologically or to learn the skills that would enable them to function as flexible, skilled, resilient adults.

The SHARE team functioned within the conventional medical model, but made great efforts to address the overall context of individuals' lives. The team staff routinely contacted family and any professionals caring for the individual outside of the hospital in an effort to evaluate and strengthen the individual's support network. The social workers scoured the city to find the programs best suited to patients' needs—for housing, addictions treatment, skills training, and psychotherapy. Medication was recommended infrequently since most problems were recognized as not amenable to this form of treatment.

By 1984, I had met hundreds of patients and felt at ease with conducting assessment interviews, administering tests, observing behaviour, and reporting on my findings. I could make a diagnosis and develop a formulation that related the person's background to the nature and origins of current problems. I understood how diagnosis and formulation provided the basis for developing management plans, including recommendations for medication and psychotherapy.

Case Study: Dr. Barnes 1984

Suppose that Mrs. Schellenberg had been referred to me at Toronto General Hospital. As I think back on my professional practice in 1984, I can imagine seeing Mrs. Schellenberg and noting that she has experienced delusions, poor judgment, fatigue, guilt, and anxiety that have persisted for several weeks and interfere with her ability to function as a mother; some of these symptoms indicate a diagnosis of some form of psychotic condition. My formulation considers multiple factors that could have contributed to the development of her symptoms and problems. If I learn of her concerns about birth control, I note this internal conflict as the basis for longer term emotional distress, that is, guilt and anxiety. Such emotional distress, together with fatigue from mononucleosis, a recent pericardial infection, and the strain of caring for her young children and ill mother, have increased her vulnerability to psychological crisis, which for her has taken the form of a thought disorder. If I learn of her uncle's long history of psychiatric care, I comment on a family genetic predisposition to psychotic difficulties. I recommend that Mrs. Schellenberg be evaluated for medication to alleviate her delusional thinking and associated distress; when her thinking and emotional state are more stable, psychotherapy is recommended to assist with conflicts related to birth control.

When Mr. Schellenberg asks about his wife's diagnosis and prospects for recovery, I am aware of complexities in responding to this question. My default position is to refer Mr. Schellenberg to the staff psychiatrist on the basis that such matters should be discussed with the professional in charge. However, if authority for such discussions has been delegated to me or if I judge that the psychiatrist would not mind me discussing such issues, I ask Mrs. Schellenberg for permission to talk with her husband. At this point in my career, I am well aware of my professional obligation to keep patient information confidential even from close family unless the patient agrees that I can talk about his or her care.

With Mrs. Schellenberg's permission, I explain to her husband that his wife has been diagnosed with a brief psychotic condition, that hospital staff are concerned about whether she might be developing schizophrenia, and that if she is diagnosed with schizophrenia, it will be particularly important for her to take medication. If Mr. Schellenberg presses about schizophrenia, I would tell him that this diagnosis means that the affected person will likely require medication for life and that the prognosis is poor because schizophrenia is typically associated with a chronic, deteriorating course. Mr. Schellenberg thanks me. I feel sad about conveying discouraging news, but confident in my expert knowledge and hopeful that my explanations and recommendations will be helpful. I do not see the Schellenbergs again.

Night Life

I enjoyed my days at the hospital and my developing professional competence as a psychologist. However, the matter of what I did after working hours left me somewhat uneasy about my professional career. In the evenings, I returned to my small, rented apartment in the Annex neighbourhood of downtown Toronto, took off the nylons and stylish Famolare sandals that my mother had given me, and hung up the skirt and blouse. I put on a T-shirt that said "A woman without a man is like a fish without a bicycle," corduroy jeans, and a plaid flannel shirt. During 1977 and 1978, I went to 342 Jarvis Street for Lesbian Organization of Toronto collective meetings; in later years, I went to the homes of friends for Lesbian and Gay Community Appeal board meetings. On weekends, I went to potluck suppers or bars or women's dances.

The impulse towards this other life had emerged uninvited when I attended a small liberal arts college in Colorado Springs, Colorado. At the beginning of my second college year, my roommate Marcie talked openly and shamelessly about her romantic advances to women on campus. I had grown up in a conservative religious American family, so I knew that such behaviour was immoral and explained this to Marcie in no uncertain terms. As a dormitory student advisor, I felt certain obligations, so arranged an appointment with the college mental health services to discuss Marcie. The psychologist explained that homosexuality was a matter of arrested psychosexual development and that little could be done about it unless the person wanted help. Marcie did not want help.

Within weeks, when I fell in love with Jan and began to explore sexually, I did not want help either because I felt more alive than I had ever been. For seven years, I thrashed in a welter of feelings. These experiences later became an invaluable reference for understanding psychoanalytic concepts and psychiatric disorder.

Projection: Attributing to other person ideas, thoughts, feelings, and impulses that are part of one's own inner experience but unacceptable, such as my accusing Marcie of immoral feelings and desires. *Reaction formation*: Developing a socialized attitude that is opposite to an unconscious wish or impulse, such as my devoting myself to maintaining high standards of morality at the college dormitory in order to avoid thinking about my own unacceptable attractions to women. *Ambivalence*: Coexistence of two opposing impulses in the same person, as when I feel both drawn to and repelled by Jan. *Euphoria*: Heightened feelings of psychological well-being I experience as relationship with Jan becomes more intimate. *Elation*: Air of confidence and enjoyment associated with increased motor activity that I experience when I'm with Jan. *Preoccupation*: Centring of thought content on a particular idea, such as my continual thinking about the significance of the relationship with Jan. *Denial*: An aspect of external reality is rejected; I have no idea what she means when my mother asks if there is anything wrong in my relationship with Jan. *Anxiety*: Feeling of apprehension due to unconscious conflicts, a common feeling when others seem to notice that Jan and I are more than "just friends."

Dependency: A state of reliance on another for psychological support, as in feeling that I cannot manage without Jan as a major part of my life. *Depression*: A morbid state characterized by mood alterations such as sadness, by low self-esteem associated with self-reproach, by vegetative signs and symptoms such as loss of appetite and sleep disturbance, and by withdrawal from interpersonal contact and at times a desire to die; what I experienced when Jan broke off our relationship. *Homosexuality*: Sexual attraction or contact between same-sex persons; this has nothing to do with what I experienced with Jan. *Suppression*: Conscious act of controlling and inhibiting an unacceptable impulse. *Neurosis*: Mental disorder characterized by anxiety.

Gradually my anguished thrashing quieted as I thought over my experiences with Jan and talked with a few carefully chosen, supportive friends. By 1976, I had reluctantly decided that romantic feelings for women meant I was lesbian. Corinne, a close heterosexual friend, went with me to hear a talk about homosexuality given at the McMaster University Medical Centre in Hamilton, Ontario, by an openly gay man from the Community Homophile Association of Toronto (CHAT). Laura, the openly lesbian sister of a graduate school housemate, explained that big-city bars and dances were where lesbians and gay men met each other and drove with me to Toronto to search for such places; she located a feminist dance where I felt both intensely anxious and immediately at home. She gave me readings from the Furies, a Washington, DC, lesbian-feminist collective. Despite enormous fear, I called the gay phone line in Hamilton and found out about McMaster University Homophile Association meetings and dances. I disclosed my sexual orientation and a new relationship to my parents; they expressed their love for me and hoped that I might someday become heterosexual. Within months, I had moved to Toronto to pursue my postdoctoral fellowship at the Clarke Institute.

As I persisted, my fears subsided and I became accustomed to being around lesbians and gay men. In Toronto, much to my surprise, lesbian-feminist groups, new friendships, and the ferment of feminist and gay liberation movements allowed me for the first time to become confident in myself as a person with a place and purpose in the world.

Although homosexual acts were removed from the Canadian criminal code in 1969, social attitudes, law, and policy were slow to change. Until 1976, Canadian immigration law and policy grouped together pimps, prostitutes, homosexuals, those living from the avails of prostitution, professional beggars, vagrants, and chronic alcoholics; though I was not, in 1979, familiar with such law and policy, I viewed being homosexual as socially undesirable, so did not mention my night life to my hospital colleagues.

I attempted to reconcile my personal and professional worlds. I learned the feminist and antipsychiatry critiques of the mental health system—that psychiatric institutions are agents of social control that function to punish men and women who deviate from social norms in respect to gender roles, sexual orientation, or political beliefs. I joined a group of Canadian lesbian and gay activists for a photograph published as part of a 1979 *Toronto Star* newspaper's Sunday magazine article on the decriminalization of homosexuality in Canada. To prepare for this publication, I disclosed my sexual orientation to Dr. Brooker at the Clarke Institute and to Dr. Alistair Munro, the chief psychiatrist at Toronto General Hospital; both men were supportive. I spent three years studying psychotherapy with mentors teaching with radical therapy and feminist approaches, and became convinced of the transformative potential of psychotherapy that addresses issues of sexism, racism, and homophobia. In the nine years at Toronto General Hospital, I matured as a clinician and researcher. I was somewhat ashamed that I enjoyed a professional career in an institution heavily critiqued by feminist activists whose values I share, but believed that hospitals, though flawed, were fundamentally a force for good.

Notes

1 Hospital records for this admission are shown in Appendix II, beginning with figure 3 (p. 244).
2 See the medical record in Appendix II, figure 9 (p. 250), for a doctor's comment "No striae gravidarum, para IV" (i.e., no stretch marks, four pregnancies with births of viable offspring).
3 Because I am not interested in singling out or criticizing particular individuals, my stories of my professional life from this point forward will use fictious characters and scenarios based on my hospital experiences and, for the case studies, on what I know about Susan's experiences.

3 Towards Healing

Those who were then governing the country knew what was really happening to it and what we later called *zastoi*, roughly translated as *stagnation*.... One of the richest countries in the world, endowed with immense overall potential, was already sliding downwards. Our society was declining both economically and intellectually. And yet to the casual observer, the country seemed to present a picture of relative well-being, stability and order.... Such was the situation in the spring of 1985 and there was a great temptation to leave things as they were, to make only cosmetic changes. This, however, meant continuing to deceive ourselves and the people.... *Perestroika* [restructuring] has enabled us to open up to the world.

—Mikhail Gorbachev[1]

SUSAN
Healing Beginnings

By the early 1980s the dysfunction in my life and marriage forced me to choose between remaining stagnated on antipsychotic drugs or risk the venture into an unknown examination of the decaying inner system that held my own false union of self together.

While wise and generous energies brought Mikhail Gorbachev to Russia's aid, I never cease to be amazed at the energies that allowed me to not only begin reclaiming the psychic realms occupied by influences I was no longer prepared to endure but to also begin a process of healing through tracking that story.

Commitment to Heal

Ten years after the event of my psychosis, life forced me to seriously question the drugs that psychiatrists had so assuredly prescribed me. Though drugged, my art spirit was kept vicariously alive from the kitchen where I could overhear the piano teacher explain music to the children. My daughter's enthusiastic renderings of lengthy Aram Katchatourian works and quickly uttered "SHIT!" at the odd missed note came, along with the music itself from the other room; the sounds reached my soul like critical counterpoints to the antipsychotic drug side effects that had grown from frustrations to physical harms then to suicidal urges.

Markedly slowed, I moved from one task to another in sedated robotic fashion gaining motivation by saying to myself, "I - m-u-s-t - l-o-a-d - t-h-e - d-i-s-h-w-a-s-h-e-r." Or "I- m-u-s-t - m-a-k-e- t-h-e - b-e-d-s." I've heard many people describe drugged thinking as walking in corn syrup. It's an accurate description. To wash and change seven beds took an entire nine-to-five workday. The bending required to make beds and load a dishwasher left me light headed, dizzy, flushed, and short of breath. I needed charts to mark when I took drugs because I forgot the minute I took them. I remained mostly silent on social occasions since I forgot what I was about to say before I spoke and was slow and stammering if I did speak. In a distant part of my mind, I worried my intelligence was severely harmed, but my drugged stupor and passivity made it difficult to question either my disabilities or my psychiatric treatment.

Without being prescribed or offered psychotherapy at any point during my years on drugs, the sole sources of counselling in our suburb that I was aware of were the family doctor to whom the hospital referred me in my sixth year on drugs and the parish priest. I was intuitive enough to know that both men had already labelled me "crazy" and how the priest would refer me to the doctor and the doctor would prescribe more drugs if I told either of my suicidal thoughts. On my own, I paid serious attention to and coped with my suicidal urges for a time but when these feelings threatened to override my fears for the children's safety, I despaired that my options were at an end.

A turning point occurred on the darkest of days around the 1980 period. I made a decision that day to fight against the rest of my being to give water to a dying houseplant. The near-death state of the plant disturbed me to the degree that the plant's survival seemed inseparable from my own survival. My depressed, leaden body caused the watering of the plant to be among the most difficult feats I have ever performed. But I did get water to the plant and through that act, not only opened the door to change but learned the importance of each small step.

Later that same day, feelings that the morning plant event triggered probably tripped a flight response and my getting out of the house. In any event, I visited an aunt at Women's College Hospital, and while there was introduced to her physician, Dr. Moon. Dr. Moon, who proved as mythic a helper as her name suggests, agreed to take me on as a patient. At our first doctor/patient visit, Dr. Moon carefully listened to my story for more than an hour, validated my wretched feelings, then referred me to a psychiatrist willing to help me wean from the drugs.

Withdrawing from Medications

My best memory is that there was a two-year spread between my husband's discontinuing the Librium he had been prescribed for anxiety and when I began to withdraw from antipsychotic drugs. Simultaneous to my decision to wean from drugs, I ended my practice of not speaking to my husband unless he spoke to me. Once I returned to expressing myself freely, he reverted to putting me down. I also started to leave my religion at this time, an action that seemed to increase my husband's anxieties that his control over me was weakening.

The psychiatrist, Dr. Ives, was an immensely kind man. To determine my husband's and my joint attitudes toward my decision to wean from drugs, Dr. Ives asked that we make an initial visit as a couple. My husband complied, but when the doctor asked how he personally felt about my going off drugs, he said, "I couldn't care less; she can do whatever the hell she wants." He then looked at his watch and signalled that our meeting with the psychiatrist was over. I ran to keep up with him as he left the doctor's office. We drove home in silence and once there his first words to me were, "I want you to be very clear, Susan, about what I am going to do if you go off your drugs. I was happy to help you with the children and house while you were on drugs but starting today that ends. You are on your own and don't expect any more nice clothes either." My husband's threats came as a devastating shock but I did not budge from my withdrawal goal.

My first withdrawal attempt was a cold turkey approach that caused me to briefly re-experience "racing thought" kinds of pre-psychotic symptoms. Discouraged that I was irreversibly ill, I resumed taking the drugs but at our next visit the psychiatrist hastened to apologize for not telling me to withdraw gradually and assured me that my adverse reaction was normal, given the number of years I had been on the drugs.

Early on, Dr. Ives also suggested I read *Ego and Archetype: Individuation and the Religious Function of the Psyche,* by Edward Edinger.[2] Memory difficulties did not allow me to retain what I read but constant rereading of the Edinger book allowed me to absorb its information intuitively. The psychiatrist's care of the larger whole of my experience gave me a sense of being safe and nurtured. The fact he suggested the book validated my intelligence when mental slowness convinced me I was otherwise. *Ego and Archetype* initiated my understanding that in leaving drugs I was setting out on an unknown journey.

I began withdrawing from the drugs Stelazine and Cogentin by decreasing the dose of Stelazine by a half-milligram till I felt stable enough to reduce it further. Because I experienced severe spasms and cramps when taking Stelazine alone, the original Cogentin dose remained constant until I reached a half dose amount with Stelazine; at that point the Cogentin was also reduced to half. After each half-milligram reduction of Stelazine, it would take me about three or four months to stabilize. The period of time needed to secure a sense of control on the new dose was also influenced by the amount of domestic stress I was experiencing at the time.

A key part of our stress from the drug-withdrawal period onward was the fact I did not have a paying job and my husband thought I should. Though I was managing a home and five teens, I was constantly told, "You do nothing." The drugs and their side effects were impossible to explain and when I tried, my explanations were viewed as excuses. The psychiatrists who had told him the drugs were good were the authority on that subject.

Early on in this battle, an acutely humiliating drug after-effect occurred when I tried to re-enter the work force and began a nursing refresher course at George Brown College. In the first class, we wrote a pretest to determine our recall of nursing. The tests were returned and our marks read out the following week. As my name begins with "S," I sat listening to grades being called out in the 70-to-90-percent range, and then heard my name and my mark of 11 percent. The shame was hard to bear. Because memory is vital to nursing, I abandoned nursing as a career option. When the next yearly nursing registration renewal arrived in the mail, I threw it in the garbage and committed to following my art and getting off drugs instead.

The first three or four days on a newly reduced drug amount were frightening. I felt psychologically fragile, close to psychosis, and as if I was standing on a powerful vibrating machine. A feeling of going progressively deeper into a never-ending series of mirrored rooms also marked those days, each entrance being navigated, tested, and won with an insight or an attitude. The mirrored rooms recalled Vienna's Schoenbrunn Castle, which I visited the year prior to my marriage. It was a terrifying experience. Every new threshold would reduce me to a state of near fragmentation. The grace that seemed to allow me to move forward was a final letting go to a trust that even though I appeared to be sinking into a deeper unknown, there was an energy that would stay and guide me out to an eventual healing. With Catholic teaching as my only source of meaning, I was often engulfed in the terror of being deluded and in league with the devil.

My husband's push to regain control of me was ongoing during the withdrawal period. In the third withdrawal year, marital tensions led me to tell Dr. Ives that I was unable to remain married and continue weaning from drugs. "I understand," was his only response. As I stood to leave his office, the sight of him writing me a new prescription was so devastating that I became angry. I said, "I am not going to promise you I will take them." He kept writing but in a whispered voice said, "Good! They are not the answer anyways."

The tardive dyskinesia effects on my ability to recall words and think quickly heightened our communication difficulties as a couple and strengthened the family myth that I was the less stable partner.

I now believe that it was my frustrated need to communicate that prompted me to study conversational French. Because students in this setting were all slow of speech, I was able to feel normal as well as benefit from the mental stimulation of a second language. Though unqualified to be a teacher of English as a Second Language (ESL), I was allowed to join an ESL group and give bread-and-butter English lessens to elderly East Indian immigrants who lived in a subsidized housing project. With the use of language instruction techniques learned at Alliance Française, and my ability to cope in a slow-speech setting, my students achieved beyond the expected norm and their friendship and regard for my intelligence did wonders for my confidence.

Speech frustrations at home were my prime rage trigger. I was ashamed of and devastated by inflicting my rages on the family. Guilt and rage Ping-Ponged with my increasing efforts to be good as I descended further and further into feeling evil. Religiously steered towards "goodness" from infancy onward and made to confess to priests the "You go tell the priest you made me angry" feelings of a mother who could not own her own anger, I know that "good" did not tolerate anger, let alone daily displays of rage.

Where my own parents had never disguised their battling over differences, their periodic confrontations allowed them to clear the air and grow closer over time. To witness people take psychological aim at their partner's jugular as my in-laws did was new to me. To realize that my husband and I were repeating their pattern was deeply shaming. Certain that I was insane and that my going back on drugs was the solution to our problems, my husband resisted couples therapy. Books like Jean Baker Miller's *Toward a New Psychology of Women* informed my struggle to change.[3] Our dynamic did shift but only into a heightened, "the smarter the mouse, the smarter the mousetrap" phase.

We reacted to the least change in the other. As my weaning from drugs progressed, my husband increasingly used foul language. As I became more aware and tried to change my passivity and neediness, he complained that I was no longer there for him and became more distant and depressed. We became more deeply enmeshed and stuck in projecting our problems onto each other.

My husband's energies were being taxed on numerous other fronts during the drug-withdrawal period. Radical and rapid shifts toward a global economy in the early 1980s caused the American parent company of the Canadian subsidiary he headed to be taken over twice in a brief span of time. The systemic business mergers and acquisitions mindset of that time stripped his parent company as well as many other companies of monies needed for the research and development of new product. The new order of business caused my husband grave concerns both for his company's long-term health and for our family's security. As a highly intuitive executive who had advanced in his company through the area of marketing, the sudden need to adapt to policies set by accountants rather than market forces as well as his need to guide his company through these new processes was an immense challenge.

My husband found little solace from this work situation at home during that time. Once his drugged and docile wife, I was now immersed in leaving my religion, giving up drugs, and exploring independence while still being dependent. Four of our children required help for varying degrees of dyslexia. The children's problems forced my husband to change his "mind-over-matter" perspective on their dyslexia to a willingness to utilize the support of child psychologists, special education, and guidance teachers. He was in his own mid-life, and the deteriorating health and care of his aging parents were also pressing concerns. My husband often insisted that my refusal to help him by going back on the drugs was proof that I did not love him. I tried to help in other ways, but my memory of the drugs never allowed me to quit the withdrawal process.

My husband's fears around my stopping my medications were also expressed through sabotage aimed at convincing me I was schizophrenic and in need of drugs. He began to call me "Schitzo" in front of the children and to increasingly undermine my system of organizing them and the house. Being belittled in front of the children was shaming but I also worried how they would be affected by witnessing such behaviour. I tried to gather knowledge on how relationships work but mainly learned everything the hard way. If my asking to discuss the children with my husband was not convenient at one hour of the day, I tried every other possible hour before realizing I needed to ask him for an appointment. My husband's rage when I did ask for an appointment was the first time I did not take blame and realized he wanted me silenced.

My system for distributing the children's weekly chores had been highly effective until this point. Each Monday after dinner, I would pass a basket that held five rolled pieces of paper, each containing the name of a household chore. Groans, laughter, and swapping deals always followed, but once the children settled things among themselves, the chores were always done. One Monday after my withdrawal process began, my husband grabbed the basket and ordered me to get rid of it and to stop making the kids do chores. The children soon realized they could play one of us against the other. They rebelled collectively and in very little time, I was stuck with a family that expected me to run a hotel. My husband said that my inability to "control" the children was solely my problem and the result of my not taking drugs.

As my withdrawal continued, we grew ever more polarized on how the marriage should work. Our respective positions—"There is a problem" versus "There is no problem"—solidified. In 1982, I went to a lawyer to seek a divorce, but my mind was still so affected by drugs I could not entirely make sense of the lawyer's instructions. Realizing that I was not yet able to cope alone, I continued in the marriage, hoping to attain a better-functioning mind and then leave. My recovery aims offered me immense incentive to change. My husband, at the height of a successful business career built on a "there is no problem" attitude had less motivation to change. His desire to maintain our status quo was also logical in the sense that doctors had clearly stated that he was all right, I was sick, and the marriage was perfect. To his way of thinking, my view that our marriage needed to change was insane.

From 1980 to 1988, when the marriage ended, our home developed an aura of sadness and carelessness that was opposite to the feeling of love in the house that *au pairs* often remarked on when the children were small. The children, then between nine and eighteen years of age, befriended one another, but their schooling, our family life, and the quality of our physical health suffered. The availability of sports and music lessons and the fact of our having two pianos, a set of drums, and numerous guitars gave the family ways to express their pain and helped prevent their getting into serious trouble. When I consider the collective pain of our five children at the time of our breakup, I become concerned for similarly stressed children today who lack access to extracurricular activities due to educational funding cuts.

My dependency issues were one thing to learn about in books but another to try to correct. When I admitted this failing and my intention to be a more responsible partner where money was concerned, my husband refused to explain and share the family money management role with me. Being quick of mind and impatient by nature, he was frustrated by my sluggish thinking. By that time, I was receiving an allowance but had become despondent and careless about how much I spent on groceries or on myself. I ceased my frugal grocery shopping habits, used pricey hair stylists, expensive cosmetics, and overspent in numerous other ways.

When I was able to respond to my husband's "You should become a dental nurse!" with "I will become a dental nurse when you become a ballet dancer!" I felt more confident in my sanity but also more panicked about money—the drug side effects lingered past the time of being drug-free and divorce seemed inevitable. Unable to do simple math, record telephone numbers accurately, or master the coordination skills needed to work a calculator, I felt capable of very little employment other than fashion modelling. My mother, who had combined modelling with sales prior to her marriage, had trained me from age eleven onwards to walk up and down stairs in heels with a book on my head and to always dress fashionably. My father and husband's expectations that I was to sparkle when with them in public also honed my fashion sense. Though I modelled for several years beginning in 1986, fashion modelling embodied ideals that I was in the process of outgrowing, and I felt humiliated that my limited memory was taxed by simple runway choreography—I didn't appear to be intelligent enough to model. It was also bizarre and enraging to have my fashion work, which consisted of putting clothes on, walking, turning, and taking clothes off, start at a pay level of $115 per hour, while my years of training as a nurse, raising children, and nursing ailing and dying parents lacked monetary value.

My husband and I began to ski and dance more frequently during these years. Dance was non-touch and disco then. We often danced entire evenings without saying more than a few words. I see now that the severity of our co-dependence and difficulty in breaking free of each other required a death ritual. Dancing, though bizarre and unconscious in one sense, gave us a gentler non-verbal way to witness and openly express our own and each other's sadness and pain.

We periodically managed to agree to couples counselling when crisis points arose but never found a mutual will for long-term work on our issues. My husband's view of mutuality was, "If you want equality, you'll have to fight for it." During the last two summers when the children's only responsibilities were their paid summer jobs at their father's company, the house sunk into greater chaos. I was expected to provide meals and comforts for family members who failed to notify me of plans to dine elsewhere or took no responsibility for the after-dinner kitchen cleanup. I left both summers for several weeks and stayed with one of the children's former sitters. Both times, I threatened divorce unless we went to counselling and adopted a better style of parenting. My husband agreed to couples therapy and even enlisted extended family members to talk me out of leaving. But once a therapist mentioned that each of us would need to explore our childhoods to save the marriage, he would quit therapy and our problems would resume and escalate.

Over the years the spiritual courage to withdraw from drugs and the marriage was greatly aided by the physical challenges of skiing. From our ski honeymoon until after the children's births, I dreaded skiing. Then, for the sake of having company on our ski vacations, I enrolled in ski schools and gradually became an average steady skier.

On our last ski holiday together in 1986, the deep sense of triumph I felt on taking a helicopter to and skiing with my husband down from the peak of Whistler Mountain in British Columbia convinced me that I could survive on my own. I always treasured the positive growth that I acquired in the relationship, but until this point I had used the positive to justify staying in the marriage.

In 1986 as my need to leave the marriage grew to be an inarguable fact even to me, my husband entered a period of inconsolable grief over his father's illness and impending death from Alzheimer's disease. Rather than turn to me for help at this time, he publicly ignored me to the point of entering the church and sitting with our daughter rather than me during his father's funeral service.

The pain of this and earlier similar events had by then forced me to accept that my husband's rejection of me was a mirror of my own rejection of self. Once anchored to this awareness, I was able to accept that divorce was not a sin and that the price for my staying in the marriage would be my agreeing to be schizophrenic and drugged indefinitely. The courage to leave took longer to gather.

Early in 1987, when my husband began to throw things in anger at my art, a lawyer advised me to get my art out of the house and to obtain a court order for him to move out. My husband's reaction to the order was again to seek my siblings' help in convincing me he would do couples therapy and change if I gave the marriage one more chance. Touched in these meetings by my husband's declarations of love and seeing all my siblings in successful working marriages, I decided on yet another reconciliation.

As the reconciliation began, I determined to be in the present and not look back. We also agreed to discuss the marriage solely in the family counsellor's presence and to organize fun events both for ourselves as a couple and as a family. It was strained in the beginning but I began to delight in our growth in abilities to agree to disagree on differences and to move from closeness to separateness without needing a fight to achieve distance. At the six-month mark, my husband brought up the matter of the court order that had been kept in place at our lawyers' and counsellors' advice in the event the reconciliation failed. We were cautioned about taking that legal step slowly. After reaching a witnessed agreement that our therapy and new coping systems would remain in place after the order was removed and on the date the lawyer would be asked to remove it, the court order was lifted.

When the lawyer's letter confirming the dissolution of the court order arrived in the mail, my husband glanced at the letter and said, "I want you to know, Susan, that I never wanted you: I wanted this court order lifted and as of now our couples therapy is at an end." A numbing frigid void enveloped and remained with me. It was October 1987. The children, now into a new school year, faced the last of our failed reconciliations. I coldly determined to ignore my husband and to keep the home and the children's lives intact till the end of their school year.

Sexual Abuse Memory

In 1987, three and a half years after I was drug free, an issue involving our daughter, who was the eldest child and close to graduating from university, triggered my first recall of a childhood sexual trauma. Our worsening marriage forced our teenaged daughter into a terrible position where she coped by taking on a mediator role to try to ease our pain and that of her brothers. She was attractive and intelligent, and her father began to ask her instead of me to fill the role I had formerly taken at social and business functions. Their socializing included dancing in discos and dining at "in" places. Her father also gave gifts to her that were similar to gifts I had previously received from him. Their activities were noticed to the extent that close friends warned me about them. Aware, but unable to be heard by my husband when I expressed my concerns, my sense of being silenced grew to the point of feeling strangled. Anxious that my leaving the marriage to correct the problem might cause my daughter to become more rather than less entrenched in this situation, I focused instead on getting her educated and out of the home. My overwhelming concern and rage over my daughter erupted one evening during a painful discussion with my husband when I abruptly shifted from a normal speaking voice to a shriek and screamed, "Stop! Don't you know my father slept with me?"

I was shocked by my words and the abuse recall. I became frantic next. My husband's initial response was one of rescue, but I could not accept his touch. I raced into trivializing the abuse and trying to protect my father's memory in my husband's eyes. Subsequent efforts to link my father's abuse to issues of inappropriate fathering as well as to our daughter's situation failed. My abuse disclosure reinforced my husband's conviction that the abuse was further proof of my mental and sexual defectiveness.

I had blocked memories of my father's abuse for thirty-two years. Though the memory may have been ready to surface with the psychosis, it took the pain of seeing my daughter's situation to bring it to consciousness. My father had slept with and cuddled me like a teddy bear from as early as I can remember. He continued to do this as I grew to be a teen. When I was about twelve, I became extremely frightened on several occasions when I experienced his erection in the small of my back. After one of these incidents, I reacted violently and punched and kicked at him till he got out of my bed. When my mother came to my room the next morning her first words were, "You upset your father last night." Years of burying this double-edged trauma resulted in my failure to protect my own daughter.

As I experienced my father rather than my mother as the prime nurturer in my life, it was difficult to examine his abuse. Several therapists tried but failed to help when they encouraged me to work through the abuse from a stance that my father was a bad man. I finally found help in 1990 with a wise shiatsu/dream therapist who allowed me to give full expression to the beautiful caring aspects of my father as well as to his offensive acts.

My resolution of the abuse recall had been blocked by my fear of parental rejection. Though both my parents were deceased at the time of the recall, I was still their daughter in a psychological sense and, as though they were still alive, I feared their rejection of me for uncovering the abuse, shaming them in front of my husband, and causing an even a deeper rupture to my already-threatened marriage. My understanding of the fourth commandment, "Honour thy mother and thy father," did not allow any circumstance to break this edict. Where I once managed abuse cover-up by idealizing my childhood and parents, the trauma recall erased that option and forced me to move further into my healing journey.

Death of Mother-in-Law

My husband's mother died following cataract surgery in 1987, a year after his father's death. My husband's "I forbid you to visit my mother in hospital" prompted me to drive to Saint Catharines early the next morning to see her on her second post-surgery day. With Anna's favourite coffee and chocolate donut in hand, I was greeted as I entered her hospital room with, "Ach, Susan, I had forgotten how pretty you were," and later as I was leaving she kissed me and told me I had great courage. Three times that same morning she mentioned how she should never have stayed with her husband but had no way to raise her children on her own. I was deeply touched by her unusual warmth and compliments and by the permission to leave her son her confession implied. Anna died the following day.

The following April, as the school year was ending and the time I decided to leave was approaching, my energies became depleted. Disconnected from my feelings and physically too weak to care about seeing a doctor, I attributed this energy loss to my other losses. It was only by good fortune that I was diagnosed with colon cancer when I was called to repeat a mammogram. Rather than just giving me a mammogram requisition, my doctor's nurse observed and became alarmed at my pallor and arranged for the doctor to see me. The next morning, I was told that my blood test results required immediate hospital admission. I received three pints of blood on admission and two days later was operated on for colon cancer.

In shutting down my feelings to stay in the marriage, I almost lost my life. By living in my head, playing god, and deciding what divorce time would be best for my children, I exposed them to more chaos than if I had left earlier. A friend who visited me in hospital and who arrived on crutches herself due to knee surgery said, as she handed me a book, "My therapist suggested I read this." It was *The Pregnant Virgin,* by the Jungian analyst Dr. Marion Woodman.[4]

After reading *The Pregnant Virgin* during my hospital stay, I was able to leave hospital with a sense of hope rather than defeat and to determine that my cancer scar would mark my initiation into a new life and into a truthful coming to terms and letting go of my past. Dr. Woodman's other books have opened numerous other doors for me since.

After three months recovering from surgery, I left the marriage and rented an apartment in the High Park area of Toronto in July 1988. My youngest son, seventeen at the time, lived with me until he began university. My daughter, the oldest, was out of the home by then, and the three middle boys, after living with their father for awhile, began creating new lives for themselves.

From the time of our separation onward, I immersed myself in learning how mind and thought affect the body's physical health. A naturopath taught me how diet, lifestyle change, and supplemental vitamins could help prevent a cancer reoccurrence. An intensive year-long period of weekly shiatsu dream therapy as well as weekly psychodrama work brought much needed support and self-awareness. Because the psychodrama group was equally composed of men and women, the listening to and acting out of stories, especially those of the men in the group, opened my eyes to men's suffering and to the toxic aspects of my conditioning to treat men as gods. In 1990 following the completion of this period of psychological work, I was further empowered by a ten-day wilderness dream workshop in the New Mexico desert.

Mind/body health promotion techniques were gaining in public acceptance close to the time my cancer occurred. Evidence that showed how some cancer-affected people were changing the course of their illnesses through regular practice of meditation and visualization inspired me to adopt both practices for my health.[5]

Although most of my mentors were advocates of Zen meditation and I was already aware of the basics of Zen meditation through Philip Kapleau's, *Three Pillars of Zen,* and Ernest Wood's, *Zen Dictionary,* my anxiety, panic, and unresolved psychosis issues made meditation a difficult practice for me.[6] Where yoga helped me to remain grounded in sitting positions, the combined standing meditation, movement, and memory work that constitutes tai chi was the most effective intermediary meditation practice for me. Tai chi sword forms, in particular, strengthened my attitudes towards physical as well as psycho-logical self-defence and furthered my ability to do sitting meditation.

Being a visual learner, I greatly benefited in my post-cancer period from learning visualization techniques. The hibiscus flower's bowl and phallic shapes came to represent for me the eternal masculine and feminine and became the image I would visualize residing in my gut, breast, or any other body area I wanted to protect from illness. Told at the time of my cancer surgery that I had a greater-than-average chance of developing breast cancer, I began to rou-tinely visualize the nipples of my breasts growing from hibiscus buds into full flower. I never cease to be amazed at the amount of tension that releases from my breast area during these visualization exercises or to be grateful for my continuing wellness.

Over time, I grew able to discern tangibly how my immune system was served by positive thought and weakened by negative mental states. With this new insight into my immune system, I became convinced that my physical survival depended on my quality of mental health. I do not expect mind/body techniques to create health for me beyond my allotted time but these tech-niques have helped me to remain cancer free for twenty years, and to cope with lesser illnesses such as shingles without a single painkiller. For these rea-sons, I trust that the practice of meditation and visualization, when used in conjunction with the best of naturopathic and traditional medicine, will sup-port quality of life throughout my life.

Learning to Feel, Learning to Think

Learning to feel and think again were processes I began soon after my drug withdrawal started. Inside the marriage it was too painful to feel and holding onto my sanity was sometimes all I could achieve, so my early attempts to understand what it meant to feel led me to the practice of yoga and to books recommended by mentors.

From childhood onward, I had split feelings into "good" and "bad" and repressed the bad or painful ones. I also split feelings into public/private cat-egories of acceptability. This public/private split made me bring multiple chameleon selves into relationships, changing myself into who I thought people wanted me to be. Anti-psychotic drugs dulled my emotions and added a new category of caution to how I sifted feelings—that is, "Was that a sane or insane feeling or thought?"

To learn how to feel, I worked at feeling outer textures such as the vegeta-bles I prepared, the earth that I gardened, and the varied other household sur-faces that I touched during the course of a day. The reward for these efforts was feeling more rage. However as "feeling" or "addiction" were the only avenues left, I was forced to trust and to continue in my struggle to undo my old repressive patterns. Yoga was central to my creating a subtler body and a stronger sensitivity for feeling. Later, body arts such as voice, tai chi, drama, and authentic movement, the art in which one listens to the body and follows it where it wants to move, trained me to observe where and how my body wanted to move and communicate.

The return of my thought processes was greatly helped by the breathing techniques that are used in drama and the body arts. My mental capabilities and ability to express myself in words were greatly assisted as well when I learned to use the computer. My immediate and extended families enthusiastically encouraged my use of the computer and kept me abreast of computer technology.

Body arts were essential as well to learning how to relax and breathe into the physical and emotional discomforts that accompanied the release of buried feelings. In addition to becoming anxious, I experienced muscle pain and cramping from a slight to a severe degree in some part or multiple parts of my body when repressed material came to consciousness. The pain was located mainly in the trauma-affected areas of my body. Sexual trauma memories caused cramping in my lower trunk and legs. Issues of being rejected or my rejecting others caused pain to radiate in my heart area and down my arms. My way of dealing with the pain prior to becoming conscious was to soak in a hot tub or distract myself with addictive behaviours.

Addictions such as excessive doing for others, socializing, and movie going were particularly insidious because they were masked by social acceptability. By not involving harmful substances or social acting out, my addictions were easy to overlook. The honesty of mentors who shared their own stories of healing from addiction, my practice of painting dreams and journalling, as well as my intentions to struggle on until I was able to live fully in and with my feelings helped me to face the physical pain involved in becoming conscious.

From 1990 onward, Shiatsu dream work gave me important new access to my body. By the time I finished a year of weekly sessions with a trained therapist, I was able to follow the process on my own. To begin, I hold a dream image in my mind while observing what area of the body is reacting to the image. This usually manifests as a cramping or twitching somewhere on the body. Once I determine where the body is responding to a dream image, I visualize the dream image on the affected body area. The final step involves my quietly breathing into the affected area and dream image while I wait for other images, dreams, or sensing of the issue to enter consciousness.

With the feeling or "coming home to myself" groundwork laid, I was ready to enter into a more conscious understanding of how art heals and into a less anxious and disturbed practice of art.

ROSEMARY
Chief Psychologist

Moving Up

As psychologist colleagues moved from Toronto General to become the heads of departments elsewhere, I questioned my own future. In 1986, I saw a chief psychologist position advertised at Women's College Hospital, a small, university-affiliated Toronto hospital. A colleague encouraged me to apply and admonished that I might remain a staff psychologist for the rest of my career if I did not take some risks. To my surprise and delight, I was offered and I accepted the position. I and my colleagues considered this a good career move.

Women's College Hospital seemed an excellent environment for me. The hospital was established during the early 1900s as a place for women physicians to receive clinical training and had a long-standing interest in women's health. I moved to address the split between my personal and professional lives by joining a small informal group of hospital professionals working to nurture feminist values in health care.

I stayed in touch with former colleagues. A year or so after I left Toronto General, the psychiatric resident's position on the SHARE team was reassigned to another program, a significant loss to Dr. Analytic because staff physicians rely heavily on the work of residents. Dr. Analytic continued with the SHARE program for a time, then resigned to set up a community practice. The in-patient beds previously assigned to crisis intervention care were reassigned to Dr. Grantholder, a psychiatrist who had been awarded thousands of dollars in research grants to study the effects of various psychoactive medications. Dr. Grantholder used these hospital beds to admit patients who met the narrow criteria for participation in his research studies. The SHARE program was substantially downsized; by the early 1990s, the program consisted of a half-time psychologist and a social worker seeing out-patients in suicidal crisis.

Case Study: Dr. Barnes 1989

For a few years, I continued to conduct assessments of psychiatric patients at Women's College Hospital. Suppose that Susan had been admitted to Women's College Hospital in 1989 and that her psychiatrist had ordered a psychological assessment. I introduce myself to her on the hospital ward, addressing her as Ms. Schellenberg and arranging to meet in my office, a spacious, carpeted room with a large window. I am wearing a grey wool skirt suit, high-necked dark red polyester blouse, a pearl necklace, pantyhose, and low-heeled dress shoes. I interview Ms. Schellenberg, taking notes about her experiences at the retreat, her sense of being the Virgin Mary, and her fatigue. I ask about her experiences growing up and note her mother's insistence on absolute obedience. I think to myself that these childhood experiences would likely have taught her that her own opinions and feelings were of little importance compared to the expectations of those in positions of authority. I ask about her being mother to four children, ages three to seven, her marriage, her care of her ill mother, and her interest in art. I note her devotion to the family, efforts to be a good daughter, wife, and mother and concern about communication with her husband and birth control. I administer psychological tests.

I find Ms. Schellenberg's fatigue very understandable given the long hours that she must work and wonder if she simply needs an opportunity to rest. At the time, I have a daughter who is about four years old, and I have often felt exhausted while caring for her as an infant and toddler. I can hardly imagine caring for four small children, even though Ms. Schellenberg mentions having the help of an *au pair*. I am sad that Ms. Schellenberg deprecates her work as a mother and am touched that she reaches out to others who are less fortunate despite her heavy responsibilities at home.

When her husband knocks at the door to ask when he can take his wife for a walk, Ms. Schellenberg apologetically excuses herself. When I note that we still have some tests to complete, she looks very anxious and asks if she can meet me in the afternoon; I agree and we set a time. Her husband directs her to go to her room, get her coat, and wait for him by the elevators. She leaves immediately. Mr. Schellenberg appears anxious but authoritative as he asks what is wrong with his wife and when she will get better. I explain that I will be talking with his wife about the results of the assessment, and that he can ask her about my feedback after I have spoken with her. I explain that I would need his wife's permission to talk with him further about the results and offer to meet with the couple if his wife agrees and he would like to arrange this after talking with her about my feedback.

What has changed since 1969? Technicalities are different. The diagnostic system has been reorganized. In 1980, the American Psychiatric Association published the third edition of the *Diagnostic and Statistical Manual: Mental Disorders* (DSM III); I learned this classification system while working at Toronto General Hospital. Ms. Schellenberg would now be diagnosed with Brief Psychotic Reaction initially and with Schizophrenia if her condition continued for six months or more. Psychological tests have been revised and I administer a somewhat different battery than what the psychologist used in 1969. Medications have been tweaked. However, none of these changes greatly alter the care provided to Ms. Schellenberg. Diagnosis and medication are still central.

However, I have changed and the social climate is changing. In 1989, I think of how the Schellenbergs are influenced by gender role socialization. To the extent that I am able, I convey my understanding of Ms. Schellenberg as an adult separate from her husband. To indicate that Ms. Schellenberg is in charge of her own health and health care, I tell Mr. Schellenberg that I will give assessment feedback to his wife and advise him to ask her about what she has learned from me and to request her permission for the couple to meet with me. When providing feedback to Ms. Schellenberg, I acknowledge her extensive care-giving responsibilities; I also note the ways in which these may have strained her and thus contributed to her acting and thinking in ways that were frightening and distressing to herself and others during her psychotic break. I express appreciation for her very evident devotion to her family. I point out how psychotherapy might help to resolve her concerns about birth control and her marriage and to develop more ways to care for herself as she continues to care for her family. I express hope that making these changes as well as taking the prescribed medication will help her to avoid a recurrence of such distress. In my report, I emphasize the strain Ms. Schellenberg faces as a caregiver in multiple roles and note the potential value of psychotherapy in helping her to learn better self-care and skills in setting limits.

I did not often attend psychiatric in-patient rounds at Women's College Hospital, but suppose that I did attend to report on my assessment of Ms. Schellenberg. I join the psychiatrist, a medical intern, the social worker, occupational therapist, and nurse in a large, carpeted, multipurpose room. The occupational therapist's craft materials are stored on shelves along one wall; a metal cart holding a slide projector rests along another wall and a projection screen is at the far end of the room. Stacks of metal chairs and a round table have been pushed to one side; the team members sit at another round table in the centre of the room. A second metal cart holds the black, three-ring binders that contain patients' medical files. This utilitarian ambiance is similar to what I recall from the Clarke Institute and Toronto General Hospital.

The staff gather for 10:00 AM rounds and sip coffee, chatting casually as we wait for Dr. Medmodel, the team psychiatrist and only male team member. At 10:08, Dr. Medmodel arrives, apologizes for being late, and quickly opens the meeting by asking about Ms. Schellenberg. Barbara Capable, the head nurse, interjects to tell Dr. Medmodel that Jane Doe, a patient admitted just an hour ago, is very distressed that she is being forced to wear a hospital gown rather than her own clothes. Ms. Doe came into the hospital voluntarily, cannot see why she should have her clothes taken from her, and is threatening to leave even though Barbara has explained the ward policy that all patients wear hospital gowns until they have been assessed by the psychiatrist and an order has been written to permit them to wear street clothes. Ms. Doe has agreed to remain in hospital during rounds on the condition that the nurse talk to Dr. Medmodel about her concerns. Dr. Medmodel says that he would like to begin with Ms. Schellenberg and will discuss Ms. Doe's situation later. He asks Barbara how

Ms. Schellenberg is doing as he takes her medical chart from the cart and flips through the pages during Barbara's nursing report.

When Barbara finishes, I say that I have completed the psychological assessment. When Dr. Medmodel nods, I note that Ms. Schellenberg is still distressed and has problems with her perceptions of reality; these problems seem to be residual aspects of her recent psychotic break and are consistent with a diagnosis of a Brief Psychotic Episode. I note that illness, fatigue, and multiple caregiving responsibilities may have contributed to her recent crisis, and I recommend psychotherapy in addition to the medication that she is receiving. Dr. Medmodel comments on Ms. Schellenberg's effort to do community work as an indication of her ongoing impaired reality testing. I say that Ms. Schellenberg does have some difficulties in reality testing, but may also feel that she is valued only because of what she does for others; poor self-esteem might explain her efforts to do volunteer work when she appears to be already very taxed at home. Dr. Medmodel cautions that too much emphasis on women as victims risks missing more serious pathology such as impaired reality testing.

Referring to a recent presentation on women's issues and mental health, Dr. Medmodel raises the question of whether Ms. Schellenberg's sense of being influenced by forces outside her control might pose risks for the safety of her children. I recall the feminist speaker pointing out that women's lack of encouragement to value their own health might contribute to health problems that could affect a woman's ability to function as a mother and wonder whether Dr. Medmodel is thinking of the same talk. I comment that Ms. Schellenberg did mention fears for her children's safety as one of her test responses, but that she seems devoted to her children and I have no other indication that the children's safety is a concern. Dr. Medmodel decides to pursue this issue with Ms. Schellenberg in an interview, which is a common procedure during rounds. Barbara leaves to find Ms. Schellenberg and brings her into the meeting room. Dr. Medmodel stands, offers Ms. Schellenberg a chair, explains that we are all members of the professional team looking after her while she is in hospital, and introduces each professional by name and professional discipline. Ms. Schellenberg looks uncertain and anxious.

Dr. Medmodel asks Ms. Schellenberg how she has been doing; she replies that she has been sleeping better and feels more rested; she thanks Dr. Medmodel for having reduced her medication dosage. In response to Dr. Medmodel's question, she says that she has not experienced hearing voices or thoughts of being the Blessed Virgin Mary for some days. When Dr. Medmodel asks her to describe these experiences in more detail, Ms. Schellenberg hesitates and looks at her hands as she struggles to find words. Finally, she says that it was like being hypnotized and experiencing herself as a passive vessel of God's imagination and thus capable of carrying out whatever she is directed to do.

Dr. Medmodel asks if she fears that she might injure her children when she is in such a state. Her colour changes suddenly and her eyes widen; she looks directly at the doctor. No, she says angrily, absolutely not. She has given everything to her family and cannot believe that he is questioning her in this way. Dr. Medmodel says that he did not mean to upset her, but it is his job to ask difficult questions. He knows that Ms. Schellenberg means to be a good mother, but is concerned about the effect of her illness. He is glad to see that she is getting better. He has no further questions, and asks if she has anything she wishes to say before the interview concludes. Ms. Schellenberg asks when she will be discharged. Dr. Medmodel says that she is doing well, but he feels that she should stay in hospital for another week or so to make sure that she has recovered enough to go home.

A brief discussion ensues after Ms. Schellenberg leaves. I reiterate that Ms. Schellenberg takes pride in being a good mother and may have found it upsetting to have her abilities questioned in this respect. The nurse points out ways in which Ms. Schellenberg has spoken fondly of her children when on the ward. However, the occupational therapist points out that Ms. Schellenberg seemed to have difficulty the day before in following directions concerning how to assemble the balloon noisemakers. Dr. Medmodel concludes that Ms. Schellenberg continues to be somewhat unstable. He writes an order for Ms. Schellenberg's medication dosage to be slightly increased, then asks Barbara to report on Ms. Doe as he returns Ms. Schellenberg's binder to the cart and reaches for Ms. Doe's chart.

I leave rounds ready to spit nails and wondering whether my assessment helped Ms. Schellenberg or her husband in any way. I have never liked bringing patients into rounds for interviews because it seems to me an unnecessarily intimidating and humiliating procedure. I feel angry and embarrassed that my exchange with the psychiatrist may have led him to question Ms. Schellenberg before the team on her ability to care for her children. I feel that Ms. Schellenberg has ensured that the children have good care despite her serious difficulties and cannot see how questioning her in this way can be in any way helpful to her. I wonder if she will feel that I used what she told me against her when I made my report to the psychiatrist. I worry that I have betrayed her trust. However, I cannot talk to Ms. Schellenberg because I told her that I would not see her again and I cannot initiate a conversation where I question the approach taken by her psychiatrist.

● ● ●

Many such experiences led me to question whether patients were helped by hospital mental health care and to worry that some were harmed. Patronizing and belittling staff attitudes interfered with patients' abilities and desires to be active participants in overcoming personal difficulties. Reliance on diagnosis and medication seemed excessive; staff's narrow focus and gender bias seemed to undermine patients' abilities to recover from emotional crisis.

I was cautious about expressing my questions and frustration to colleagues; after various conversations, I decided that the psychiatrists were unlikely to be supportive and that other staff had mixed reactions to such incidents; some shared my distress while others felt that the situation had to be understood from the doctor's viewpoint. I felt unable to make a strong stand on a controversial position where I had uncertain support. I had already begun to avoid the psychiatric services as much as possible. Colleagues accepted that a department head would attempt to expand services, so I branched out to take part in the Sexual Assault Care Centre, the first program of its kind in Ontario. I developed and led a psychosocial support team for people hospitalized with AIDS and HIV-related conditions. I assigned the psychiatric services to another psychologist.

For some years, I saw these problems as aberrations amenable to correction through reform. Like the scientist and activist Dr. Ursula Franklin, I believed that leaders were well intentioned and poorly informed and thought about how to correct this situation.[7] I attended numerous meetings and had long discussions with feminist colleagues about reading the tea leaves of hospital politics. I helped with the development of the Brief Psychotherapy Centre for Women and the Women's Health Centre, both programs that use a feminist approach to care. I worked with colleagues to help develop a professional advisory committee so that professionals other than physicians had a basis for more visible leadership roles within the hospital. I participated in hospital-wide efforts to develop a philosophy of care and was delighted that day-long discussions with several hundred staff led to a statement of core values that included empowerment of women, accessibility of programs, broad definition of health/holistic care, high-quality care, collaborative planning, and innovative/creative approaches. I felt that applying these values to the psychiatric services might help to resolve the problems I saw, for example, with Susan's care I also learned more about the law and funding arrangements that govern hospitals.

Hospitals are organized around the practice of physicians. Only a physician has authority to admit and discharge a patient. Organizationally, physicians are entirely different in terms of pay and accountability from every other staff person in the hospital. Physicians govern themselves within the hospitals through the hospital medical advisory committee and report directly to the hospital board of directors. The hospital president has the authority to hire, evaluate, and fire other professional staff, but not physicians. Physicians are paid by government funds that are outside of the overall hospital budget. All other professional staff report, through various administrative lines, to the hospital president and are paid within the hospital global budget.

These differences have practical, day-to-day implications. Dr. Medmodel arrived a little late at rounds probably because he was seeing outpatients in his office for which he bills the government health insurance program. He can bill for patients discussed in rounds, but the possible billing amount does not increase when discussions are longer, so he is motivated to keep discussions short so that rounds are not prolonged and he is free to return to his office where he can resume seeing outpatients for whom he bills. To compensate for the loss of income resulting from time in rounds, administrative activities, program development, or teaching, Dr. Medmodel is provided with a fixed annual stipend known as a sessional fee. However, such fees are ordinarily not increased if he devotes more time to teaching or other activities. If Dr. Medmodel commits a great deal of time to activities other than seeing patients for whom he can bill his professional services, he is lowering his income. Dr. Medmodel is apt to feel frustrated by expectations that he attend administrative meetings, particularly time-consuming events such as day-long staff retreats or planning sessions, since this takes him away from other paying work.

I, on the other hand, am on a fixed salary, not directly tied to the number of patients seen or time devoted to other activities. More prolonged discussions at rounds, involvement in teaching, or seeing more or fewer patients have no direct impact on my income, though my boss may give me a poor performance evaluation if I use time in a manner not in keeping with organizational goals and priorities. I consider an event such as a day-long planning session to be part of what I am paid for and sometimes a welcome diversion from routine activities. I am frustrated when Dr. Medmodel arrives late, leaves early, or does not show up at all for such a meeting.

Complex interdependencies motivate professional staff to find ways to work with one another. Dr. Medmodel understands that the smooth functioning of the multidisciplinary psychiatric team is important to his patients' care, and wants to secure other staff's cooperation. I want good relations with Dr. Medmodel because his support or opposition will have a large influence on the patients whom I see and any proposals I have for changing psychology services or developing new programs. Most staff are, like me, decent, caring individuals who find the work meaningful, so we share a personal commitment to good patient services.

As I work on various initiatives, I come to understand more clearly the arrangements that shape the hospital. Although mission statements speak very broadly of health care, hospitals are essentially places for physicians to practise, for example, to diagnose injury and disease and to provide treatment. Other professional groups such as nurses, physiotherapists, social workers, and psychologists are viewed as providing auxiliary services that assist the physicians. Law, policy, and funding arrangements ensure that approaches other than the medical model for care are not central to what hospitals do. As a hospital board member once commented to me, "We will decide on the programs that our physicians feel important to develop, then deploy our other resources accordingly."

Dr. Medmodel was trained as a physician so he is committed to the hospital approach to mental health care. The basic framework, particularly for individuals with serious mental illness, consists of emergency, in-patient, and clinic services. Primary emphasis is placed on detection of individuals with emotional disturbance, accurate diagnosis, protection of individual and public safety through hospital admission, and careful medication administration—in short, a medical model. These services are considered the indispensable framework around which mental health care is organized, just as the steel chassis provides the basic framework for construction of a car. The basic framework is usually the first to be established when mental health programs are begun and the last to be diminished or closed when funding is reduced.

Programs that emphasize other methods of evaluation and intervention are typically considered specialized or secondary. While they may be highly valued in certain times or settings, they are, in my experience, highly dependant on funding trends and on the personalities and professional preferences of their leaders. Dr. Medmodel knows that other interventions, including psychotherapy, occupational therapy, art therapy, meditation, and so on, are helpful and provides psychotherapy to some of his patients. He regrets the limited availability of other services, but has neither time nor interest for developing programs in such areas. Most psychiatrists feel as he does, with the result that these programs are treated as luxuries, like the additional styling features of a deluxe car which one will buy if they suit personal taste and are affordable. Such programs are particularly vulnerable to cutbacks when the interests of hospital leaders change and budgets are reduced.

Neither Dr. Medmodel nor any other psychiatrist participated in the hospital-wide brainstorming that developed the hospital's statement of core values. He does not mind the statement so long as it does not interfere with his ability to work in the way he always has. He attends educational presentations on women's mental health issues, but does not attend a meeting of mental health staff working on ways to implement the newly stated values into the mental health program. He is concerned that in-patient beds are being cut and is involved in the discussions about a program to assess trauma patients referred by a government workplace insurance agency; this program will provide new billing opportunities and help make up for budget cuts in the psychiatric in-patient area.

As I understand hospitals more clearly, I no longer feel that leaders are well intentioned and poorly informed but come to believe instead that they are well informed and poorly intentioned; I begin to doubt the prospects for reform. I also wonder what else is happening when I attend all these hospital meetings. During the week that I meet with Ms. Schellenberg, I attend a department heads meeting, a mental and community health program heads meeting, the HIV/AIDS Psychosocial Support Team rounds, the hospital quality assurance committee meeting, and a day-long workshop on a new performance management system. I participate in three candidate interviews as a member of the hiring committee for the Brief Psychotherapy Centre for Women. I conduct two four-hour assessments, prepare reports on these assessments, have three meetings with psychotherapy clients, meet with the psychology intern who has just begun work with our department, have my monthly meeting with my boss, prepare the departmental budget, and work on the report that I am preparing concerning program implementation in the new Women's Health Centre. I leave by 5:30 on most days because my daughter must be picked up from the daycare by 6:00. I bring paper work to do after I have made her dinner, helped her to brush her teeth, read her a story, and tucked her into bed. Though I share these responsibilities with a very supportive partner, I am usually rushed and often tired. The psychiatrist asks if I can see Ms. Schellenberg for psychotherapy as she has told him that she appreciated my feedback and would be willing to meet further with me. No, sorry, don't have time.

When I believed that my efforts at reform would make things better for Ms. Schellenberg, I could justify not seeing her for psychotherapy. However, as I lose faith in reform, I increasingly miss clinical work. Finally, I become lost. My ability to live with the split between my feminist values and professional career commitments erodes as I am increasingly unconvinced that my time, creativity, and energy are supporting what is most meaningful to me. I feel cynical, exhausted, and angry about my apparently successful career and this also confuses me. I am, after all, chief psychologist at a prestigious, university-affiliated hospital where I am highly regarded. I have a nice home, a loving partner, and a beautiful daughter. What could possibly be wrong?

Susan's Hospital Experiences

When I read Susan's clinical records in 1992, I recognized her mental health care as standard. The records suggested recovery in that Susan remained largely symptom-free and resumed her responsibilities as a wife and mother; most mental health professionals would describe her hospital care as a success on this basis. However, Susan's account of her life thirty-odd years later told a different story. The hospital admission and years of follow-up treatment led to depression as well as marital and family problems. Suicidal thoughts and impairments in speech, memory, and mental acuity all developed, yet remained unidentified and untreated until after Susan committed to healing. Restoration of speech and mental faculties, improved family relationships, and development of emotional balance occurred only after Susan gave her own sense of well-being priority over the direction of those in authority. She worked hard for many years with tremendous success to end her use of psychoactive medication, achieve greater control over her life, and nurture her creative abilities, in the process profoundly reorganizing her life and sense of self. By the time I was reading her records, she was well advanced in healing, but little thanks was due to the mental health care she had received for so many years. The mental health system failed to mobilize her enormous potential for recovery and growth.

Here were the dilemmas that I faced when thinking of Susan's experiences. There was the reality of a person in undeniable and overwhelming distress. Some anti-psychiatry writing argues or implies that mental health treatment causes serious problems where none existed, and mental health interventions does occasionally greatly worsen relatively minor problems.[8] This kind of abuse does occur, but I did not see much of it during my years of hospital work. Many individuals and families have experienced something like what happened to Susan. National surveys indicate that one million Canadians live with a serious mental illness, and international statistics indicate that mental health problems account for five of the ten leading causes of disability in terms of productive years lost.[9] Susan herself, her family, and friends faced overwhelming problems that were beyond their ability to resolve despite great effort to do so. When admitted to Lakeshore Psychiatric Hospital, Susan was experiencing visual and auditory hallucinations and behaving in ways that made no sense and were very disturbing; she was obviously in crisis and in need of sanctuary. Hospital admission provided a respite from heavy responsibilities as daughter, wife, and mother and medication that reduced the intensity of emotional distress. Hospital care relieved her frightening symptoms and allowed her to resume functioning as a mother and wife to the family she loved deeply. What went wrong?

Some individuals who need professional assistance receive services that are tragically harmful due to accidentally or maliciously substandard care. Wendy Funk, for example, describes going to a family physician fatigued and with a bad sore throat, being diagnosed as depressed, and then receiving a series of increasingly intrusive and debilitating treatments, including involuntary (i.e., legally forced) hospital admission and repeated electroconvulsive shock therapy.[10] She explains that her treatment was not in any way appropriate to the nature of her problems and caused her to become seriously, perhaps permanently, disabled. As another example, some individuals in emotional distress have been seriously harmed when the health professional providing care initiates sexual relations; Phyllis Chesler's classic critique describes this abuse as one of the most serious perpetrated against women in emotional distress.[11] Survey studies in the 1980s indicated that between 3 and 7 percent of male mental health professionals reported initiating sexual contact with clients.[12] Abusing professionals advance sexual relations with patients by a variety of means including force, drugging, deceit, flattery, and manipulation[13] and serious psychological harm is caused by such professional misconduct.[14]

It is easy to agree that grossly substandard care and assaults against vulnerable individuals are deplorable. Regulatory and legal remedies, though cumbersome, are available to redress such harms. Funk, for example, mentions that she is progressing with complaints to the professional licensing body and a civil suit against her treating physicians.[15] The information provided in her book indicates that legal action is a highly appropriate response to grossly substandard mental health services. Changes in law and regulatory practices mean that licensing bodies and courts now take patient concerns about professional sexual misconduct far more seriously than was the case in years past.[16] Moreover, threats of lengthy, expensive disciplinary complaints and civil suits offer an important incentive to both individual professionals and institutional settings to adopt policies and procedures that respect and enforce the patient's right to appropriate care. Continuing vigilance is essential to protect the civil liberties of individuals held against their wishes for mental health evaluation and treatment.

However, the failures of the mental health system in Susan's case were more subtle. Although she was admitted as an involuntary patient (meaning that she was legally required to stay in the psychiatric hospital for a time), Susan never indicated that she felt the physician's decision to arrange admission on this basis was inappropriate or that this authority was abused. I found no indication in the clinical records that Susan's care was substandard or inappropriate. Susan's clinical records were detailed, complete, and indicative of thorough and conscientious professional work. The quality of the professionals' work met or exceeded the standards of the day. Moreover, although some technical terms, concepts, and medications have changed, the clinical methods and treatment goals applied to Susan's difficulties remain widely used. Susan's experience reflected the mental health care system functioning normally.

Notes

1 Nobel Lecture, 5 June 1991 Available at http://writespirit.net/inspirational_talks/mikhail_gorbachev_talks/nobel_peace_lecture/.
2 Edward F. Edinger, *Ego and Archetype: Individuation and Religious Function of the Psyche* (New York: Putnam, 1973).
3 Jean Baker Miller, *Toward a New Psychology of Women* (Boston: Beacon Press, 1976).
4 Marion Woodman, *The Pregnant Virgin: A Process of Psychological Transformation* (Toronto: Inner City Books, 1985).

5 Joan Borysenko, *Minding the Body, Mending the Mind* (Reading, MA: Addison-Wesley, 1987).

6 Philip Kapleau, *The Three Pillars of Zen: Teaching, Practice and Enlightenment*, complied and edited with translations, introductions, and notes by Philip Kapleau. Foreword by Huston Smith (New York: Harper and Row [1966, c. 1965]).

7 Dr. Franklin mentioned her early belief that leaders were well intentioned and poorly informed as well as her later view that leaders were well informed and poorly intentioned when describing the evolution of her approach to political activism. She gave this account as part of her talk at a Women's Legal Action and Education (LEAF) Persons Day breakfast I attended in Toronto, Ontario. Unfortunately, I was not able to retrieve the date of this event.

8 See for example, Peter Roger Breggin, *Toxic Psychiatry* (New York: St. Martin's Press, 1991); Wendy Funk, *What Difference Does It Make? The Journey of a Soul Survivor* (Cranbrook, BC: Wildflower, 1998).

9 Scott Simmie and Julia Nunes, *The Last Taboo: A Survival Guide to Mental Health Care in Canada* (Toronto: McClelland & Stewart, 2001).

10 Funk, *What Difference Does It Make?*

11 Phyllis Chesler, *Women and Madness* (New York: Avon Books, 1972).

12 Kenneth S. Pope, "How Clients Are Harmed by Sexual Contact with Mental Health Professionals: The Syndrome and Its Prevalence," *Journal of Counseling and Development* 67 (1988): 222–26.

13 Gary Schoener et al., eds., *Psychotherapists' Sexual Involvement with Clients: Intervention and Prevention* (Minneapolis, MN: Walk-in Counseling Center, 1989).

14 Pope, "How Clients Are Harmed."

15 Funk, *What Difference Does It Make?*

16 See for example Andrew W. Kane, "The Effects of Criminalization of Sexual Misconduct by Therapists: Report of a Survey in Wisconsin," in *Breach of Trust: Sexual Exploitation by Health Care Professionals and Clergy*, ed. John C. Gonsiorek (Thousand Oaks, CA: Sage, 1995), 317–37; Melissa Roberts-Henry, "Criminalization of Therapist Sexual Misconduct in Colorado," also in *Breach of Trust*, 338–47.

4 Strengthening through Structure, Healing through Art

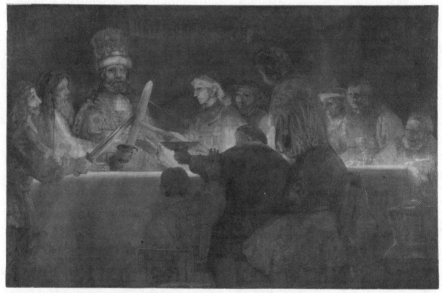

REMBRANDT, *THE CONSPIRACY OF CLAUDIUS (OR JULIUS) CIVILUS*. CANVAS, 71.25 × 121.75 INCHES (CUT DOWN). PHOTO: THE NATIONAL MUSEUM OF FINE ARTS, STOCKHOLM.

> The table at which the freedom fighters are gathered is symbolic of the oath that will hold them together until the last one of them has sacrificed himself for the cause.
>
> —Angela Greig, 1983

In 1984, when I lacked the words to make sense of my inner war or the strength to face my choices, my resolve was reinforced through warrior images. One such image, Rembrandt's *Conspiracy of Claudius Civilis,* inspired courage when I lacked it most.

SUSAN
Introduction to Art and Structure

MENTORS GAVE ME THE COURAGE to make art and the structures that would enable me to heal from mental illness through artistic expression. If my parents and teachers had been conditioned to guide children according to their interests and skills, my art training would have begun in my teens. From an early age I excelled in art at school, was drawn to artistic images in the family's *Books of Knowledge,* and habitually visited the Royal Ontario Museum's Elizabethan costume, medieval armour, and North American Native displays. But art became as split off in me as in my Depression-influenced mother and the socially controlling church that conditioned me to regard artmaking as an occasion of sin and capable, especially in the case of women, of turning me/us into debauched free thinkers.

In 1979, after a ten-year absence from painting, I resumed artmaking. The practice of art heightened my religious-based fears of art, as well as the chaos and terror triggered by my unresolved psychosis. These feelings often snowballed into paralyzing fear of a repeat psychosis. Due to this reaction, I could only paint for short periods. When I was most afraid yet most in need of art, the warrior archetype reflected in film, dream, or art depictions of Joan of Arc repeatedly resonated for me during this period and strengthened my determination to remain on my art journey.

I met with a kind YWCA career counsellor to determine how, given the drug side effects, I might develop my past nursing and art skills into a new career. In a warm and validating manner, the counsellor advised me to "say yes to everything," and to try volunteering in a hospital occupational therapy department with a view to some day filling an art-related staff position.

Inspired, I met with the head of volunteers at St. Joseph's Hospital. After explaining my goal to work in the hospital's occupational therapy department, she handed me a large manual and told me that *she,* not I, would decide where I would and would not work. My immediate response to the director's tone was anger at the thought of her terrorizing other empty-nested women who came to volunteer freely at the hospital. I next asked the director in my most rejecting fashion to direct me to the hospital's employment office. As I wrote out an employment application, I could see I was unemployable but also recognized for the first time how many skills I had developed during my child-rearing years.

As I left the hospital's employment office, I knew that I wanted to do art more than anything in the world. That afternoon, a long-held urge triggered by my anger at the hospital's volunteer director pushed me to find and rent a studio in Parkdale. My delight in having an art space of my own and in the many friendships I found in this building strengthened me. Where the prolific pace of the other studio artists emphasized my slowness, I felt accepted there and when I was not painting, I used the studio to organize other work I had said yes to, namely volunteer community TV production and the presidency of an art club.

The start of my volunteer work in community television began close to 1982 when Maclean Hunter asked me to produce an arts talk show. If the station had selected me for this TV-hosting role on the basis of my short well-prepared talks at local art openings, they did not know how rehearsed or how concentrated my breath work was when I delivered those talks or how impossible it would be for me to create the same effect *ad lib*. In declining Maclean Hunter's offer, I did suggest that the station needed English literature programming for Etobicoke students who were visual learners. When the station asked me to produce this type of programming instead and assured me I would not be in front of the camera, I accepted. During my first two years with Maclean Hunter, I involved Etobicoke secondary students as well as drama and English teachers in the creation of programs that discussed plays in the school curriculum and allowed secondary drama students to perform excerpts from the plays being discussed. My skills at bringing people together far exceeded my knowledge of literature, but work on these programs did open me to learning more in this area.

Close to this time, the actress partner of one of the studio sculptors openly expressed her concern over my speech difficulties and asked if I would like her to connect me to a speech therapist. Speech therapy threw me headlong into feelings of being in love with the male therapist. I judged these feelings to be wrong because I was married and I struggled to repress them. But the more I tried to repress, the more overwhelming the feelings became to the point that severe emotional disruption ensued and brought me to the brink of another psychotic episode. The fear that I would need to go back on drugs resulted in months of silent inner struggle. Eventually, my psychiatrist described my being in love with the speech therapist as a transference. I took his use of the term *transference* to mean that "falling in love" reflected a normal reaction to the speech therapy process. The psychiatrist's explanation and having a word as remote as "transference" to name this experience helped to lessen the shame I attached to these feelings.

As I reached 1983 and a desperate state of fear that I was about to experience another psychosis, my daughter's former teacher Angela Greig, vice-principal of Thornton Hall (a Toronto private secondary school), invited me to attend her school for a year of anatomical drawing and Rembrandt studies. Angela's invitation, "You must study with me or you will never be anything but a Grandma Moses," inspired me to give up my studio and begin my most exciting year of learning ever.

Daily two-hour art sessions involving multidimensional renderings of the skeleton and its parts were followed by an hour-long lecture on Rembrandt. The content and structure of my year, as well as the person of this exceptional scholar, artist, and consciously feminine woman, enabled me to bridge my Catholic past to the beginnings of a more Jungian outlook. Although Angela's art history classes never involved moralizing or psychological theorizing, she imparted Rembrandt's genius both as a painter and dramatist when describing the psychological moments captured in his works.

My year of being fully engaged with art studies allowed me to put aside the psychological work that began but was never completed with the speech therapist. Though I continued with a drug withdrawal form of therapy, it would be years before I was able to face the issues that drove my transference in speech therapy. Shortly after my sessions with the speech therapist ended, my husband and I went spring skiing at Whistler in British Columbia. One morning after breakfast, as we began walking through the streets of Whistler towards the chairlift, I saw the speech therapist in a yellow plaid shirt and jeans and peaked cap walk towards us from the chairlift area. The speech therapist looked directly at me, then walked past us on my right. In disbelief, I looked behind to see if it really was him. He was leaning with his body facing left against a waist-high street planter and his head facing toward me. In terror, I kept walking with my husband towards the chair and as we went up the mountain I became convinced an eclipse of the sun was also taking place. The transference issue was key to my clearing of the core trauma memories that triggered my psychosis but in 1983, I was incapable of facing that work.

The timing of my art studies was doubly auspicious because some months prior, I decided to stop taking all antipsychotic drugs. With this decision and at psychiatrist Dr. Ives' suggestion, I went on a lesser tranquillizer called Ativan and began another withdrawal from it. When I reached but remained stuck at a one-quarter milligram maintenance dose of Ativan, I recognized how, despite the insignificant amount of Ativan I was taking, it represented an outside "power or thing" that would keep me safe and sane.

Ativan's safety-net role was largely replaced by my daily art practices, observations, and connection to Angela. Despite the fact that I studied

Rembrandt during the most highly self-centred period of my life, his magnificent series of self-portraits forced me to see the openness and complete vulnerability of another human being and artist. Rembrandt's ability to create art in spite of crushing personal losses and setbacks also touched my heart during a time when losses left me barely able to feel my own life, let alone any other person's.

Encouraged to read Albert Lubin's, *Stranger on the Earth: A Psychological Biography of Vincent Van Gogh*, I found much-needed permission in this account of Van Gogh's life to explore my own background and to change a long-held belief that my psychosis occurred because I was derelict and chronically ill.[1] Rembrandt and Van Gogh's lives reinforced my commitment to leave an art record of my mind as it healed and my will to persevere with overcoming my art difficulties.

I took my last dose of Ativan immediately following an art history exam on Rembrandt that I was not required but that I chose to write with the other students. Exam anxieties, drug-related memory problems, and hand tremors resulted in my condensing a multiple question exam into one long outpouring of a sentence. Yet, my compassionate teacher phoned later that same day to say I had written a "superb" exam and to invite me to come and discuss my paper with her the following morning before class. My elation at having written and survived the Rembrandt exam was such that I was able to decide against taking my drugs that night.

My first night without drugs was marked by a powerful dream in which I stood on the peak of a large mountain on a starless night. As I looked into the darkness, my hands were anchored to my hips in a gunslinger pose. Then, out of the darkness a gigantic predatory bird many times my size came charging at me with extended talons and scooping wing movements. I stood my ground and repeatedly roared, "NO!" at the bird until it finally backed off and drifted from sight. I then fell into the most exquisite sleep that I have ever slept. The dream occurred in 1984. I have been drug free since. The day following this dream, my teacher went over my exam and gave me a short unforgettable lesson on how to write. "Remember, Susan, one idea per sentence." I wrote better exams as the year progressed.

Attention to care, or what Angela called a "morality of form," was core to every aspect of my studies, even the washing of my paintbrushes. It was no small matter to learn care when depression caused me to swing between the carelessness of enthralled states when I believed I was a great painter and times of low self-worth when I destroyed my art. Daily lessons on how to discern the care that marks fine art while having my own art given both the greatest care and rigorous critiquing seeded my being with new concepts of care. My studies empowered me with new seeing and saying *no* to the loss of care in my marriage and home life. Care as a core theme continued in the lessons I gained from each of my subsequent mentors.

I learned as much about life from Angela Greig's presence that year as I did from her teachings. Her hourglass Great Mother figure, magnificent clothes, conscious and dramatic physical presence, facility with words, ability to be forcefully tough as well as nurturing and fun with her students, and the fact she was a "real" rather than a "super woman," imprinted a powerful new image of the feminine on my soul. I felt stronger and coped better after that year of study than I had ever felt before.

As my studies ended, I returned to the studio I previously rented and began to volunteer-produce a different series of educational programs for Maclean Hunter community TV.

Barry Duncan and Bill Smart were English teachers, authors, and co-founders and leaders of the Association of Media Literacy; they each wrote two programs of a four-program series called *Myths: Patterns to Live By*. The required research for these programs introduced me to the ancient and present mythologies of childhood, ritual, women, and the hero as well as to the scholarship of Joseph Campbell, Claude Lévi-Strauss, Bruno Bettelheim, Marshall McLuhan, and others.

Concerned that I was abandoning my art to TV production, I wrestled with these doubts until a day when the television crew, teachers, and I gathered in a primary school classroom to record a storytelling performance by Helen Porter. Helen, in a periwinkle blue suit, white Victorian blouse, and matching blue heels, cast a chic modern Mother Goose spell on the children as well as on us as she entered the class. Her work with the children and an on-camera interview about the importance of story to children's development were inspiring enough in themselves but later when she relayed off camera an Inuit tale called "Skull in the Snow," it so mirrored my life at that time that I ceased to worry that I was in the right work.[2]

The speaking required for the meetings and shoots with the show's guest professors and storytellers as well as for my public-speaking role as an art club president was aided by breath techniques I had picked up in speech therapy and drama classes. Despite the fact that I was unable to retain learning in ways that allowed me to discuss myth on any level, I was privy to endless discussions on myth as well as to superb teachers who welcomed questions. Added opportunities to work closely on the paper and video edits, to gather program visuals, and to create the programs' poster reinforced my confidence and anchored me to new understandings of myth.

For an unskilled producer with a drugged mind, the constantly repeated manual and visual tasks and research that went into the two-year production and promotion of these programs, in addition to the kindness and acceptance of all those I worked with, provided me an education on myth that would have been impossible for me to absorb in a classroom. My 1984–1986 work on these programs meshed perfectly with my past Rembrandt studies and the dream studies that would follow soon after. The wonder and synchronicity of this unsought flow of near-magical assistance gave me courage to remain on my journey when everything else in my life was in chaos and decline.

Each of my mentors advocated a sanity of structure rather than unbridled expression. Most appeared to base their practice on a system that, whether in art, drama, voice, movement, or dream, I understood as being in some way related to story and the work of Carl Jung. The focused and relaxed repetition of some simple practice in one of these arts usually allowed an archetypal movement, sound, or image to come to a conscious level where its truth could be studied. An example that comes to mind is the meticulous pencil rendering I was required to do of a skull that took me weeks to complete. I could not work that intimately with a skull without first learning the shapes of the skull for the purpose of art and, second, opening to the issue of my mortality. It was not important to know how the art was affecting healing; it was only necessary to do it and, as they say, let it cook.

Restructuring Internal Self

As the deconstruction of my fractured self-concept as a father's daughter, a man's wife, and children's mother and my restructuring as an individual and as a woman unfolded, the process also revealed that I could go only at my soul's pace: rather than being a magic product, the work would be an ongoing life process. Like dream and fairy tale, the images that resonated for me during that time could take minutes, months, or years to become fully conscious.

The unconditional acceptance and non-judgment that was common to all my mentors also supported my ability to gain comfort while painting. Their approval contrasted with the marginalizing, silencing, and shaming effects of my illness and offered an alternative to the culture of putting down others, particularly women, that I had internalized. I tried to imitate the mentors' affirming behaviours initially and over time the repetition of positive affirmations became more authentically integrated into my ways of relating to my art, to myself, and to others.

Back in 1981, after complaining to Dr. Ives about my speech difficulties and asking if they were treatable, I was referred for testing to the Department of Speech and Language Pathology at the University of Toronto. The tests I received offered my first understanding of psychoactive drugs and how the long-term antipsychotic drugs had damaged my speech centre. I felt relieved that my difficulties in this area were legitimate, but remained discouraged for a time that I might be at an "as-good-as-it-gets" point.

Official validation of my drug-harmed speech centre proved helpful when Angela, in order to explain Rembrandt as a dramatist, introduced me to the writings of contemporary dramatists. This area of study inspired me to explore drama classes. By utilizing the breathing techniques used by actors and continuing to force myself to speak in public, I was able to gain comfort while speaking. My former halting speech and rapid eye twitching are noticeable now only if I am tired or under extreme pressure; they were originally pronounced.

Angela Greig, whose own background included studies with English dramatist Peter Brook, encouraged me to read Brook's work, *The Empty Space*.[3] She also suggested that I read Constantin Stanislavski, Jan Kott's *Shakespeare Our Contemporary*, and the writings of French dramatist Antonin Artaud, *The Theatre and Its Double: Essays*.[4] Each dramatist helped me understand my body/soul/voice connection more. Drama studies also allowed me to develop a deeper understanding of the universal gestures which, whether applied to my figurative painting, appreciation of theatre and film, or to gaining self-awareness, provided another tool for observing my body in its various psychological states. I also benefited from drama workshops in movement and improvisation; I have found psychodrama, which combines aspects of drama with therapy, to be very helpful. Although I tried a little performing, I think drama was meant mostly for my own pleasure, the way music is for people who sing in the shower.

Actors such as the late Sir Alec Guinness, who overcame childhood trauma to the degree he was able to bring an immense integrity to roles as diverse as Hitler and the Ben (Obi-Wan) Kenobi in *Star Wars,* inspired my goal to achieve that range of awareness in my own humanity.

My intention to express a feeling in any art was what allowed growth; this intention was as important as the level of mastery I possessed or the actual work that I produced. The more I learned to create within artistic structures rather than go into the subconscious empty handed, the more I was able to sustain periods of creativity. The volcanic psychic eruption of repressed feelings that a Lakeshore Psychiatric Hospital psychologist had labelled a "cauldron of snakes" got tamed and trained to mainly come up with one dream or manageable feeling at a time.

Restructuring of Catholic Self

To do the work of healing—to locate, trust, and not break and split away from my inner self—it was also necessary for me to let go of all of the images and external manifestations of the Higher Self as it was understood by formal religion. Too fragile to hold the concept of a god on an altar and one in me simultaneously, or of assigning the masculine but not the feminine to this mystery,

I was unable to enter a church without some degree of feeling split off from the new self I was trying to construct.

As a member of a large extended Catholic family, I found it physically as well as mentally difficult to attend family funerals and weddings. As my understanding of the feminine became more developed, I would spend entire services trying to get relief by translating the liturgy so that the godhead, which I could refer to only as the "universe," held feminine as well as masculine meaning.

I initially experienced the erasure of all the familiar energies and meanings that surrounded Christian symbols as a death. However, at the point when meaning seemed totally lost, mentors furthered a gradual new awakening to what I considered an enriched interpretation of these symbols. From that time onward my past and present forms of spiritual understanding began to knit into a new whole.

From the time I was drug free until the end of my marriage, my efforts to remain sane were greatly supported by another recommended book, *The Bible for Students of Literature and Art*.[5] Taken from the King James version of the Bible, the work contains the biblical stories that have most informed art and literature throughout history. The Bible's art context, in bypassing hierarchical church meaning and dogma, offered an important connection to my past. I would rise early every morning to read and gain comfort from the book of Job. The same experience of reading the Old Testament countered my early school conditioning where teachers set a closed Bible on my desk while cautioning me against interpreting the Bible on my own or opening it to any other than the assigned study page. I sense now that I needed to physically own, read, and freely interpret the Bible in order to separate from my religion.

Other pivotal reading guides through this process of change included Joseph Campbell's *The Hero with a Thousand Faces* and Erich Neumann's *The Great Mother: Analysis of the Archetype*.[6] *The Great Mother*, a work several mentors had encouraged me to read, was for many years incomprehensible to me. But I was greatly drawn to the book's pictorial section of Great Mother art. The images describing her evolution as an archetype in the art of diverse cultures allowed me to intuit an understanding of Neumann's book and to evolve with that knowledge over the years. The more I understood new symbolism and saw how the central message to heal oneself and to love self and others remained constant, the more I was able to separate from my past.

My sense of needing physical distance from all things Catholic along with my then totally dormant sense of humour were both shaken by the kindly Jesuit art historian, Peter Larisey. Peter, who was a member of the May Marx building where I rented studio space, offered the following koan-like response to my question, "Why does art heal?" He said, "Some atrocities defy forgiveness; art teaches forgiveness."

Many years of pondering this response prefaced my eventual understanding of its truth.

Work with Artist Paul Hogan

When I asked Peter Larisey on another occasion if he knew of any artist who might have ideas about designing themes for hospital fundraising campaigns like the one my sister-in-law had recently asked me to give thought to, he suggested Paul Hogan. When I met Paul, he was the director of the widely acclaimed Spiral Garden at the Hugh MacMillan Rehabilitation Centre in Toronto (currently Bloorview Kids Rehab). Paul's garden concepts allowed Toronto artists, disabled children who lived at the rehabilitation centre, and neighbourhood children to participate together in story through the arts and the care of the garden.

At the time we met, Paul's acceptance or total ignoring of my 1980s corporate wife–artist split was affirming, especially when the same split was proving a growing irritant to many people on both sides of my divide. I found Paul's understanding of art and its potential to heal to be the largest and most realized vision I had come in contact with then or since. His concepts were often ahead of his time. For example, he envisioned an entire hospital staff planning a costumed ritual that would begin with a giant stork landing by helicopter on the hospital roof, then travelling through all the hospital's floors; the funding campaign would receive its official kickoff when the stork and procession arrived in the hospital lobby. But his work came to fruition in a different form for a 1992 hospital event that I will discuss later. Suffice to say here, Paul became a powerful mentor and friend who would change the course of my life.

Structures for Dream Art

My inner critic was prone to naming my commitment to paint and record my inner journey as grandiose. Dream work helped me to overcome this thinking and to accept the frailty of my artist self in the 1980s. Structure was a critical need. To draw strength from giants like Rembrandt and Van Gogh and from a deep sense of purpose helped me to remain sane in the marriage and to do my coming to consciousness work later.

The New Mexico dream workshop I attended in 1990 broadened my dream interpretation skills and ability to express my dreams in art. Led by American counsellor, teacher, and artist Alexandra Merrill, the workshop featured a method of dream interpretation called Percept. The Percept approach offers a way of speaking and writing a dream that allows one to own each part of the dream and, through that experience, to claim separateness and individual reality. The three basic steps to writing a dream in Percept include:

STEP 1. Writing the dream in present tense. For example, the following was a recurring New Mexico dream:

> *I dream that I am in a New Mexico desert. I look left and see a nun riding a horse. The nun and horse approach, then pass by me and ride away to my right.*

STEP 2. Rewriting the dream in Percept. In the second stage, one rewrites the dream using the words "part of myself" after each noun, verb, and adjective that appears in the dream text. This practice ensures that every word is identified as part of the dreamer's self. I write this phrase in full here to illustrate the method, but when I journal a dream now, I either use POM as an abbreviation or automatically own each dream aspect as I journal.

> *I am the dreaming part of myself, in the New Mexico part of myself and the desert part of myself. I am the looking left part of myself and the seeing part of myself of a nun part of myself who is the riding part of myself of a horse part of myself. The horse part of myself and nun part of myself are the approaching part of myself, then the riding away part of myself to the right part of myself.*

STEP 3. Discovering dream meaning through word associations.

For the third percept step, I take each word in the dream and enter them in a left column in my journal. I then write what each word means to me. If the word "desert" reminds me of "hot," I note it, then return to the word "desert" rather than proceeding to write what "hot" means to me. I continue associating with "desert" until one particular word association resonates with greater energy that the others, such as, dry, hot, *journey*, barren, lost. In the case of this dream, the word "journey," as in the biblical sense of a "journey into the desert" is what the word "desert" meant to me.

Because this particular dream kept recurring with differently coloured horses, when I came to paint the horse, I felt I could choose any colour of horse I wished. However, as I researched horses, I was pulled against all other preferences to render the horse as a pinto. Discouraged but obedient to this impulse, I was later thrilled when I discovered that *pinto* in Spanish means painting. The combined journalling and painting of this dream reinforced that my life journey or the nun part, the woman who is true to herself, was that of a painter.

Socially Engaged Art Structures

When dream teacher Alexandra Merrill came to Toronto to give an early 1992 workshop, she thrust her own copy of art historian Suzi Gablik's *The Reenchantment of Art*[7] into my hand and said, "You need to read this!" Gablik discusses significant late-twentieth-century art projects that reflect new global trends towards socially involved art practices. (Canada's R. Murray Schafer is among the artists Gablik talks with.)

One week after receiving the Gablik book, invitations to participate in socially engaged forms of art began to occur. I was asked by writer and storyteller Helen Porter to join her and other artists in a socially engaged art project slated for December 1992. A month or so after Helen's invitation, Paul Hogan invited me to join in the Rat Plaza street ritual being planned for June of 1992.

The June street event Paul was developing involved a group of Toronto artists known as the Chong. As a process, the Rat Plaza involved the six-month planning and creation of an enacted story in parade format. The Chong artists gathered in a series of garages located in a downtown Toronto alley that ran west of McCaul Street, just north of Dundas. In these garage spaces, the artists created the costumes and artifacts that would eventually embellish a series of parade altars meant to honour diverse "cults" that over the years had defined the Chong's existence. Altars to the cake, the rat, sardine, "Mother Ralph" (in the form of a bearded Elvis Presley bust attired in nun's headdress), as well as other entities gradually came to life with their individual daises, canopies, costumes, and related totem items. My drugged slowness was somewhat improved at the time of the Rat Plaza, but I still failed to recognize that the casual clothes (Holt Renfrew warehouse-sale items) I wore to the Chong garage meets would set me apart in the alley. Foreign in appearance as well as in my yet-to-be-converted corporate-wifeness, my alley visits resulted in feelings of being different and less-than. Despite the stresses of our external differences, the essential kindness that arose from the Rat Plaza's meditative art practices allowed me to co-exist with the Chong and to "be" and persevere in the Rat Plaza process.

In the end, Rat Plaza's scale and the artists who animated its themes were so aimed against the norms of the culture I was attempting to shed that to participate and survive the event helped minimize my fears of rejection where my life and creativity were concerned.

● ● ●

I might never have considered exhibiting my dream art and accompanying text at the 1992 *Never Again: Women and Men Against Violence* event at Women's College Hospital in Toronto if it had not been for Alexandra's introduction to Suzi Gablik's book. The hospital agreed to host what became an art/medical partnership event that marked the anniversary of the 1989 mass killing of women engineering students in Montreal's École Polytechnique. *Never Again* also marked the first time a Canadian hospital addressed violence as a health issue.

When the hospital also asked me to help convene and gather a committee for the event, I asked Paul Hogan to create a joint art exhibit with me and to participate in shaping the project. Paul created a magnificent backdrop that transformed the hospital lecture hall into a theatre space for the troupe of storytellers Helen Porter gathered to present daily storytelling performances as well as for the event's televised daily lectures on violence.

We obtained permission and a space next to the hospital cafeteria to create a Native healing room with walls decorated in plain brown paper from ceiling to floor on which visitors painted clay-coloured cave-like paintings. The floor in the centre of the room held a circular altar with a living ten-foot profusion crabapple tree in its centre. The healing room came to life under the direction of Paul, Native artist/healer Shirley Bear from the Tobique Reserve in New Brunswick, and theatre artist Jan Makay, who created a fabric vagina-shaped doorway that led from the cafeteria into the healing space. My contribution to the healing room was to organize the donation of the tree and the hospital's permission to use the space, and to survive a lone walk with the Sheridan Nursery delivery person and the immense tree through a seemingly endless hospital corridor gauntlet of perplexed and irate stares. The tree professes its innocence to this day.

As a hospital/artist go-between, the nurse part of me was concerned for the practical needs of the hospital and how the staff would perceive art's expression as a healing room or as the liberty taken when the large Paul Hogan painting called *Our Lady of The Gutter* replaced the photograph of Queen Mother Elizabeth that overlooked the hospital's main entrance for the duration of the *Never Again* event.

At the hospital as with Rat Plaza, the art collaboration acted like a homeopathic cure—both created the sense of a more enormous outer split than the one I was dealing with internally.

By the end of the event week, the only doctor to comment on my art told me, "I have come to this art exhibit every day and with each visit found a feeling of peace." The week-long event ended with an excruciatingly counter-hospital-culture ritual where the tree was ceremoniously drummed, chanted, and taken by the artists from the healing room to be planted in front of the hospital. A year later, this tree's beauty and profusion of blooms drew thanks from others on the hospital staff.

Art Structures Expand to Include Writing

The *Never Again* event drew criticism from artists who felt my show was not a proper use of art but opened several new doors as well. Lina Chartrand, artistic director of the Company of Sirens, encouraged me to write a play. My sister-in-law Gail Regan, president of Cara Operations Limited, offered her company's funding of a permanent exhibition of my *Never Again* art if it became accepted by a psychiatric teaching facility. The challenges of finding a psychiatric facility willing to accept my art as well as writing an accompanying wall text for each painting in the exhibit and writing the play furthered my belief in self by forcing greater exploration of my story.

In 1998, the majority of the paintings from the Women's College Hospital show as well as several new works were renamed the *Shedding Skins Dream Art and Text* and were mounted as a permanent exhibit in the main lobby of the Centre for Addiction and Mental Health (CAMH) in Toronto.[8] Between the time when I heard that CAMH had accepted my art and the time the art was installed at the centre, Rosemary suggested I write a book to accompany the exhibit. I had not yet obtained my psychiatric records and I had learned from the play that my most honest efforts still lacked objectivity—I felt the stirrings of a yet-to-be-expressed story but not the words. My intention for the hoped-for words was that they would, in addition to honouring my story, be respectful of my involvement with the CAMH. Although aspects of the story were critical of psychiatry, I wanted the story to be both balanced and hopeful. Fortunately, I asked and Rosemary agreed to enter into the co-writing of this book and the process that the work eventually became.

Structure Takes Root

My *Shedding Skins* dream works at the CAMH were painted between 1984 and 1992. The art records key dreams and my growth during that period. The works also represent one cycle in my ongoing coming to consciousness. During those years, I was plagued by my old conviction that I was not doing enough and was judging my art practice less worthy than nursing or other helping professions. Doubts about my sanity and whether my dream art would hold meaning for others were also constant.

Kept on course by a life that became confused when I was not painting, an arm that literally refused to execute subject matter other than dreams, and the support of mentors and friends, I gradually achieved ways to work past self-defeating messages that surfaced when I painted. The wellness that resulted from painting my dreams was a gradual unfolding. My earliest awareness of dream meanings evolved from knowledge I acquired in books or that I worked out intellectually. Head-oriented understanding of my dreams persisted until I gained the psychic strength to embrace my dreams as felt and lived knowing.

Dream, peace, and art become one reality for me now through an escalation of the sensual aspects of paint and colour. As the sensual takes over, my resistance to a dream's meaning dissolves into permission to follow the dream's insight threads out to its truth. Learning how to ride the chaotic dark of art, dream, and feeling towards a dream's intended light evolved slowly with mentors' help. Over time, living with and painting my dreams, has created improved states of peaceful coexistence between my inner and outer worlds and allowed me to come home to myself more fully.

My art practice in the early 1980s took place in brief two-hour morning periods per day. Despite the persistence of my psychosis issues and my total lack of dream knowledge during this time, the act of expressing my dreams in art was key to holding onto my sanity. When low self-worth caused a continuing sense of imminent annihilation, the power of the painted dream to mirror my soul and confirm my existence was no small matter. The mirroring of my existence bred an added trust, as in, "I exist; therefore some inner entity must love me if I am able to paint this beautiful work."

I gave much thought and time then to choosing the one image from a dream that would tell the entire dream story best. Once chosen, my planning and execution of the image was focused on a faithful rendering. Told in a 1997 dream that I should begin to work in egg tempera, I later realized the wisdom of this dream when I needed the structure and slowness of the egg tempera medium to support a deeper, more rigorous clearing in analysis of the issues that caused my psychosis. What evolved from 1997 onward was my current ability to paint for full days and to clear rather than become overwhelmed by shadow materials that arise as I paint. In addition, I am able to approach a blank paint surface with a dream rather than its totally formed image and to enjoy working consciously with received impulses as I work.

Art and life further intersected for me when I read Suzi Gablik, who argues for art's interconnection with all life disciplines in order to save the planet. In this context, I believe now that my dream journey echoes the radical individual offering to world-making that Gandhi described when he said, "Be the change you want to see in the world."

From the time I had cancer onward, I was aware that thought becomes chemistry within and beyond our person. I believe that individuals, along with their communities and environment, benefit when someone consciously sheds a limiting or harmful behaviour and replaces it with one that brings them closer to compassion for other and self. Unlike the media that can trigger feelings of being small and powerless, dream and art carry the potential to emphasize our oneness and ability to create change by changing ourselves.

From the mid-1990s until 2003, "connection" as an expression of the inner masculine–feminine became uniquely alive for me through artistic collaborations with Toronto dancers Viv Moore and Dave Wilson. To see Viv and Dave interpret some of my dreams in dance, and to intimately feel the dance as I rendered nudes of their gestures, allowed a rare exploration of my dreams and an ongoing meditation on the meaning of wholeness.[9]

Time has also convinced me that my once-unconscious urge to express inner/outer connection did not occur in a void, but rather in a culture where diverse disciplines increasingly research mind/body and earth systems to determine humanity's potential to better interconnect and balance its varied life structures.

Notes

1 Albert J. Lubin, *Stranger on the Earth: A Psychological Biography of Vincent Van Gogh* (New York: Holt, Rinehart and Winston, 1972).

2 "The Grandmother's Skull," in The *Serpent Slayer and Other Stories of Strong Women*, retold by Katrin Tchana, illus. Trina Schart Hyman (Boston: Little, Brown, 2000), 61–65.

3 Peter Brook, *The Empty Space* (London: MacGibbon and Kee, 1968).

4 Constantin Stanislavski, *Creating a Role*, trans. Elizabeth Reynolds Hapgood (New York: Theatre Arts, 1961); Jan Kott, *Shakespeare Our Contemporary*, trans. Boleslaw Taborski (London: Methuen, 1965); Antonin Artaud, *The Theatre and Its Double: Essays*, trans. Victor Corti (London: Calder and Boyer, 1970).

5 G.B. Harrison, *The Bible for Students of Literature and Art* (New York: Doubleday, 1964).

6 Joseph Campbell, *The Hero with a Thousand Faces* (Princeton: Princeton University Press, 1949); Erich Neumann, *The Great Mother: Analysis of the Archetype*, trans. Ralph Macheim (Princeton: Princeton University Press, 1963).

7 Suzi Gablik, *The Reenchantment of Art* (New York: Thames and Hudson, 1991).

8 The works in the *Shedding Skins* series are reproduced in the colour section, which follows page 230. See plates 1–16.

9 The Moore and Wilson artworks are reproduced in Appendix I, in figures 1–8 (pp. 231–34), and, from the *Casting a Vessel* series, in the colour section, in plates 23, 25, 27, 29, and 32.

5 Conversations on Mental Health Care

Walk into your worst fears.

—Angela Greig, 1983

What "seething cauldron of snakes" had become uncovered during her late actively psychotic episode, has again been lidded, but has not necessarily disappeared.

—Lakeshore Psychiatric Hospital Patient Record,
Psychological Report on Susan Schellenberg, 17 September 1969

SUSAN
Obtaining the Clinical Records

IT WAS 1995. I WAS ALONE in the Queen Street Mental Health Centre medical records office. As a condition of my obtaining my records, the attendant instructed me to read my Lakeshore Psychiatric Hospital records in her presence. Within moments of opening the records, I began to feel again the shame and disturbing chemistry of my original hospital experience.

Later that same afternoon, chance organized that I was scheduled to visit my naturopath. Perplexed by the fact that each of my wrists showed a different pulse rate, the naturopath, when informed I had just come from reading my psychiatric records, concurred that my reliving of the split most likely produced this temporary physical reaction. The opportunity to have the naturopath witness and confirm my body's reaction so soon after reading my records normalized and assisted my letting go of a difficult experience.

My decision to obtain my psychiatric records was much like my decision to divorce. I did not want either at the time but lacked workable alternatives. In the case of the records, I wanted to write this book and the book's integrity would not be possible without the records. I did not need the records to confirm I had been mentally ill but I did need them to confirm how factually off the mark both my husband, who gave the hospital my history, and the psychiatrists, who planned my treatment based on that history, had been.

When I first asked Rosemary to read my records, I doubted my right to complain about my psychiatric treatment. Since my 1969 psychiatric hospital admission, I knew the drugs were a godsend in the beginning because no act of will allowed me to break out of the psychosis. I also had recognizable facts that reinforced that some part of me was not yet right: I had come close to another psychosis in the early 1980s when I was in speech therapy; I had an inability to relate in marriage; I struggled to paint without becoming overwhelmed; and I frequently recognized that people saw me as "strange" when memory, speech difficulties, or rage lessened my ability to express my ideas. Without knowledge of the mental health system or how it regarded and treated women's mental illnesses, I lacked reasons to complain. The records and Rosemary's balanced view of them helped me attain more objectivity on my illness and treatment. Endless writing and rewriting, and reading and rereading of the records strengthened my ability to trust that although my psychiatric treatment may have been excellent in terms of what the psychiatric model offered, its gender biases and non-listening to my story or our story as a married couple were damaging to my family and me.

There is a history of mental illness on both sides of my family. My mother's sister, a national buyer for a large department store chain, was in her early forties and on her way to Paris when she became catatonic. After long-term hospitalization, she was lobotomized and then lived out her life in a series of nursing homes. My father's nephew, the son of soldier who had been badly gassed and permanently hospitalized after World War I, was sent by his mother and his parish priest to study for the priesthood to avoid being drafted into military services in World War II. His mental illness began in the seminary and he was hospitalized many times before being lobotomized. A major shame surrounded my father's brother, whose existence and mental illness remained secret until 1995, when exploring that gap in our family story became important to my writing this book and the text that accompanies my *Shedding Skins* dream art. A family-assisted search for my uncle's records resulted in our receiving a synopsis of my uncle Leo Marrin Regan's life from Kingston Psychiatric Hospital (see Appendix II, p. 241).

Besides allowing this forgotten man to become more integrated into my siblings' and my histories, the added family story found in my uncle's history opened me to a deeper understanding and compassion for the grieving, denying, and shamed parts of my father and how they had marked his life and mine. My father's childhood had been haunted by the deaths of three siblings, by the accidental scalding death of another brother, and by his own father's death when my father was age fourteen. From the time of his father's death until his mother's death six years later, my father had also been the caretaker to a grief-filled mother and his brother Marrin. To be such a young family member responsible for committing a brother into psychiatric care that became a life-time incarceration had to be doubly painful to my father. In this light and given his own childhood wounds and background, my father's efforts to hide a mentally ill brother made tragic sense. Increased awareness of my father's story also gave meaning to why he and his family often attempted to live ide-alized lives rather than the ones they were living. From this insight, I was able to examine and change how I lived these same behaviours and acted from sim-ilar fears of death and impending disaster.

As my perception of my father became more fleshed out and human rather than godlike, his choice of my strong-willed, practical mother for a partner and his failure to interfere or protect us from her harsh discipline became tem-pered by a historical, if still flawed, logic: I suspect that my father probably equated my mother's care of us as opposite to the care his dead siblings received and therefore thought of it as critical to our physical survival. My father's unre-solved need to bury his own painful childhood memories, as well as to undo a cultural conditioning that defined my siblings and me as his property, weak-ened his ability to discriminate or set boundaries when it came to his relating with me. Each historical insight on my father gained from my uncle Marrin's history loosened the hold my father's abuse had on me. I became more able to live with the paradox that my father was both a good, loving, immensely charitable man, yet also very human and flawed.

ROSEMARY
Conversation with Dr. Seeman

Around the time that I read Susan's clinical records and we agreed on writing together, Susan furthered my meagre art education by giving me Suzi Gablik's *The Reenchantment of Art*, a book that describes a historic shift as a growing number of artists break from the observer-recorder role that existed before the Renaissance and move to roles as partners in their communities.[1] In a later book, *Conversations Before the End of Time*, Gablik converses with individu-als immersed in art about whether the current approach to art is sustainable in a world facing unprecedented ecological and political crisis.[2] Gablik's way of demonstrating respect for sharply differing perspectives inspired us to ini-tiate a series of conversations on mental health and healing. For this purpose,

Susan and I arranged a series of conversations with six individuals in mental health, the arts, and business; I acted as the moderator of these conversations.

I suggested talking with a psychiatrist knowledgeable about schizophrenia because Susan's understanding that she was diagnosed with schizophrenia had an enormous impact on her life. The clinical records state that Susan was diagnosed with a condition known in 1969 as "acute schizophrenic reaction." This diagnosis implied that she had experienced psychotic symptoms but did not show indications of the more chronically debilitating condition of schizophrenia. I wondered if Susan's symptoms had ever justified a diagnosis of schizophrenia. I was also interested in the quality of care Susan received and whether an individual with similar difficulties would receive different care twenty-five years later. With these questions in mind, Susan and I approached psychiatrist Mary Seeman for our first conversation.

Dr. Mary Seeman had devoted her professional career to understanding and providing care to individuals with schizophrenia. At the time that we conversed with her, she held the Tapscott Chair in Schizophrenia Studies at the Centre for Addiction and Mental Health in Toronto and was a professor in the University of Toronto Department of Psychiatry. She had served as Chief of Psychiatry at Mount Sinai Hospital in Toronto. She had published close to two hundred papers and authored or edited seven books on various aspects of schizophrenia, including language and communication; safe and effective medication; individual, family, and group approaches to intervention; the personal subjective experience of schizophrenia; experiences of the families of people with schizophrenia; and the relationship of schizophrenia to parenting, aging, depression, and suicide. She had worked closely with the Schizophrenia Society of Canada and its regional affiliates. The University of Toronto Department of Psychiatry had commemorated Dr. Seeman's influence and ability as a teacher of medical students, interns, and residents studying psychiatry by establishing a prize in her name which is awarded annually to the resident whose work best exemplifies the integration of science and the humanities. In 1995, Dr. Seeman was awarded the prestigious Joey and Toby Tanenbaum Award in tribute to her research into gender differences in schizophrenia.

We met with Dr. Seeman in her office at the Clarke Institute of Psychiatry (now the Centre for Addiction and Mental Health) on 7 February 1996. On the walls of the office were several original art prints; from the ceiling over the desk hung three full-size wooden canoe paddles. On both sides of the blade of each paddle were paintings of animals: wolf, cat, raven, leopard, lark, and fox. Towards the end of our conversation with Dr. Seeman, our discussion refers to these paddles and the artist who created them. Dr. Seeman had an opportunity to review Susan's clinical records but had not seen her art prior to our conversation.

Dr. Seeman, Susan, and I struggled with the question of diagnosis from early in the interview.

ROSEMARY BARNES: From the information that is available in [Susan's 1969] records, what diagnosis do you feel would be appropriate in the current diagnostic system?

DR. MARY SEEMAN: I would not be able to answer that question, actually, without ticking off the various symptoms. What we have now in our diagnostic system is an attempt to look not at etiology but to make sure that any two psychiatrists sitting down with symptoms will arrive at the same diagnosis. It's an attempt to create a system that everybody uses in the same way. The system is very operational, so that you check off if you have one, two, three symptoms. If you have those symptoms, they have to exist for a certain period of time, and they have to be associated with certain deterioration of functioning in order for the diagnosis to be made. Meeting these operational definitions is what constitutes schizophrenia in 1996.

In 1969, the whole philosophy of diagnosis was actually quite different. Schizophrenic Reaction was based on a Meyerian philosophy.[3] Meyer's idea was that illness doesn't exist per se but is a reaction to—and it was actually quite a loose notion, so that there's nothing inherent in the person as being ill—the stresses of life. In the Meyerian system, you could have a schizophrenic reaction, an affective reaction, or some other type of reaction, to a common stress.

Whereas now, we're back, in a way, to the old system where illness exists within oneself. It's more of a medical model approach now, where the illness is presumed to be inside the person. If you express certain symptoms, then, you have the illness, although there's no blood test, no x-ray, or anything that will confirm the diagnosis. So the diagnostic approach now is only based on symptoms, and everybody recognizes that symptoms don't mean very much. They're just a way of people agreeing that, "Yes, this is the same description. This person fits that same description that this other person did." That's basically what diagnosis is, for reliability purposes; it is not to imply that there's something about that set of symptoms that is associated with etiologically caused disease. They do not allow an inference, in other words. I don't infer anything; I just check off.

For instance, if I saw someone today who told me that they thought they were the Virgin Mary, I might just note that and say "Well, this is a delusion, and that's one of the symptoms of schizophrenia." Period. Back then, if I saw someone who told me that they thought that they were the Virgin Mary, I would infer, in my mind, "Oh well, they have a conflict about purity," and I would then try to engage them along those lines. I would, in my mind, think

"Yes, this was a schizophrenic reaction, but it was a schizophrenic reaction to *something*, to a conflict, that troubled their sense of purity."

Dr. Seeman agreed that the 1969 records might be used to determine a diagnosis, but did not indicate what she felt the diagnosis might be. Susan continued later with the matter.

SUSAN SCHELLENBERG: What I increasingly find as I do this project is the importance of meaning. The meaning of my diagnosis is important. When I trained as a nurse, we were taught to observe, not to diagnose. For that reason, I am not writing into the wall text for the painting that "I am" or "I am not" schizophrenic.

MS: Sure, because that's not what counts.

SS: Well, it does count. But I feel that someone who is trained to say it officially should be the one to say it. I myself feel that if I go on saying "I'm not," when I am, then I am not accepting my reality. And if I say, "I am," and I'm not, then I'm doing something else to myself.

MS: When I say it doesn't count, I mean it in this sense: If you become ill with something, let's say pneumonia, then at the time when you have it, it's very important that the people who are treating you know the right bug so that they know what kind of treatment to apply. If it's a viral pneumonia, and they're treating it as a bacterial pneumonia, then obviously, you're in trouble. You want to be very sure that the physicians have it right. But, at some point, later on in life, when you no longer have the pneumonia, when you're over it, does it matter? Probably not.

SS: I don't think there is the stigma and cultural labelling in the case of pneumonia that there is in the case of schizophrenia.

MS: What is the difference? I guess that's what intrigues me. What is the difference. Does it mark you for life?

SS: Yes. I think that the culture adopts a different attitude about your competency as a human being.

MS: You felt that?

SS: Absolutely. After my break, my goal when I dressed was to appear normal. The suburbs viewed artists as outside the norm in those days. Being schizophrenic was right off the charts. I think meaning was also important, given there had been a prior family history of schizophrenia. My aunt and my cousin presented very extreme behaviours and that's what I began to relate myself to. I think it is doubly important as well where the possibility exists of a well partner sabotaging the ill partner's recovery.

MS: I would hope that there would not be any difference between a psychiatric illness and any other kind of illness. It's something that you get, are treated properly for, and quickly, hopefully, are over it. Then it's behind you and has no more meaning than that. But you're saying that you don't see that is going to happen any time soon.

SS: Oh, no. I suppose because I've been left with some drug side effects to memory and speech that my illness isn't totally in the past. There is a kind of hangover from the experience as well that came from not knowing of the exact diagnosis. That diminished my confidence in my sanity.

I recently read an antipsychiatric book called *Still Sane* in which the stories of the ex-psychiatric patients were so filled with the pain of their psychiatric treatment experience that I rarely got a sense of the person's ownership of their illness.[4] I've written a story, I've painted a story, and because I have taken ownership of my illness, I find that my diagnosis is an important ingredient to my story. The ritual of diagnosis appears to me to be as important an element to the story of an illness as hearing the words "It's a girl" or "It's a boy" the minute you give birth to a baby. It anchors you to the reality of your experience. If I hear that I am schizophrenic, it's not going to mean that I am suddenly going to be different—I am just going to know who I am a little better. Now that I am this involved in the story telling, the diagnosis is important for me to know.

MS: Of course, it won't affect how you are today. But do you want a diagnosis as of 1969, or do you want a diagnosis as of 1996? Because the diagnosis per se will change. And the diagnosis of 2006 will be probably quite different again. I'm not sure I've put it clearly but we don't know what schizophrenia is. Nobody knows what schizophrenia is. It's not a *Thing*. The way we conceptualize it—now anyway—it's a group of symptoms. And you probably had those symptoms. Whether you had them for six months or not, I don't know; I mean, those are the 1996 criteria. But, you know, there's nothing about a diagnosis that defines you in any way. You may feel it does. But that's my point of view.

I asked Dr. Seeman about Susan's 1969 experiences in relation to technical criteria used in the then-current psychiatric diagnostic system (fourth edition of the *Diagnostic and Statistical Manual* [DSM-IV]):[5]

RB: The records indicate that other people began to be concerned about you, Susan, when you were at the religious retreat, which was in the third week in August 1969. Then a series of events preceded the hospital admission on September 3, 1969. Apparently, from the notes, the delusions and the difficulties that you were experiencing disappeared fairly quickly during the hospital admission.

MS: Before the six-month criterion. [Rosemary's note: According to DSM-IV, one of the conditions that must be met in order to make a diagnosis of schizophrenia is that "continuous signs of disturbance must persist for at least six months."]

RB: Yes, the symptoms disappeared during the hospital admission, and are not noted again at any of the follow-up visits for some years beyond the time of the admission.

MS: So, the illness did not fit the six-month criterion.

RB: Yes. So it appears that it was a fairly brief period of a few weeks, maybe a month at most, when Susan had the highly unusual experiences which concerned other people and are documented in the records. These difficulties would now, in the current diagnostic conceptualization, be taken as signs of a psychotic experience.

MS: The condition would be called, probably, "schizophreniform disorder," which is under the six months. Or, if it's below three weeks, then the condition is called a "brief psychotic episode." However, just to add a little twist, the condition has to last six months unless it's treated. Susan was treated. So, the question is still there. Would it have lasted six months, had you, Susan, not been treated? Nobody knows. We don't know that. So it still remains a bit of an open issue.

I was quite surprised that Dr. Seeman refused to rule out the possibility that Susan might have been suffering from schizophrenia. I had learned, as Susan did in her nursing training, that schizophrenia was a condition where the affected individual is incurable and will experience a lifelong downward trajectory of ever-deteriorating function and poorer health. From time to time, I had heard psychiatrists speak with some sadness of their inability, despite years of research and clinical practice, to offer much that was of lasting benefit to individuals with schizophrenia. I found it hard to believe that Susan could be seen as ever suffering from this condition because she had never experienced another psychotic break, continued to function as a wife and mother even after her hospital admission, and clearly experienced ever increasing well-being and capability.

Our conversation closed with me asking about how an artist might approach the creative process.

RB: Creating art requires a going within one's self, often in a deep, intensive way, to be able to access images that can then be represented in whatever medium the artist uses for her/his work. How does an artist do this safely? Is there a risk to an artist, psychologically, in this creative process?

MS: I don't know that I can answer that. I have a number of artists in my practice. Their art is very important to them and I would say, as a general rule, their art is probably more important than their so-called sanity. Not all of them, but perhaps the majority, would sooner be a little off-balance in their mental state and still able to create, than to be very, very, very sane and unable to produce.

RB: Susan talks about structure being very important to her in her healing work and in her resumption of her art. Would it be your sense as well, that structure is what adds to the safety?

MS: I think so. You're quite right. It hadn't actually occurred to me until you said it, but yes.

RB: [referring to the animal portraits on Dr. Seeman's collection of painted canoe paddles] So, it's the fact that the artist's images painted on these paddles are images of animals. The animals have a real shape and real anatomy that he has to respect in creating these works. It's that structure that makes it safe for him, as well as makes it safe for you, Susan, when you're creating your work.

SS: I work mostly with the figure. Though I tend to be quite literal, I know I still go into that deep place where you do art. I feel much safer now because of the studies I've done on the bones and the anatomy. I have tools to express what needs to be created. And yet, even if I'm doing a series of similar works, I face a new creative experience, as in a sense that I must begin again to learn how to paint with each work. So structure has not reduced the art to a formula or mechanical process. It is an art process, and I feel extremely lucky that I met art mentors who were able to impart this freedom.

ROSEMARY
Serious Mental Illness and Mental Health Care

Many people believe, as Susan and I did, that a serious mental illness such as schizophrenia is chronic, irreversible, and degenerative. However, as I read more, I realized that experiences vary greatly, even among individuals with the same initial problems or diagnoses. Moreover, scientific findings indicate that many individuals diagnosed with schizophrenia actually improve substantially over time.[6] Sometime after our conversation with Dr. Seeman, I found that she and psychiatric colleagues explain schizophrenia like this:

> Most patients worry that they'll be "locked up forever." This is a historical holdover from times when severe mental illness led to indefinite, sometimes permanent, hospitalizations. This no longer happens. There are people with very

severe forms who, for many years, seem not to recover. In general, the first 5 to 10 years are the most severe for these people. After that, improvement does take place, even among the most ill. For those whose illness seems to be taking this severe, chronic, unremitting course, it is important to remember that there is a light at the end of the tunnel. Schizophrenia weakens its hold in the 40s and usually by the 60s formerly very ill people may feel quite good. This may seem too long to wait, but in contrast to other illnesses, it is actually quite optimistic. Most illnesses get worse with time and more debilitating. This is not the case with schizophrenia.[7]

I found that many of my professional colleagues as well as friends and family shared the mistaken beliefs that Susan and I held about the outlook for individuals with schizophrenia and other serious mental illnesses. These misconceptions are quite destructive. When one believes a situation to be hopeless, the bleak outlook negates commitment to overcome difficulties and interprets any improvement as a temporary aberration. Such an outlook is not justified by what is currently known about mental disorders, even serious mental illness. Numerous therapeutic approaches are helpful to individuals with emotional disturbances and excellent scientific outcome studies indicate that even seriously mentally ill individuals improve substantially (see chapter 8). Susan explains the powerful healing capacity of the arts, alternative therapies, and many other activities available beyond the perimeter of conventional mental health services.

Dr. Seeman commented on the variety of treatments used in mental health settings, and the possibility that had Susan been hospitalized elsewhere, a different approach might have been taken. Perhaps another facility might have been more attentive to the psychological and social aspects of Susan's emotional disturbance. The absence of a single, universal approach was underscored by a physician who had worked in an Ontario hospital in the 1960s and reviewed an early draft of our book manuscript. The Meyerian theoretical approach mentioned by Dr. Seeman theory did not, in this physician's experience, play a significant role in the diagnosis of individuals in Ontario hospitals at that time; this physician felt that schizophrenia was seen by psychiatric staff as a serious, long-lasting, potentially dangerous illness. Dr. Seeman confirmed that Susan's care was appropriate by the standards of the day, and that it is still common for mental health services to consist entirely of the medical model of care that Susan received.

There is much to appreciate about medical-model mental health care. Round-the-clock emergency services, skilled diagnostic evaluations, places of refuge, and medication provide quick help in understanding the problem, reducing painful symptoms, and creating order and security for individuals in emotional distress and for their families. I was proud to contribute to these hospital services and, in some ways, continue to be glad such services are available.

Some progress has been made. For example, a serious and longstanding criticism of conventional care, is that serious, sometimes irreversible damage results from prescribed treatments.[8] In Susan's situation, she was seriously debilitated by the side effects of her prescribed medication. She suffered from tardive dyskinesia, a disruption of muscle functioning that is a well-known side effect of antipsychotic drugs. Long-term use of the medication resulted in seriously impaired speech, loss of mental acuity, and inability to feel her emotions. As Dr. Seeman noted, approaches to selecting medications have been refined since then. But newer antipsychotic medications have different, though still potentially serious, adverse side effects. Changes in law, clinical practice, and public dissemination of health information have made the risks of long-term use of psychoactive medications more accessible. Individuals and their families can better weigh the benefits and risks of medication, which is a matter of particular importance for the many individuals using antipsychotic medications that can cause such debilitating, sometimes irreversible side effects.

Other harms (discussed later) may befall the individual receiving mental health care in the conventional medical model. However, any harms that individuals might sustain would be more tolerable if mental health services could demonstrate that they were successful in meeting the deepest need of the distressed individual, their families, and society—namely to heal. By healing, I have in mind not "cure" of the illness condition since this is not always possible but rather fostering growth in the ability to love and forgive self and other, to cope, to feel pleasure, to engage in meaningful activities, and to follow the psyche's inner direction towards greater wholeness.

What was increasingly disturbing to me during my hospital career is what is underscored dramatically in Susan's experience of emotional breakdown and healing—medical-model mental health care commonly does not foster healing. It can seriously interfere with healing. As a fellow member explained in a psychotherapy group that I attended for several years, hospital care pulled her out of the water when she was drowning, but it failed to teach her to swim. The skills and services offered by the medical model do not improve life any more than life guards teach swimming. They save the drowning but cannot teach swimming. Improved techniques such as better medications and improved patient access to information about medication risks are highly desirable because these changes reduce the danger that lifeguards will routinely injure significant numbers of drowning persons in the course of executing rescues. However, these improvements still do not address the most basic issue, namely the failure of medical-model mental health care to foster healing.

This failure is particularly frustrating because the medical model often preempts other possible perceptions or understandings in public discussion of emotional distress and mental health.[9] It is as if the only approach to public participation in water sports were to spend all available money on lifeguards and rescue facilities, while giving little or no funding or attention to instruction in swimming and water safety skills or any policy or design initiatives to make water sports safer and more enjoyable.

I had tried, for some years, to change this state of affairs – long discussions with professionals sharing similar concerns, and time and energy devoted to projects that would promote healing. I felt rage and despair when change failed to materialize in the ways and at the pace that I desired and I gradually drifted towards feeling depleted and cynical. Finally, I realized that I was childish to allow my personal well-being to be contingent on institutional willingness or capacity to reform to suit my wishes. I accepted my responsibility for and power over my own life and the limits of my ability to change others. I reflected on my career and realized that clinical work with patients was what I found most deeply satisfying. Around the time that Susan and I agreed to work together on a book, I resigned my hospital position to begin a clinical practice in the community.

In the early years of my community practice, I was relieved to be free of the need to support an institution that I found hostile to my own well-being and that of my patients, but I also felt like a failure for abandoning a prestigious career path. A few respected colleagues left hospital work around the same time; we talked, agreeing that it was good to escape stressful workloads, frustrating internal politics, and a disappointing lack of organizational commitment to improving patient care. Despite such conversations, I continued to wander emotionally, troubled about why I chose as I did and what I might have done differently. I realized gradually that I was working with Susan because of my own need to reconcile the long-standing separation between my work as a psychologist and my commitment to the values underlying feminist and antipsychiatry critiques of mental health care. Healing required collecting the disparate and conflicting fragments of my personal and professional experiences and fitting them together to form a new story of my life's work.

Conversation with Feminist Doctors Toner and Malone

I was very familiar with the idea of feminist analysis as a healing medium connecting individual and community. Indeed, the slogan of 1970s feminism, "The personal is political," urged that women's dilemmas and distress be addressed not as private matters, but as personal manifestations of inequality and injustice originating in the larger social arena. Radical feminist therapy of the 1970s argued that psychotherapy should teach women that personal problems resulted from social injustices, raise awareness of suppressed hurt and anger, and teach skills for expressing angry feelings constructively in political activism.[10] Phyllis Chesler's *Women and Madness* stimulated explorations of how social expectations and institutions influence women's experience of emotional disturbance, including the damaging impacts of gender role stereotypes and of physical and sexual violence against women and children.[11] The daring ideas of the 1970s became the research hypotheses of the 1980s, then the scientifically verified understandings of the 1990s.[12]

We were interested in discussing Susan's clinical records, experiences, and art with women knowledgeable concerning feminist analysis in mental health. We sought out psychologist Dr. Brenda Toner, head of the Women's Mental Health Program at the Centre for Addiction and Mental Health (CAMH) and Associate Professor in the Department of Psychiatry, University of Toronto. Dr. Toner had taught courses on gender issues in psychology at the University of Toronto and was internationally known for her research on chronic bowel disease.

We also approached Dr. Margaret Malone, a sociologist, counsellor, health promotion activist, and Associate Professor at Ryerson University's School of Nursing who had many years of experience working as a university teacher in both sociology and women's studies programs and as a public health nurse. In 1993, Dr. Malone was awarded the Ruth Wynn Woodward Postdoctoral Research Fellowship in the Women's Studies Program at Simon Fraser University. Her research concerned the social construction of marital separation with a particular focus on gender, emotions, and knowledge regarding social change.

Susan, Dr. Toner, Dr. Malone, and I met in Dr. Toner's office at the Clarke Institute (now the CAMH) on 14 February 1996. The mood gradually evolved from tentative and apprehensive to a passionate yet warm and funny sharing of views and experiences. Both Dr. Toner and Dr. Malone had reviewed Susan's 1969 clinical records, and we all expressed frustration and disappointment with patriarchal institutions.

DR. BRENDA TONER: They [Susan's clinical records] were striking in terms of the worst of the medical model—how your voice was not heard, how information can be distorted and misused based on what the therapist thinks is the explanation of the phenomenon. I noticed a clear lack of appreciation for Catholicism, for the rich, symbolic information and metaphors that, in your interpretation of what was going on internally, made sense from any person's perspective. That piece was not appreciated.

The therapists used a specific theoretical model of what schizophrenia was—a medical disorder—and concluded that you needed treatment with medication. The notes were organized around the schema—the therapist schema—that your problem was a biological disorder; we've got the medication for a biological disorder, so let's proceed accordingly.

ROSEMARY BARNES: When I read Susan's clinical records, I was struck by how detailed they were. Yet, this very rich information doesn't seem to be integrated into the formulation. What should have been included in the formulation?

DR. BRENDA TONER: Data do not speak for themselves. I would advocate that a way of getting a richer conceptualization is through qualitative information rather than coming in with a specific theoretical orientation. That is, we should listen to the words and interpretations of the client, then put themes on them after, rather than coming in a priori. If the clinician comes in assuming it's a medical condition, for example, a biochemical problem, any information that the clinician hears that's not consistent with the original hypothesis will be filtered out—it's selective attention. A way to avoid this problem is for the clinician to come in with more of an openness—listen to the information, listen to the interpretation, and put themes on it *after* listening.

However, this kind of analysis cannot be done without some further understanding of social and psychological issues. For example, consider gender role socialization. If the clinician has no awareness that there are power differentials in our society, he or she is not going to pick up on it with a client. The clinician needs to understand that these rigid gender roles are very restrictive to women and men.

DR. MARGARET MALONE: Structural-functionalism [a sociological theory of family organization] is represented and reinforced through the Catholic church.[13] I was raised as Catholic myself. When we were going through marriage preparation in the early 1960s, we were given two books. The woman got a book called *The Wife Desired* and the man got *The Man for Her*.[14] The woman is to please, to be available, to do all this hard work, to raise her children, and to support her husband no matter what. As a wife, I remember trying to do this, then thinking as time went on, "Wait a minute. There's nobody supporting me in this whole process." So structural-functionalism is reinforced by the hierarchical and patriarchal Catholic Church.

It is clear, in Susan's medical records, that it was her husband's voice that was being heard—not hers. He had the authority to speak for her. When reading the medical record, I was struck by how beautifully he's described as this very nice-looking man who cares for his wife. Over and over the notes say how close they were. I thought to myself, "So close that you don't have to hear her voice, too?" This piece created a lot of anger in me as I was reviewing the records. I was thinking, "How is it that they only heard his voice and not her voice?" when Susan's talking about the trauma, the incredible workload of raising four children, one after the other. I have a little grandson in my household now, and think to myself, "Gee, one child is hair-raising enough to care for, but four in a row?"

An individual can become crazy because people don't hear her voice. The less you're heard, the crazier you become, because you keep trying and failing to have your perspective listened to or validated.

➤ RECORD EXCERPT

At the hospital, the nurse told him that the patient was deeply disturbed emotionally and was schizophrenic and was to see a psychiatrist at 2:30 PM; it was then 2:10. As soon as he saw the patient he knew she was in trouble but felt strongly that she would recover better at home with the family and he took her home.

—Lakeshore Psychiatric Hospital Patient Record,
Social Record, 5 September 1969

SUSAN RESPONDS

My psychiatric records illustrate how the negative aspects of my husband's caretaking behaviour were ignored while the positive got praised. My husband told psychiatrists how he resisted getting me medical help even when people like the director of the retreat and the emergency-room nurse at Queensway Hospital told him I was in need of help. When my husband told the psychiatrist how he took me home without treatment from the Queensway Emergency and continued to keep me at home for three more days trying to get me well on his own, his husbandly devotion blinded their judgment. Psychiatrists failed to see how his working like a litigation lawyer and attempts to straighten my psychotic thinking signalled our extreme codependence and control issues. Rather than recommending the aid of couples therapy they praised our pathology.

BT: What you are saying is specific to you, Susan, but very important elements will ring true for a lot of women and men. When you talked about professionals listening to your husband's voice, I was thinking, "Yes, to some extent this is true, but also, his voice wasn't being heard either."

SUSAN SCHELLENBERG: They failed to validate the story of a human man by making him larger than life.

RB: What do you feel wasn't recognized or heard in the position of Susan's husband?

BT: The need that he had to solve it, to take care. He was the man; he needed to make it all right. He would take Susan home and try to get her thinking straight. That was how he was raised. That was the essence of masculinity.

In a relative sense, his voice was heard more than Susan's voice, but his voice was not heard from a socialization point of view. The clinicians were not interpreting his words in any way that reflected the possible difficulties of being a man in our society, and their failure distorted his voice. When there were words like "good behaviour on the part of my wife" and "I'm the head of my family," it would have been helpful and healthier for health professionals to challenge the male voice, his voice, by asking what are the positive and negative consequences for adhering to such a rigid view of masculinity. They should have challenged rather than assuming that the traditional masculine role was helpful for him. As it happened, the clinicians were hearing her husband's voice and taking it as relatively more authoritative, but he was losing out as well.

➤ RECORD EXCERPT

The Physician's Application stated that she was apathetic, imitated all movements of her husband, related recent visual and auditory hallucinations during a religious retreat, feels that she is about to die, and at other times she is the Virgin Mary.

— Lakeshore Psychiatric Hospital, Conference Report,
18 September 1969

SUSAN RESPONDS

The figure of the Blessed Virgin was the most powerfully instilled image of the feminine in my home, church, and Catholic schooling. As myth, I believe the "Blessed Virgin" had great nurturing value for young children who, like myself, had experienced maternal deprivation. But my later experience of her meaning became increasingly limited by a religion that idealized women, reduced them to things, and denied they were equal to men in all respects. My lifelong devotion to the Virgin had actually ended when I was in labour with my first child, seven years prior to my breakdown. The story of Mary's birthing of Jesus that I gathered from priests was that she did not suffer labour pains and was restored to her virginal state the minute she delivered. Mary ceased to be real as my labour contractions intensified. I pitched my rosary into the drawer, never to use it after that time. So my delusions were not coming from the place of fanatic devotion but from the "who am I?" question of a fractured feminine self who knew herself only as a wife, a mother, a daughter, a Catholic, and as *bad*.

Rather than seeing my delusions in terms of an identity issue, the hospital compounded my inner conflict by addressing my birth control concerns with disapproval of my multiple pregnancies. The hospital's failure to assist me with resolving my birth control dilemma during my time in hospital or when I was an outpatient trivialized a major source of my stress. For psychiatrists to instead invest my husband with greater authority by telling him that I should not have another pregnancy ignored the fact I carried sole responsibility for birth control in our marriage and that my husband experienced the *no* in the Catholic birth control "rhythm" method as an aphrodisiac, a signal to chase. The church's dictate that a wife was never to refuse her husband added to the stress of living with their condemnation of birth control.

A pharmacist I contacted in the early 1990s confirmed that the dose of estrogen in birth control pills prescribed in the 1990s was approximately one-hundredth the amount contained in the birth control pill I was given in the late 1960s just after the Pill was introduced. I am convinced that the Pill's hormone dosage was another contributing factor to the breakdown.[15] The drugging of my story by psychiatrists was as negating to my essence and sexuality as were the church's attitudes towards women and sex.

> **BT:** Women in Catholicism especially have been dichotomized as either good—the Virgin Mary—or as evil. I was taught by nuns. I could get a 100 percent mark in religion, so I thought I knew everything. [Laughter] I knew it was a virgin birth, but I didn't know [until this moment in the conversation] that in terms of giving birth to Jesus, there was no pain, and Mary's hymen wasn't broken, that everything went back to normal.
>
> **MM:** So the story goes. [Laughter]
>
> **BT:** I didn't know that. [Laughter] . . . I remember the wonderful part of your writing about when you were in labour, and you thought, "Forget Virgin Mary. She's been dethroned from my existence." The fear of women has to do with the mortal sin of questioning this teaching because by even questioning, you are considered evil. No shades of grey are allowed.
>
> **MM:** Another aspect of this has to do with women's anger. One of the teachings of the Catholic church is that anger is classified as a cardinal sin, that is, one of the worst sins. So the church's teachings silence anger, along with lust, and everything else that's pleasurable in life. When your sense of outrage at how you're living is devalued, when you aren't allowed to voice it, when you're told it's sinful, then the status quo is reinforced and upheld in another way. So the status quo gets reinforced in so many ways and in so many places.
>
> **BT:** It's like putting a lid on any challenges.
>
> **MM:** That kind of collective anger and outrage about our lives should really be voiced.

➤ RECORD EXCERPT

DOCTOR: "The life event with the greatest impact was ..."

SUSAN: " ... my husband," because "he has educated, loved, forgiven, and stayed with me over all the problems that have lead me to grow as a woman." Her main interest in life, "Husband, children, and art." (The latter seems another obsession, inner bid for approval, greatness and recognition).

—Lakeshore Psychiatric Hospital Patient Record,
Psychological Examination, 17 September 1969

SUSAN RESPONDS

The attitude to art and why I did art that is implied in this psychological report ridicules rather than celebrates my drive for self-expression. Though I had enormous needs for approval, I did not seek or get "approval" from doing art. I was able to study art because I fell in line with the family myth that my husband had given me permission to do art. I did not obtain "approval" for making independent decisions. In regard to my "bid for approval" elsewhere, my memory is that my friends, who at that time were mostly from nursing, found my art studies somewhat eccentric. A neighbour reacted to my art with a harsh scolding, saying that his mother would never have studied art. The church's view of art, as I understood it from my student days at a convent school, was that the making of art could lead to freethinking and should be considered an occasion of sin. My choice to study art was authentic. It came from my gut after I had spent nine months happily in my body during my fourth pregnancy. So contrary to the "bid for approval" statement, I had actually experienced further isolation rather than approval when I chose to study art. I sense ridicule in this psychological assessment and feel that the writer's "bid for approval" comment is perhaps a greater indication of his or her bias towards either art or young mothers than it is a reflection of my truth.

MM: Yes. He frames her art as if it is abnormal—that Susan's doing art is done to get approval, and to be known as great in the process of doing it. Rather, these interests are just being a part of who she is, the work she does. I wonder how a man's interest in architecture and drafting would have been perceived? I wonder if a woman who cares for children and paints is somehow less important than a man doing very similar kind of work within a different kind of constructed area.

There's a whole history to these kinds of incidents that have happened to women over time. Charlotte Perkins Gilman's short story called "The Yellow Wallpaper" describes what's believed to be her own life of being medicalized.[16] In a television drama broadcast on Masterpiece Theatre in about 1989, Gilman's story is shown: her husband is depicted as a doctor using the theories of Dr. Silas Weir Mitchell, a leading neurologist of the time. Dr. Mitchell recommended that when women are disruptive, are challenging the system—which is essentially what Charlotte Perkins Gilman did—then they should be given "the rest cure," that is, isolated and removed from all the important creative parts of themselves. Charlotte was a writer. So as part of the "rest cure," she was not permitted to write. Eventually, she became well known in the U.S. as a public lecturer; she wrote a lot about economic theory, women's issues, and all that sort of thing. She wanted to write and to share her ideas.

Gilman's experience is sort of like Susan's. Susan wants to paint, to create something out of what's going on, and the health professionals say that's not okay. It was the same with Charlotte Perkins Gilman, with Virginia Woolf, with Sylvia Plath. They're all creative women who saw what their lives were like, and tried to represent it in some kind of form, and then they were labelled as mentally ill.

➤ RECORD EXCERPT

In conference, the patient was cooperative but under visible strain as she answered questions well, although revealing florid psychopathology and weak ego defences. It was decided that she was suffering from an Acute Schizophrenic Reaction but had had disturbing thinking for some time. It was felt the prognosis was guarded, especially if she were to undertake another pregnancy, which has been considered by her and her husband.

It was felt that she could be permitted to go out this weekend ... but that medication should be recommenced, and that an explanation should be made to the husband of the serious responsibility she took when she was alone with the children. She was advised to be followed in after-care for some months.

—Lakeshore Psychiatric Hospital Patient Record,
Conference Report, 18 September 1969

SUSAN RESPONDS

During my Lakeshore Psychiatric Hospital stay, I was present at a conference where the other places were filled primarily with male health-care personnel. The presiding doctor stated that some of the staff thought I was schizophrenic and some of them did not. Referring to a recent and highly publicized incident where a Leaside mother had murdered her four children, he declared that they were all worried that I was going to kill all my babies. I remember screaming, "How dare you!" at the whole group and telling them they had no right to say a thing like that to me, especially when I was in a weakened position.

Following this confrontation, I was told that I was not stable enough for permanent discharge and would have to remain in hospital another week. This enraged me further and seeing myself mirrored in this state by a large group convinced me that it was I who was defective, not them.

Doctors never explained why they thought I might kill my babies nor did they ask me if I was thinking about doing so. They did not put their statement about the killing of babies in my medical records. Although this destructive type of thinking about the children had never entered my mind during the psychotic crisis, I went home terrified that this was something I might possibly do. The doctors also warned my husband of this possibility, which created enormous unneeded anxieties for him. Our relationship, already entrenched in an alternating rescue/victim dynamic, was cemented further by doctors telling my husband to guard me against harming, perhaps killing, the children. The doctors implanted a terror that I might kill the children, which shamed and frightened me throughout my children's childhoods and on into my grandchildren's lives until the writing of this book brought it to full consciousness.

➤ RECORD EXCERPT

Drawing on past clinical experience and considerable probing of her most bizarre thinking, delusions and behaviour whilst actively psychotic, the writer [hospital psychologist] considers her condition at such times to hold a serious element of potential danger particularly to a family of 4 small children (now ranging in age from 3 to 7). This revolves around the religious core of her psychosis, and the ascertained fact that at such times she feels totally controlled by other forces (or hypnotized), being a "passive vessel of God's imagination" and thus carrying out anything as directed without being able to exercise any volitional powers.

DOCTOR: ". . . greatest fear is . . ."

SUSAN: ". . . is that the children will be hurt by or in a car."

—Lakeshore Psychiatric Hospital Patient Record,
Psychological Examination, 17 September 1969

SUSAN RESPONDS

If doctors were connecting my fears about the children to their concerns about the possibilities of my killing them, they were wrong. My fears about the children were based on realities that had given me nightmares for a year or longer prior to my break. But no one probed for the origins of my fears about the children.

Our home originally stood on a safe, dead-end street, but shortly after we moved in, the street opened to through traffic for a new subdivision. When the road expanded, teen drivers began racing their cars up and down our street. This resulted in three of the neighbours' children being hit before our borough added new stop signs. Though our youngest children stayed in our garden, the older ones played with neighbouring friends. I was constantly aware of and unnerved by the sound of revved-up cars racing by the house and even more terrified by the frequent screeching of brakes. Waiting to see if it was nothing or, worse, anticipating hearing people cry out that a child had been hit, was a daily stress.

Another terrible concern was trying to get added safety locks for the back doors of our car prior to the time when cars were legally required to have seat belts and automatic locking systems. As I had no money to get car locks on my own and experienced two incidents where the children had opened the back door while I was on the highway, I was constantly terrified of the possibility of their getting hurt this way as well. My husband installed car locks after I became sick.

> **BT:** At the meeting where the health professionals interpreted your behaviour, Susan, as associated with being harmful to or possibly even killing your children, I found it so powerful when you responded by saying, "How can you say this when I am so weak?" What the professionals had said was unhelpful. When you're feeling vulnerable and self-esteem is low, it's particularly hard to reach down inside, to take every ounce of courage to question, and challenge the status quo for the sake of your own sense of self.

> **MM:** Another important issue concerns the hospital staff's reference to a newspaper account of a woman who killed her children. Without any evidence to support this from Susan's history, the staff seemed to assume that harming the children was something Susan might do. I found this incident particularly disturbing because Susan was in such a vulnerable state—hospitalized, drugged. And while she was in this state, the health professionals suggested that she might, in fact, kill her children. Within yourself, you may say, "No, I wouldn't do that." On the other hand, when a professional says this could be a possibility, it can create self-doubt. A patient might think, "They're the knowers. If they think that could happen, what am I going to do when I go home? What if I did harm the children?" It may not have been or was not a concern for you initially; it was a concern created by others in the hospital context.

> **BT:** So, the health professionals' lack of appreciation of the impact of what they were saying set up even more rigid stereotypes. Your husband was

expected not only to care for you but also to worry about the children. His being given that responsibility diminished you further, made you more childlike and left him with a greater burden. Neither of you were heard, nor were you offered an opportunity in therapy to express your feelings and concerns so that you could come closer together.

➤ RECORD EXCERPT

Susan's statement to the hospital psychologist that she was trying to be a "passive vessel of God's imagination." (See Psychological Examination excerpt on p. 108.)

SUSAN RESPONDS

My statement that I was trying to be a "passive vessel of God's imagination" rightly added to the doctor's concern that I might harm the children. But the writer's lack of questioning me on my "passive vessel" thinking, as well as his unexpectedly presenting his own extremely biased interpretation in the conference setting, seems unconscionable to me still. I also experience the hospital's omitting that they suggested I might kill my babies from the records as cowardly.

The retreat, given by an avant-garde layperson, exposed me to a concept that was revolutionary compared to anything I had been taught previously—the concept of obedience to the Self rather that to priests. My "passive vessel" statement was the verbatim metaphor used by the retreat master to describe this new type of obeying. The idea of becoming self-directed had appealed to me, but my years of institutional obedience were too ingrained for me to change in the course of a brief retreat. As an isolated housewife with no other structure to replace old beliefs with, the new "passive vessel" was an easy-to-hold visual image. As an image and concept, it held a vague hope and potential means for me to live in peace with a religion when my only other option was damnation if I left the church.

My religion and culture conditioned me to take trust away from Self and place it absolutely onto customs, dogma, and powerful hierarchical governing systems. The doctor who found inherent danger in my "passive vessel" thinking admits to forming this judgment in the context of his past clinical experience. His assessment was obviously divorced from my story or an awareness of how to help women who are negatively impacted by religion. A medical model that held similar expectations of obedience from patients as the church did from its members was not ready at that time to see my illness in the context of the larger patriarchal pathology.

MM: The psychological report refers to "the religious core of her psychosis" as being associated with Susan's experience of being "the passive vessel of God's imagination." Therefore the religious core is associated with what has been labelled a "psychosis." But there was no reference to the religious context in which Susan was raised, that is, her very strong, ideologically based, Roman Catholic background.

When you are raised as Catholic, you are expected to live according to the direction of the authority and religious instruction. You are not encouraged to analyze critically the ideology underlying the teaching doctrines of the church. You are encouraged to accept it, foster it, and live it from the time you are a young child.

The reality is that women at that time when Susan was young were expected to give over to the "divine power." So, to interpret surrendering to that power as a psychotic manifestation without an understanding of Catholic religious instruction is very misleading. Again, context is important. If there's no context, the person's experience can be labelled in very misleading ways. If you remove the relational context between Susan and her husband, their shared religious understanding of marriage, and their relation to the structural-functionalist idea of marriage, then it looks as if Susan is crazy. But in fact, Susan is acting out and struggling with a discrepancy between what she was told was to be her life, and what in fact, was her experience.

➤ **RECORD EXCERPT**

He said he and his wife are very close to each other and have complete trust and confidence in each other. They have their arguments but he always treats her as a lady and they do everything as a family; family unity is very important. He is the head of the family, though; they complement each other.

—Lakeshore Psychiatric Hospital Patient Record,
Social Record, 5 September 1969

SUSAN RESPONDS

My "history," which professional staff gathered from talks with my husband, gives several clear indications that our relationship contained a pathology; yet those areas were not brought to our attention as a couple or made the subject of any prescribed therapy treatment. By appearing to be as accepting of our outwardly idyllic marriage as we ourselves were, the health professionals added to our craziness.

MM: Susan's husband says, "We are very close; we're really a loving couple," when Susan is in the hospital having tremendous difficulty; this statement denies the reality of what's going on. Yet, his denial went unnoticed by the professionals. There's a discrepancy between what he is saying, and what is, in fact, happening between him and Susan.

RB: When Susan's husband said, "We're very close," were hospital staff not considering what it might mean to him for her to be very debilitated and in hospital? That they were denying or overlooking his pain?

MM: No, that isn't what I was thinking. I was thinking that it might reflect badly on Susan's husband if his wife is having difficulties. What does it say about him as a man if his wife is having difficulties? When he said, "We're getting along really well. We're really a loving couple," he is saying, "We're really okay. I can look after this." For example, he took Susan home after that first attempt to go to the hospital and kept her isolated, thus implying, "I can look after you." But he couldn't. When he went to the hospital and said, "We really are very close," the health professionals did not recognize that what he said might not be the reality. They did not seem to consider that something is happening that clearly creates a problem for Susan as well as her husband.

RB: So you think the health professionals took him at his word—"We are very close"—rather than looking more deeply and thinking "Maybe this relationship is not so close." Perhaps, the relationship had difficulties for him as well.

MM: Yes. It's an interactional issue. If one person is having difficulty in a relationship, then the other person's having difficulty, too. At the least, one person may be having difficulty in relation to the other's problem. In the medical records, Susan is the identified problem, and no one else has a problem. But we don't live in isolation—we live in relation to other people. What happens to one person will inevitably have an effect on others.

➤ RECORD EXCERPT

Patient was accompanied by her husband this afternoon. She was looking rather well, and claimed to be feeling well. Husband gave examples of her good behaviour over the last few months, and expressed his own gratitude for the supervision and care she received here. She is sleeping well and her household is operating better than it has for many years, as long as the second or third year of their marriage, according to her husband. Patient was given an appointment three months from now and will not be taking medication for that period.

—Lakeshore Psychiatric Hospital Patient Record,
Outpatient Services Clinical Record, 14 July 1970

SUSAN RESPONDS

My husband comments to the doctor that our home was running better than it had for awhile, now that I was drugged. Though this statement shows the value my husband placed on my being docile and manageable, doctors also overlooked it. I have since put the time of my husband's thinking the home was starting to run less well close to the time that I decided to study art.

MM: The health professionals seem to say to Susan, "If you just do what you're supposed to do, everything will be just fine. We'll give you a few drugs to soften the edges, you can perform your role a little better." The health professionals, in effect, took this approach rather than challenge the structural-functionalist model or the ideology of the nuclear family.

BT: He commented on the good behaviour as if you were a child. Actually, I try not to take this approach even with children!

It was very striking that your good behaviour was further evidence that the status quo was fine. Your exploding in rage at the professional conference meeting was further evidence that things were not fine. Expressing your anger was healthier for you. Your "good behaviour" was unhealthy.

So what was healthy for you was interpreted as further psychopathology. It's fascinating! I think that this still goes on today. Health professionals still use the term *secondary gain* in a disapproving way to refer to, for example, a patient's need for approval and—in your case—your interest in art.

➤ **RECORD EXCERPT**

Mr. Schellenberg, a well set, tall, neat and attractive, clean-shaven young man with brown eyes and hair and an honest open face, was seen in an office interview on September 5, 1969. He said he and his wife are particularly close, so he is very concerned about her condition and has been trying to delve into the retreat she attended to find out just what did happen there.

—Lakeshore Psychiatric Hospital Patient Record,
Social Record, 5 September 1969

SUSAN RESPONDS

The writer's description of my husband's brown eyes is a small point but he actually had striking and unmistakably blue eyes. In contrast to the extensive history my husband gave to the medical staff about my family background, his brief account of his family alluded to the fact that he and his family were normal, well functioning, and without problem. From my limited knowledge of psychology, I find it hard to comprehend how mental health professionals could observe our dynamic as it is shown in his recorded words and unquestioningly accept this one-dimensional view of my husband's family. Besides showing bias to well persons as opposed to those who are ill, this perspective sanctioned my former husband's denial of facts that were pertinent to our changing the way we related as a couple. The records diminished his family's struggle with prejudice as first-generation German immigrants during the Second World War and discounted my husband as a total human being. The history-taking process reinforced for my husband the adverse cultural messages for men to be in power, in control, and cut off from feelings when an opposite attitude was needed to improve the mental heath of our family.

RB: Both of you have seen Susan's records from Lakeshore Psychiatric Hospital and have read Susan's writing about these experiences. You have both worked as health professionals. How does the mental health system function now compared to how it functioned then?

BT: Over the last twenty-seven years, how much of healthcare practice has changed in terms of a greater appreciation of the social context, and more listening to the voice of the patient? I've been to Grand Rounds where I've thought, "Where have people been in the last thirty years?" because I see the same reductionistic type of thinking in terms of formulation and treatment. However, I've also been very struck by individual health professionals who have been able to integrate the social and cultural factors in the lives of women and men into an understanding of a variety of psychiatric disorders—if you want to call them "psychiatric disorders." We've got a lot of work to do, but there has been some movement by some people within the health profession. It's not universal … We need to educate health professionals very early on, to provide some very intense mentoring about the importance of listening to what the client is saying. We need to teach clinicians to appreciate that individuals are the best experts on their own metaphors and symbols.

Gloria Steinem in *Revolution from Within* writes that we all have veils; we—especially women—are walking around in veils and we need to lift the veil.[17] It's a level of awareness that we need to communicate. Education, repetition, creative ways of expressing the phenomena will lead to some real changes within the system. One important approach is to take the very good information from the communities of self-help—feminist ideas and theories and the like—and to bring it within a scientific arena because then you gain credibility.

MM: Well, has [the mental health system] changed, or has it not changed?"
I think it's clearly changed. Number one, we're talking about these problems, which is a difference. Number two, Susan, you're in a position to
present your story in this special way. That came through a lot of hard
work from a lot of other people, who came before you or along with you
too, to facilitate this kind of thing.

However, when I am teaching in the classes, I'm still hearing young
women talking about what happens when they go to the doctor with depression or some other emotional problem. For example, a young woman in
one of my classes was talking last week about having seen the doctor for
an eating disorder. She said, "That's all he could hear about me. I came in
another time with a sore throat, and I was 'the anorexic.' He couldn't just
treat my sore throat. It had to be related to this label."

My students' experiences speak to what's happening with younger
people who are challenging the ways in which their lives are organized.
One young woman in my class has endometriosis. Again, her label has
defined her to her doctor – she talks about this frequently in class. She
started a support group where she found that how she's been treated is not
much different than for a lot of other people. So there's commonality. The
group members are not isolated anymore, but are collectively seeing that
the ways that health professionals are looking at their lives are very similar. So what's the similarity? Often it's that the women's complaints, the
women's voices – and often even the men's voices – aren't heard. Everything
else gets filtered through the label.

ROSEMARY
Conclusions

Medical Model Care

Doctors Toner and Malone, and Susan and I all expressed yearning for more
sensitive and compassionate care for both women and men. Doctors Toner
and Malone point out that the medical model is prone to problems that recur
so commonly, they must be regarded as systems failures rather than the shortcomings of any individual practitioner.[18] One problem is narrow focus as
explained by Dr. Toner: "The cultural or societal factors, that is, the problems
of living, gender role expectations, and social context ... were considered very
little, if at all, in either formulation or treatment, at either conceptual or intervention levels ... The therapists used a specific theoretical model of what schizophrenia was—a medical disorder—and concluded that [Susan] needed
treatment with medication."

A second problem is bias in respect to sociocultural experiences such as gender, race, religion, or sexual orientation where clinicians fail to appreciate the complexity or meanings associated with, for example, traditional male and female roles, religious background, immigration, or the straddling of more than one culture. Dr. Malone notes, for example, "in Susan's medical records, that it was her husband's voice who was being heard—not hers. He had the authority to speak for her ... I was thinking, 'How is it that they only heard his voice and not her voice?' when Susan's talking about ... the incredible workload of raising four children, one after the other."

Bias heightens the risk that the clinician will understand patient problems poorly and intervene in inappropriate or harmful ways, for example, failing to question whether Susan's or others' expectations of her as wife and mother were in any way detrimental to her mental health.

A third problem is patronizing and belittling attitudes; such attitudes substantially interfere with development of the trusting and mutually respectful patient/professional relationship that is essential to accurate assessment and effective intervention. One example of the detrimental impact of such attitudes is the clinical decision that Susan might be at risk for harming her children, a decision made without asking Susan about the basis of her fears for the children's safety. Other examples include the derogatory comments made in the psychologist's report about Susan's interest in art and the assumption that this interest represented a misguided effort to secure approval and recognition from others.

A fourth problem is failure to nurture the patient's desire to heal, that is, to be a primary author in overcoming personal difficulties and improving quality of life. For example, clinical staff failed to see or pursue the constructive and healing possibilities of Susan's artistic interests or efforts to challenge the status quo of her relationship to her husband or those in authority. As Dr. Toner explained in our conversation, "Your exploding in rage at the professional conference meeting was further evidence that things were not fine. Expressing your anger was healthier for you.... What was healthy for you was interpreted as further psychopathology. It's fascinating! I think that this still goes on today."

In other words, the routine functioning of the hospital in-patient ward and outpatient clinic caused Susan to experience multiple harms. Health professionals focused narrowly on diagnosis and treatment and failed to recognize the contradictory and repressive role expectations that Susan faced as a woman, young mother, and devout Catholic. Susan was subject to patronizing and belittling attitudes that were evident in the denigration of her interests in art and community needs, as well as in the view that her concerns about her children's safety were indicators of pathology rather than realistic worries.

Susan's desire to heal was undercut by professionals' tacit acceptance of the status quo of her marriage and beliefs that she suffered from an incurable and disabling mental illness for which medication offered the only hope to prevent relapse. Despite regular psychiatric appointments, none of the professionals providing care identified Susan as profoundly worried and unhappy, harmed by antipsychotic medication, and having serious difficulties in her marriage.

It is as if the lifeguards to whom Susan and her family turned to rescue her when she was drowning focused entirely on diagnosing the category of her drowning crisis, presumed that the crisis had nothing to do with community views that girls should not learn to swim, criticized Susan for attempting swimming, and accused her of wanting to drown her children as they pulled her out of the water. To keep with the analogy, they performed artificial respiration long after the point when she was able to breathe independently, using techniques known to put the victim at risk for permanent breathing difficulties, and never mentioned the benefit of swimming or water-safety instruction even though Susan came to the beach to check in with the lifeguards repeatedly for some years following her near-drowning crisis.

Dr. Malone notes that gender role problems are now more widely recognized and individuals themselves are better informed and taking steps to find support from others. Dr. Toner notes the progress that some clinicians have made in developing clinical analyses and interventions that consider the adverse effects of traditional gender roles. She proposes a broad program of research on women's mental health issues. Neither Dr. Toner nor Dr. Malone believes that the health care system reliably addresses the concerns outlined here. As a group, mental health "lifeguards" have probably become somewhat more helpful and resuscitation techniques, for example, medications and patient education have improved; but lifeguards still vary greatly and a drowning person often risks rescue in a narrow-minded or belittling manner that discourages learning to swim.

The Feminist Alternative

Narrative therapy, a relatively recent approach to psychotherapy, understands feminist theory as one of the socially subjugated bodies of knowledge that offer alternatives to a society's dominant stories.[19] Susan as a wife and mother was performing a dominant story—acting on knowledge and practices widely known and accepted in Canadian society of the 1960s and 1970s. Socially subjugated knowledges are those that are either written out of the generally accepted historical record in deference to a more widely established preferred perspective or those that are circulated only within confined, marginal locales or groups.[20] At the time of Susan's hospital care, feminist critiques of traditional female roles were socially subjugated that is, not easily accessible, for both of these reasons. In the 1960s and 1970s, the thinking and accomplishments of the late-nineteenth and early-twentieth-century feminist movement were either excluded or included only peripherally in widely circulated accounts of North American and European history. Feminist thinking and political activities unfolding during the 1960s and 1970s tended to be narrowly circulated among groups of women considered marginal to the dominant North American social institutions. Narrative therapists prize such socially subjugated knowledges as alternatives to consider when dominant stories are failing to incorporate vital aspects of individual experience.

What Susan found helpful about feminist analysis seems to be consistent with this understanding. Dr. Malone's explanation of the structural-functional model, for example, clarifies the dominant story of the ideal husband and wife and suggests how this story failed to incorporate Susan's vital lived experiences—her concerns about repeated pregnancies, her interest in work as an artist. Feminist thought offered stories that increased Susan's confidence to value her vital experiences that were not incorporated into stories of herself as wife and mother, observant Catholic or, somewhat later, as mentally ill patient. In this way, feminist and other sociopolitical analyses, such as analyses of racism, homophobia, religious prejudice, and so on, offer understanding on how a dominant story is failing and offers some possible alternatives.

Since Susan's hospital admission, feminist perspectives are now more available within the dominant culture so that individuals can more readily identify problems such as a narrow focus on diagnosis and can locate alternatives such as joining support groups or raising concerns with caregivers. The more the dominant culture can accommodate such diverse stories, the more the collective well-being of the community is enhanced.

Some caveats must be kept in mind. The feminist movement, for example, led in identifying and addressing issues such as violence in the lives of women and children and entrenched biases against women. Nevertheless, feminism, or indeed any ideology applied as a rigid rule, can be as insensitive and harmful as the medical model. Had Susan in the 1970s been directed to understand her distress as due to repressive social and religious institutions and to express her anger by joining political protests, such an approach would likely have undercut her ability to heal just as surely as the medical approach did. Professionals who impose a formulaic approach close the door to the individual's initiatives to locate his or her own vital experiences and incorporate such experiences into personal life stories. Sociopolitical analysis imposed without respect for these processes encourages the individual to adopt a passive "victim" role, just as the medical model, used badly, encourages the individual to accept a passive "patient" role; such approaches invite the individual to be regarded by themselves and others as possessing no personal authority.

Both Dr. Toner and Dr. Malone point out that equality between men and women is not particularly attractive if women are to give up the traditional feminine role simply to adopt the traditional masculine role with the resultant denial or devaluation of the feminine in both men and women.[21] Such an approach denies men and women their individual feelings, preferences, strengths, and weaknesses—in short, their humanity.

Values and Process at the Heart of Feminism

What Susan found healing, the way she learned to swim, was respectful interaction with people who listened to her, who encouraged her gently to reconnect with her body, feelings, and abilities and to develop an understanding of the world, a story of herself, that was consistent with her own values and vital experiences.

Susan's experience of healing and the present conversation brought to mind my discussions with feminist colleagues during the 1990s. When feminist professionals tried to articulate what defined feminist health care, what emerged was not specific knowledge, ideology, interventions, or programs but rather a set of values and a process for implementing them.[22] The value/process framework that emerged was less exclusive to women's issues and experiences and more able to honour the feminine, and thus the humanity of both men and women. Threaded through the present conversation, we noticed all four of us similarly pointing to the importance of values and processes.

First, a *holistic, contextualized approach* is sought as the basis for understanding problems and developing solutions. Dr. Toner, for example, points out the importance of teaching clinicians to understand patient's difficulties within the broad sweep of their lives, family, community, and society. Dr. Malone describes the importance of challenging the structural/functionalist conception of marriage. These comments point to remedies for the narrow focus and bias of the conventional medical model.

Second, *collaborative relationships* are valued, that is, relationships where responsibilities and pleasures are shared cooperatively with mutual respect. Every story needs characters and an audience and we can participate in one another's stories in many ways. Dr. Malone describes support from others as the basis for understanding and gathering the strength to take action on personal concerns. Dr. Toner notes the importance of teaching clinicians to "listen to the words and interpretations of the client, then put themes on them after, rather than coming in a priori … to appreciate that individuals are the best experts on their own metaphors and symbols." As well, when problems and solutions are understood in broad and complex terms, it is unlikely that any one person or approach will be able to address every area. Diverse people sharing with one another in a spirit of mutual respect are likely to foster healing most effectively within both individual and community.

Finally, *respect for individual voice* is fundamental. From the beginning to the end of this conversation, Doctors Toner and Malone repeatedly emphasize the importance of listening carefully. This listening extends beyond understanding words, beyond even recognizing the undercurrents beneath the words, to responses that affirm the individual's right and responsibility to be fully involved in making decisions and taking steps to improve their lives. As Dr. Malone notes, "When people's voices are really heard, it is incredible where they can move with their lives." Respectful listening nurtures the individual's desire to heal, provides the garden in which the healing process can unfold, and offers the antidote to patronizing and belittling attitudes.

So at the heart of the feminist analysis is a valuing of holistic, contextualized understandings, collaborative relationships, and respect for the individual. Women's College Hospital in Toronto was founded by women physicians in 1911. Interestingly, the hospital's motto is *Non quo, sed quo modo*, "Not what we do, but how." Apparently, the idea that women think of their healthcare work as defined more by process and values rather than by product is at least several generations old.

SUSAN
Conclusions

More than any other event, Rosemary's and my conversations about my records with Dr. Seeman, Dr. Toner, and Dr. Malone provided the insights necessary to end my cycle of long-term rage towards psychiatrists. As new awarenesses on my psychiatric treatment arose, I moved from being a raging, stuck, shame- and guilt-filled victim into an owning my own role in a psychiatrist/god and patient/victim dynamic. With this growth, I was free to express justified anger at how gender biases in my and other cases can and did distort psychiatric judgments and abilities to diagnose and treat mental illnesses. With insights gained from our conversations on the records, my isolated focus on my own story grew more in sympathy with mental illness sufferers in general. The rare opportunity that our conversations allowed me to gain in wellness furthered my desire to write this book and to share the benefits of these conversations with others.

My records were written prior to the legislation that permitted patients the right to legal access of their hospital records. Whether that fact influenced how my caregivers wrote about me in the records, I cannot say. But I am certain that my ability to conceive of very real people writing real thoughts about me in the records, was as important to my healing as their medical data. Without that core of authenticity, the records would not have allowed me to recall and release negative caregiver projections that had remained with me since my time in hospital. By projections I mean, for example, that when the psychologist thought, wrote, and named my psychosis a "cauldron of snakes" in the records, that same energy passed from him to me at the time and those same energies remained in my body until my reading the records allowed me to clear them. I experienced numerous instances of similar negative energies being physically released from my body as I worked with the records.

Whereas psychiatrists' overprescribing and my past conditioning to hand my power over to doctors influenced my choice to remain silent in the past, the ability to write a response to the records allowed me to make new sense out of old non-sense. As I gained new meaning from my records, my wellness increased.

If I had faced recovery from my mental illness in a less auspicious way, I believe that I would still have been luckier than the many who are being told today that their mental illnesses are rooted in chemical imbalance. I have no trouble believing that chemical imbalances and brain malfunctions occurred during my mental illness but psychoneuroimmunological studies that prove how the emotional system is an interdependent partner with all other body systems and provide evidence that thought can and does become chemistry, validate my belief that, in my case at least, the chemical imbalances resulted from my diseased emotions rather than the other way around. Though I cannot speak for other cases of mental illness, I am grateful that I was spared a diagnosis that implied my illness was due to a genetic or chemical imbalance and beyond my control.

Any story that reduces my experience to the part of me that can be placed in a test tube or seen under a microscope would negate an immense part of me that was fully engaged in the psychosis. The part that I have been taught to define as my soul or my psyche was moved during and by my experience to the point of allowing me to change the direction of my life and the value I place on my existence.

Notes

1   Suzi Gablik, *The Reenchantment of Art* (New York: Thames and Hudson, 1991).
2   Suzi Gablik, *Conversations Before the End of Time* (New York: Thames and Hudson, 1995).
3   Adolf Meyer, *The Collected Papers of Adolf Meyer*, ed. Eunice Winters. 4 vols. (Baltimore: Johns Hopkins University Press, 1948–52).
4   Persimmon Blackbridge and Sheila Gilhooly *Still Sane* (Vancouver: Press Gang, 1985).
5   American Psychiatric Association, *Diagnostic and Statistical Manual of Mental Disorders*, 4th edition (Washington, DC: American Psychiatric Press, 1994).
6   See, for example, Richard P. Bentall, ed., *Reconstructing Schizophrenia* (New York: Routledge, 1990); Robert D. Coursey, Joseph Alford, and Bill Safarjan, "Significant Advances in Understanding and Treating Serious Mental Illness," *Professional Psychology: Research and Practice* 28 (1997): 205–16; Courtenay M. Harding et al., "The Vermont Longitudinal Study of Persons with Severe Mental Illness, I: Methodology, Study Sample, and Overall Status 32 Years Later," *American Journal of Psychiatry* 144 (1987a): 718–26; Courtenay M. Harding et al., "The Vermont Longitudinal Study of Persons with Severe Mental Illness, II: Long-Term Outcome of Subjects Who Retrospectively Met *DSM-III* Criteria for Schizophrenia," *American Journal of Psychiatry* 144 (1987a): 727–35; Courtenay M. Harding and James H. Zahniser, "Empirical Correction of Seven Myths about Schizophrenia with Implications for Treatment," *Acta Psychiatrica Scandinavica* 90 (suppl. 384) (1994): 140–46; Courtenay M. Harding, Joseph Zubin, and John S. Strauss, "Chronicity in Schizophrenia: Revisited," *British Journal of Psychiatry* 161 (suppl. 18) (1992): 27–37; and Patrick A. McGuire, "New Hope for People with Schizophrenia," *Monitor on Psychology* 31 (2000): 24–28: Larry Davidson, Courtenay M. Harding, and LeRoy Spaniol, eds., *Recovery from Serious Mental Illness: Research Evidence and Implications for Practice*, Vol. 1 (Boston: Center for Psychiatric Rehabilitation, Boston University, 2005); Larry Davidson, Courtenay M. Harding, and LeRoy Spaniol, eds., *Recovery from Serious Mental Illness: Research Evidence and Implications for Practice*, Vol. 2 (Boston: Center for Psychiatric Rehabilitation, Boston University, 2005).
7   J. Joel Jeffries et al., *Living and Working with Schizophrenia*, 2nd ed. (Toronto: University of Toronto Press, 1990), 76.
8   Peter R. Breggin, *Toxic Psychiatry* (New York: St. Martin's, 1991).
9   For discussion of this issue in relation to psychiatric diagnosis, see Jonathan D. Raskin and Adam M. Lewandowski, "The Construction of Disorder as a Human Enterprise," in *Constructions of Disorder*, ed. Robert A. Neimeyer and Jonathan D. Raskin (Washington, DC: American Psychological Association, 2000), 15–40.
10 Popular in the 1970s were the following: Hogie Wyckoff, *Love, Therapy and Politics* (New York: Grove, 1976); Hogie Wyckoff, *Solving Women's Problems* (New York: Grove, 1977).
11 Phyllis Chesler, *Women and Madness* (New York: Avon Books, 1972).
12 See, for example, Dean G. Kilpatrick and Heidi S. Resnick, "Posttraumatic Stress Disorder Associated with Exposure to Criminal Victimization in Clinical and Community Populations," in *Posttraumatic Stress Disorder: DSM-IV and Beyond*, ed. Jonathan R.T. Davidson and Edna B. Foa (Washington, DC: American Psychiatric Press, 1992), 113–43; Diana E.H. Russell, *The Secret Trauma: Incest in the Lives of Girls and Women* (New York: Basic Books, 1986); Gary R. Schoener et al., eds., *Psychotherapists' Sexual Involvement with Clients: Intervention and Prevention* (Minneapolis, MN: Walk-in Counseling Center, 1989); and Judith Worell and Pam Remer, *Feminist Perspectives in Therapy: An Empowerment Model for Women* (Toronto: John Wiley and Sons, 1992).

13 Talcott Parsons and Robert F. Bales, eds., *Family, Socialization and Interaction Process* (London: Routledge & Kegan Paul, 1956).

14 Leo J. Kinsella, *The Wife Desired* (Teckny, IL: Divine Word Publications, 1957); Leo J. Kinsella, *The Man for Her* (Oak Park, IL: Valiant Publications, 1957).

15 K. Thompson, A. Sergejew, and J. Kulkarni, "Estrogen Affects Cognition in Women with Psychosis," *Psychiatry Research* 94 (2000): 201–9.

16 Charlotte Perkins Gilman, "The Yellow Wallpaper," in *The Charlotte Perkins Gilman Reader*, ed. Ann J. Lane (New York: Pantheon, 1980), 3–20.

17 Gloria Steinem, *Revolution from Within* (Boston: Little, Brown, 1992).

18 Breggin, *Toxic Psychiatry*.

19 Good introductions to this work include Jill Freedman and Gene Combs, *Narrative Therapy: The Social Construction of Preferred Realities* (New York: W.W. Norton, 1996); Michael White and David Epston, *Narrative Means to Therapeutic Ends* (New York: W.W. Norton, 1990); Michael White, *Narrative Practice and Exotic Lives: Resurrecting Diversity in Everyday Life* (Adelaide, South Australia: Dulwich Centre, 2004); Michael White, *Maps of Narrative Practice* (New York: W.W. Norton, 2007).

20 White and Epston, *Narrative Means to Therapeutic Ends*.

21 Others who make this point include Gerd Brantenberg, *Egalia's Daughters: A Satire of the Sexes*, trans. Louis Mackay (Seattle, WA: Seal, 1985); Marilyn French, *Beyond Power: On Women, Men and Morals* (New York: Ballantine, 1985); Worell and Remer, *Feminist Perspectives in Therapy*.

22 See for example, French, *Beyond Power*; Worell and Remer, *Feminist Perspectives in Therapy*; Sheryl Ruzek, "Feminist Visions of Health: An International Perspective," in *What Is Feminism?* ed. Juliet Mitchell and Ann Oakley (London: Basil Blackwell, 1986), 184–207.

6 Conversations on Story, Art, and Healing

We used to wonder where war lived, what it was that made it so vile. And now we realize that we know where it lives, that it lives inside ourselves.

—Albert Camus, *Notebooks*, entry for September 7, 1939[1]

SUSAN
How Story Influenced Healing

STORY HAS BEEN PIVOTAL TO MY GAINS in wellness in the years following my psychosis. Story was natural to my visual and auditory ways of learning since childhood. Whether story involved the reminiscences of elders at family gatherings, narrative images in our encyclopedia the *Books of Knowledge*, the church-imparted Christ story that circled the seasons of my growing up, my Joan of Arc comic book, the drama of innumerable Irish wakes, or 1940s films where the cost of admission, an old aluminium pot, went from the theatre to a war munitions factory, I felt safe in the presence of story. Story replaced the lost inner and outer excitement that resulted from my conditioning to repress and suppress my own feminine story.

Around 1989, prior to writing my story, my younger brother, who was gathering family stories for his children, asked me to write about my experience growing up as a Catholic woman. Prior to writing about my Catholic experience, I had a degree of exposure to feminist concepts, but I had not yet embodied them. Writing my story lent more importance to feminism and enlarged my ability to recognize the breadth of the patriarchal self-concept I was battling. In my later discussions with my brother on what I had written, my former sense that we shared similar childhoods as siblings dissolved. I love and am deeply appreciative and admiring of each member of my extended family, but the writing of my story shifted my ways of recognizing myself in the larger family setting. Familiar enmeshed ways of relating as sibling, aunt, and in-law or as seeing myself as the groups' "broken one," underwent stages of change. I began with experiencing myself as a stranger in the group and later with seeing them and me as whole but separate people bonded by history and memories.

Encouraged in 1992 by theatre artists who had seen my art at the Women's College Hospital *Never Again: Women and Men Against Violence* event, I began writing my story as a play. During the writing of the play, my late friend Helen Porter (who was also a storyteller and writer) would ask, "Are you going mad, Susan, because you are not writing unless you are going mad?" Helen's humour, encouragement, and role as dramaturge helped me build a much-needed permission to feel and normalize the turmoil of writing.

In 1994, I workshopped *My Old Movie of Dreams* 1994 play after writing, producing, and collaborating on it with the Company of Sirens and a cast of four. Though play character names were changed, the play was based on my story. A refined version played in Toronto for two weeks in 1996. Both experiences aided my growth as an artist. My work with the play's collaborators, which placed my life on public view and subjected my work to the director's, the dramaturge's as well as the critics' knives, was new and challenging. The play received enough positive audience feedback for me to feel it was a worthwhile effort, but the critics were unimpressed. After the *Toronto Star* panned the play, I cocooned with the film *Apocalypse Now* until the difficult lesson that reviews are one of art's risks took hold.

In the past, my favourite story experiences when I trained as a nurse were the mandatory daily readings of patient histories. This same preference influenced my initial decision to present my story in the form of a case study when Rosemary and I began writing the book. Hindsight shows I also chose this writing style for the added distance it gave me from the emotional work of remembering my story. I retain an appreciation for the caution and wisdom in this first approach to sharing my story, but I gained a more wholesome distance from my past with each revision's unearthed feelings.

Story has been critical to my process of change not only through writing but in the many ways I learned my story through hearing or reading other peoples' stories. When my mind was most fragile, and the power and distance afforded by simple tales like "Beauty and the Beast" was all I could handle, I was still able to gain insight on my need to embrace and transform my inner beast from that level of story.[2]

My beastly inner seriousness also needed the sacred story in humour. At the lowest points, when I could not draw on my own humour, it was the gentle humour in classic *Bugs Bunny* cartoons and shows like *The Muppets* that would bring me relief. Woody Allen's remark "I am giving my psychiatrist one more year, then I am going to Lourdes" restored my perspective on numerous occasions.

As Rosemary and I planned conversations on mental health and healing in 1996, I felt Helen Porter and Gail Regan would have much to contribute. Helen was a storyteller, writer, and dear friend whom I had known since the mid-1980s. Helen's friendship, genius, and stories brought grounding and delight to my immediate post-withdrawal years and to my later going public with my art and writing. Helen's personal journey and growth uniquely inspired and encouraged my healing.

Gail Regan is my sister-in-law and has been a dear supportive friend for over fifty years. Before meeting Gail, the women in my circle mainly followed the traditional paths set out for women by the Catholic Church. Gail's habit of acquiring a university degree with each of her pregnancies as well as her continuing studies throughout her life were foreign concepts initially but over time became extremely informing for my growth. In addition to Gail's business, hospital, community, and academic achievements, she has given vast energies over the years to creating nourishing ritual for our large and still-growing extended family. In addition to being vigorous in how she lives her own story, Gail has devoted much of her life to understanding the stories that drive health, business, and government institutions and to learning how the stories of diverse cultures can enlighten and improve our own. I felt our book would be enhanced by Gail's original mind and ways of knowing story and I hoped that she in turn would enjoy the mental and emotional stretch that conversation with Helen Porter was bound to provide.

·

ROSEMARY
Conversations on Story and Healing

Gail Regan was influential in blocking the merger of Women's College Hospital with a much larger university-affiliated hospital during the years I worked at the hospital. Gail served as chair of the Women's College Hospital board of directors and encouraged the hospital to take a unique advocacy role in relation to women's health. Gail was a corporate and community leader, president of Cara Holdings Limited, vice-chair of Cara Operations Limited, and president of Langar

Company Limited. She held a doctorate in educational theory and a master's in business administration. She had served on the board of directors of Energy Probe and the Council for Canadian Unity.

I had been a rapt audience member at her performances before meeting Helen Porter personally. Helen was a Canadian storyteller whose thirty years of professional work included performances at the Blythe Festival, the National Arts Centre, Roy Thomson Hall, Young People's Theatre, the St. Lawrence Centre, Factory Theatre, and Tarragon Theatre as well as in radio, television, and film. She had written three plays. *I Love You So Much It Hurts* toured Ontario in 1995 with great success. *Biblical Tales of the Nineties* was written for Vision Television. Many of her short stories had been broadcast on CBC Radio and published. She produced and hosted the *Oh! Canada* gala for the Art Gallery of Ontario, an event featuring Canadian artists.

I was delighted to meet with Gail and Helen. They were both involved with preparations for Susan's art to be installed as the *Shedding Skins* permanent exhibit at the Clarke Institute (now the Centre for Addiction and Mental Health) and with production of her play, *My Old Movie of Dreams*. I wanted to learn about their perspectives on Susan's hospital care and healing, why the hospital failed to support healing, and the role of story in healing. Gail, Helen, Susan, and I all met in Gail's warm and elegant office at Cara Operations Limited in downtown Toronto on 21 February 1996.

ROSEMARY BARNES: Helen, when the Clarke Institute committee first gathered to discuss Susan's paintings and play, you opened the meeting with the story "The Goose Girl," from *Grimms' Fairy Tales*. This story tells of a girl who journeys to claim her bridegroom but is tricked by a servant along the way and loses her sense of herself. The servant is then taken as the bride when they arrive at the new kingdom. The young girl feels she must remain silent about her story until eventually she tells the king's stove. The king listens as she tells the stove her story, recognizes her as his true bride, and marries her. Why did you choose to tell this story to the committee setting out to prepare public presentations of Susan's work?

HELEN PORTER: "The Goose Girl" is a beautiful old tale about identity, both female and male. The story is based on the fact that most of us begin life with a sense of who we are, then go through a time of betraying our true selves. The false servant betrays the goose girl, takes her identity, proceeds to the next kingdom, and takes the intended husband away from the real princess. This servant represents a part of the goose girl's self, a false self that takes over and dominates until the goose girl goes through the process of dealing with nature. Remember the goose girl's horse was murdered and its head put up on the gates of the city. Every time the girl goes out of the city to mind the geese, she looks up and the horse speaks to her. Through this, she is reminded and learns to trust her instincts—her instinctual self—and to let go of this false social self that has so betrayed her. The king falls in love with this goose girl after he begins to notice how lovely she is. He says, "What's happened, why can't you speak and tell us who you are?" She replies that she can't speak or tell anyone what's happened. So he says, "Tell the stove; the stove will keep your secret." So she tells the stove and the king is listening on the other end of the stovepipe.

I feel that Susan's story is similar to that of the goose girl in that she was raised in a Catholic system of religion and education where she put on the mask of young womanhood, as she was instructed, and married the bridegroom. But that wasn't the true Susan who was marrying the bridegroom; it was the Susan who was wearing a false mask created by rigid religious, educational, and social training. Susan lived with this bridegroom, her husband, and they had their four children. Then she began to awaken through the agents of her instincts—through the four children and through the love of this man. Even though her husband was loving the mask, his love brought her alive. Gradually, out came the true Susan's face and voice, very frightened, very much a part of nature, scaring herself and everybody else. It was lidded by the doctors with medication. But through dream work—which I think is instinctual life—her true self emerges. The dreams are like her telling her story to the stove in the fairy tale. They helped her to share her story consciously with herself and with others, until she reached the point of being able to tell the world. Telling the story is uniting with the true bridegroom: her inner sense, her inner intelligence, and wholeness become apparent.

So I see Susan very much following the goose girl's journey, which is wonderful and the reason I used the story that morning at the Clarke Institute. The Clarke was also playing the role of the stove by being willing to hear and share this story with the world, and accept it through the paintings and through the images. I thought this was marvellous, that the Clarke was willing to take that on and share this tale with the world.

I just want to say one more thing. I think that a lot of these old fairy tales, such as "Cinderella," "The Goose Girl," and " Snow White" are about the fact that all of us come into the world with our true soul; then a negative, or a proper social self takes over, and robs us of our soul. That proper self is represented in "Cinderella" by the two wicked stepsisters, and the stepmother, who are the parts that block the soul. But all the fairy tales tell us that the soul will win out if we go with our instincts.

GAIL REGAN: I was just wondering how the instruments of social order get us to forget our true selves. I think there must be suppression of story to do that. The way there are grades could be an example of that; for instance, you were in grade six, but now you're in grade seven, so you don't have recess any more. This change in the schedule has nothing to do with you—that you had a pattern and tradition of having recess with your friends; now you're just one year older but that doesn't happen anymore. It's a suppression of story because we're graded, we're not a continuous flow of experience. I'm sure there are other devices that break our story.

HP: Just being graded. By being graded A, B, C, D, you begin to identify as an "A" or a "B" or a "C" and you lose your whole sense of self. Children start out with the potential to be a Picasso. At five, we have this incredible creativity, we are open, we're curious, we're exploring, and then by grade three, by eight years of age, most of us have lost that ability to think artistically, to create, to be curious. One of the things that appears to me to stop that creativity is grading. You begin to think of yourself as good or bad or fair and your parents read your report card and they start to see you as those marks; some teachers even start to look at you as those marks.

RB: Those are both changes imposed by an institution. Is there something about institutional structure that suppresses story? You're raising the very important question of how one's own story comes to be suppressed. What are the reasons, why does this happen in our society?

GR: When I'm telling my story, I'm telling my construction of my experience. Susan and I have attended workshops where we learned to use "percept language;" this language allows me to be fully aware of and responsible for my experience.[3] I think that society, hierarchy, and function depend on—or at least have depended on—giving away one's own experience. One does this in order to do assembly line work all day, or to do data processing all day, or to do the accounting on somebody else's books all day long. Being able to tolerate alienation and also to fit into a very abstract conceptual world is work that's got to be done; it's work that doesn't come easily to human beings. So there is the necessity to get out of my story and to learn the consensual validation, the concepts that bind us together.

RB: So the suppression of story happens when the individual sets aside personal story for the sake of meeting the needs of an institution. One example is the child learning to set aside his or her own story for the sake of meeting the needs of the hierarchal institution of the school.

GR: Certainly it's how I experienced school. Endless tedium that had nothing to do with me. I experienced school as a suppression of my story. The school was certainly not interested in me. They were interested in my submission to learning the curriculum.

RB: Which wasn't necessarily your curriculum; in other words, the curriculum didn't arise from your story, particularly, or from your own needs. When we began the committee meeting at the Clarke you made a very strong statement about how you saw Susan's story touching other people.

GR: This was my reaction to the play. I was very touched. The play was so powerfully done that my reaction was, "This is Susan's story. This is her story. Wow! This is *her* story."

RB: You are thinking of the performance of *My Old Movie of Dreams*?

GR: Yes. One reaction was "Wow! This was Susan's story." It's so clear and powerful. But I also had the sense of "This could be my story." Or, if I told Susan the events in my life, she could write a play similar to this one; really any person with proper help and guidance could write his or her story in this way. So, I had this sense of being hit in the gut. This is Susan's story, but it's also my story. Or if it were my story, Susan would have the same reaction.

RB: Did hearing Susan's story give you a stronger sense of your own story? Or a sense of power to tell your own story?

GR: It gave me the sense of having a story. "Oh! I have a story too." Yes, I have constructed my reality. I'm not just a little stamp that the school system churned out.

RB: I know you were saying at the meeting at the Clarke that one of your hopes for this project was that others would come in contact with Susan's story and have a similar kind of sense that, "I have a story. We all have a story."

GR: Yes. Yes, but I think what that does is … when you're a conceptual person and you've learned to classify yourself … It could be a grading like A, B, C, D, but it can be other things like Myers Briggs, where one of the dimensions is extraverted/introverted.[4]

RB: [Laughs] Psychologists are big on those things.

GR: According to that test, I'm introverted. So if I'm introverted, that means I'm not extraverted; when I'm "A," that means that I'm not, "not-A." It's a matter of Platonic logic—categorical. I think of myself as being in certain categories, which means that I'm not other categories. So if there are extraverts around, I can say, "I'm not like them. They go to parties all the time, whereas I go to a few parties, and only for the sake of social politeness; but I'm educated and I just stay home and read a book."

The next step after categorizing is we/they thinking, invidious judgments, then the we/they set-up. "They" are those folks who need to be governed. "We" need to provide prisons for "them" or "we" need to provide public transit service for "them." The "we" provides for the "they," rather than all of us as a community building what the community needs. What evolves from this is that you can get the most dreadful programs in prisons and in schools, because they weren't designed by anybody who intended to use them.

RB: So story offers a very different way of thinking about self and relationship to community as compared to thinking in terms of "we" and "they."

GR: Yes. Thinking perceptually in terms of story has a different impact than thinking conceptually in terms of categories. After watching Susan's play, I think, "Oh, gosh, she had a psychotic break—I'm really lucky I didn't have one." I no longer think, "Oh, she's one of *those* people who required help for mental health problems, and I'm not one of *those*. Now, I just think, "Oh, I was lucky."

RB: So Susan's story may encourage a shift in consciousness from a we/they, hierarchical, power-over frame of mind where decisions are made on behalf of other people to something different. The story invites a shift towards a consciousness where we think of ourselves as interdependent and working together to create solutions to shared problems.

GR: Yes. I think the story shifts the frame of reference from the first, the power-over approach, to the second view of interdependence.

RB: Helen started off by talking about healing within the individual which takes place in the telling of one's story, as when the goose girl told her story to the stove. What you describe, Gail, is the potential for healing within listeners, as we become aware of our own personal stories, and recognize ourselves within Susan's story. We as listeners are then in a position to relate to society and social issues differently, as story shifts our consciousness towards recognition of our interdependence and shared problems.

HP: Bettelheim shows that children who are raised on fairy tales grow in a different way than children who aren't raised on them.[5] Folk tales, and particularly fairy tales, are able to name for a child their unconscious story in a safe and supportive way. The fairy tale tells it. Goethe and Tolkien support Bettelheim's theory. Our own Robertson Davies said that a child who doesn't have fairy tales is like a child deprived of mother's breast milk.

These stories contain the archetypes that feed a child's basic self. A child absorbs those fairy tales—unconsciously takes them in—and uses the archetypes in the stories as a foundation in her imagination. Later, that child—just from unconsciously having taken in those stories—is helped in her dealings with issues of injustice, falsehood, choosing right from wrong, knowing who she is and who she is not, and resisting what society puts on her, especially as a teenager. Fairy tales make a difference when you're a teenager and you're choosing sexually, finding your identity. A teenager gets all these images coming at her; it's a very hard time. It's when we are most weak; we just take in what's coming at us. The fairy tale can give a teenager this inner sense of, "Something is not right here; this doesn't feel that it fits." So, I think stories work that way in a child's life in the beginning.

I think a child who can tell her story fairly openly to her family, to her church, to her school, or to her camp is a child who is much better off when the time comes to find authority as an adult. But I think very few children ever get a chance to tell their stories, because I see it. As a storyteller, I see parents constantly limiting their children. Can I give you some examples? I was invited to a boy's birthday party and was asked to do stories for his sixth birthday. "Don't tell any fairy tales," the parents said, "because we don't have them in our home. No Grimms' or any old fairy tales, because we're very careful about what we give the children. So there is no story told or read that is hurtful or scary. We don't want anything like that." I said, "I don't know what I can tell then, because you want me to tell stories that have no real power." Many well-meaning parents today do not want their children to have any stories that have blood in them or any violence or anything that smacks of pain. They're robbing their child of a certain kind of archetypal education, one among a number of the things that support the personality.

RB: Is this a need only for children? If a child heard many fairy tales, would that child have no further need for fairy tales in adult life? Are fairy tales for children or do we need to hear them also as adults?

HP: If you didn't get to hear fairy tales as a child, you can start reading them again as an adult. But there is no comparison to hearing them as a little child. As an adult, you're going to try to understand them, whereas little children don't try to understand them.

RB: They just take them in.

HP: Children never say, "What do the three little pigs mean, mommy?" No. They know intuitively what it means. But a thirty-three-year-old person reading "The Three Little Pigs" will learn that the big bad wolf came and blew her house down; the adult will then be struggling and saying, "What does it mean? Like three, what does three mean? And the big bad wolf, like, would that be my dad, or my boyfriend, or who is that?" So, understanding fairy tales is very hard for adults. They have to go back and do some inner work.

If you have heard the fairy tales when you were little, it makes a difference in your basic security as a person. I think it makes you a better reader, probably; you understand your culture better. I think you have a jump ahead, because you've absorbed unconsciously a lot of things such as those numbers—three, seven—and the names—stepmother, stepfather—and all those issues, justice in particular. This knowledge gives you a sense of confidence deep inside.

I want to say one more thing about the repression of fairy tale and imagination that's going on today, in terms of parents being afraid of the violence in these tales. Some parents feel they should protect children from fairy tales. In a lot of homes where there's no anger, there's a lot of fear of death, or fear of violence. As the father of the six-year-old boy said to me, we don't have anger in our home, it's not something we have. I've had a lot of people tell me that there's no anger in their home. Well, that says to me that three-quarters of my story can't be told if I can't talk about anger, but the reality is that every day people are knocking me down in some way. Kids go to school, where there's always going to be a bully or a giant—like the teacher who scares you or someone else who is going to upset your applecart. So you come home and if you can't really deal with that, then your story is cut off. A lot of this depends on the family's openness.

In Susan's case, it's very interesting, because it sounds like the fairy tale in her life was Grimms' "Ashenputtel" (Cinderella)—the wealthy father and the mother who was a bit of a wicked stepmother—a good mother, a good physical nurturer—but also a wicked stepmother in her control of the family; she was getting lost in those two roles. I saw the wicked stepmother really take Susan under with her tasks. I see Susan's story very much as the wicked stepmother putting her into the grey nightgown and wooden clogs and saying, "Start cleaning! Start scrubbing! No, you're not going to the ball. You're going to stay and scrub. You'd shame us if you went to the ball." So that Susan's been cleaning and scrubbing and doing all that work. Until—I'm sure through having the babies and looking after them—the birds start to come to her and speak to her, and she's rising up out of the ashes where she's been sitting. Her breakdown with those nuns and priests— at the religious retreat where the psychotic incident happened—seems like the awakening of that self through all the scrubbing and cleaning. It comes up like, "Aaaaaagh!!!"—kind of wild and snaky. Because it's so deep down and so new, it comes out as weird. But there, I think her true story and her true tongue is speaking. And unfortunately those people couldn't recognize what was happening, didn't know their stories, didn't know the soul in themselves.

RB: Who was it who didn't recognize Susan's story?

HP: The doctors didn't know their fairy tales. Their response was, "Let's just put the lid on it." It was scary, I know, when the husband comes in with a young woman and there are four babies, four children under the age of seven and she's talking about being the Virgin Mary and all these things. I guess they have a pragmatic response, "We've got to control this so the family can get back to normal." But I felt that they weren't taking into account the fact that this woman's been calm up to this point. This is the first time that it's happened—they don't seem to stop and think about that. It wasn't like she'd had a breakdown at seventeen; there was no history of mental breakdown in that woman. It's curious and I thought very odd that the health professionals did not stop and say, "Why is this happening now?" That's what's missing to me in those records. There's no sense of her life story in those doctor's records. How come a lovely woman, who's subscribed to all the expectations of a lovely woman's life up to that point, suddenly has this breakdown and they don't even ask, "What's going on here?"

GR: Because they can't bear that it would happen to them. There, but for the love of God, go they. This could be me tomorrow.

RB: When we were talking a little earlier, Gail, you were raising issues similar to the ones that Helen is asking here. You were commenting about why everyone came to regard Susan as suffering from schizophrenia. Schizophrenia is not the final diagnosis recorded at the conclusion of the hospital admission, but it seems to have become the diagnosis that Susan, her husband, and the healthcare professionals used to understand her situation. What are your thoughts about why everyone adopted this idea?

GR: I had started to read R.D. Laing, about how psychiatry is really an instrument of social control.[6] He was exploring schizophrenia, actually, but he wrote about how people who get stressed out from double binds will appear to be schizophrenic. He argued that it's really their social milieu that has to be adjusted; the double binds have to be cleared for them to recover. I was reading all this at the time that Susan had her psychotic break, but you're so helpless.

I'll use an analogy: Suppose you were in childbirth. You couldn't give birth at home and you had to go to a hospital—this was before Semmelweis, and the hospital had a very high rate of childbed fever.[7] So you know it's going to be extremely risky to go to the hospital, but you've got no place else to go. Those were my feelings about Susan. I know this is all wrong, but that's the only system that exists. I didn't have the skill myself to criticize her doctors or the procedures. So I had the sense of abandoning her on the one hand, but being forced to on the other.

RB: By not having any alternatives, anything better to suggest, any other way to respond to her distress.

GR: Yes. Questioning the hospital's approach would have met enormous resistance too. To suggest that this might have been a marital problem—well, then you're going to have to deal with that perfectionist husband of hers. Or to suggest this might be a self-differentiation problem, that she had to work things out with her mom—well, that would not have set easily with Mrs. Regan, and these two people are the helpers. So, you just have to hold your nose, and jump off the diving board. At that point, you're helpless to help.

RB: You commented earlier that everything seemed so perfect—the marriage was perfect, there were four healthy, beautiful children—that it was inconceivable to those trying to help that there could be any explanation for what had happened other than mental illness, other than schizophrenia. I was quite struck with this explanation of why everyone latched on to the notion of schizophrenia and stayed with it for such a long period of time. Susan's life seemed so perfect on the outside that it was inconceivable for there to be a story underneath the story on the surface.

GR: Everything seemed so perfect that therefore the problem had to be a mental illness. Because it couldn't possibly be a difficult marriage or Mrs. Regan's parenting. The children were charming, and there were enough financial resources so how could a thing like that possibly happen?

My mother would have been a little different. If I had been living Susan's life, I would have had a phone call from my mother every morning, saying, "Aren't you bored? Isn't it dull, looking after your children, not going out? Why don't you hire a babysitter?" My mother's voice hasn't been exactly helpful to me, in terms of the standards of care I've given my kids; but I think I would have had more of an out. Whereas Susan was more thoroughly socialized to the role than I have been; she's very quick in the kitchen and produces lovely children's gourmet meals. There was more enthusiasm for the role in her than there was in me. So, her own behaviour would have added to the mystification.

RB: The puzzlement over how a problem could have developed.

GR: How could it have happened? Lovely mom, lovely husband, making it financially, four beautiful children. Helen, you feel it is the lack of fairy tale in us. When the snake emerges, we fail to say, "Ah-ha, there's the snake!"

● ● ●

Helen's explanation of fairy tales as psychological maps for facing challenge and maturing profoundly changed my understanding of these stories. Gail described Susan's story as preventing a they/we perspective, encouraging a realization, "This could have been me," and helping to name a snake when we see one. I began to think more about the stories in my own life. Around this time, perhaps because of our conversation, I read Clarissa Pinkola Estés's *Women Who Run with the Wolves*, a powerful and humorous Jungian analysis of fairy tales as maps of women's psychological development.[8]

Susan and I journeyed through life dramas that differ in many respects. Yet at the fundamental level that Helen and Gail described, I recognized the milestones of my own stories in Susan's experiences. I thought of my experience of coming out as a lesbian, for me a profound journey in search of self. I recalled trudging along, being "normal," pursuing the life course set out by my upbringing, wondering if this is all there is. Ah yes, there is the Slough of Despond (I thank John Bunyan[9] for the names of particular milestones), full of the doubts and fears I encountered when I let myself slow down enough to reflect on how unhappy I felt. And there is Hill Difficult, which I took after committing within myself to make things better; though I looked for another way, I could find only a steep, uphill route where I made frustratingly slow progress only by small steps. And there is one of my mentors, Laura, just come from the United States for a short visit and, coincidentally, an open lesbian willing to talk freely of her experiences. I confide in her that I think I also am a lesbian. "Good luck," she says. "You'll need it. It's not an easy life."

And there is the Valley of the Shadow of Death, which I entered as I realized with more certainty that I was romantically attracted to women, meaning that my existing understanding of myself had to die to make room for the new Me who made a first appearance as a monster labelled "Pervert," "Sicko," "Unnatural," and "Doomed to a life of twisted sexual preoccupation." And there is another mentor, Corinne, a friend who is very loving when I tell her I feel I might be a lesbian, and who gently encourages me to find out more and accompanies me to the lecture about homosexuality at the university medical centre. Yes, and the Valley of Humiliation where I struggled with decisions about coming out to family and friends and received my mother's anger and efforts to make me change my mind and heart. And at last, the Celestial City where I met a large number of happy, intelligent, funny lesbians and gay men who were proud of themselves, enjoyed loving relationships, and worked to create a positive place for their lives in the larger world. Celestial City turned out to be unavailable as a permanent residence but was rather a way station where one rested and chose, often without awareness, the road for the next journey.

My coming-out story was very similar to Susan's story of struggle with psychosis at the level of its deep structure in the psyche. The bones of our stories are the bones of a basic maturational drama that we all experience.[10] Each patient, each health professional, each janitor, each manager, each computer technician, secretary, fireman, housewife, mother and father, son and daughter has at least one and likely many stories similar to those which Susan and I describe: stories of growing up and leaving home, of immigration, of illness, of betrayal, of loss, of births and deaths and rebirths, situations where the normal rules do not apply and growth occurs only by reaching deep within to find new truths and expanding outwards to learn new skills and perspectives. I quite agreed with Helen's observation that health professionals who know their own stories are more likely to recognize and respond constructively to their patients' stories. This conversation and *Women Who Run with the Wolves* helped me to identify my work with Susan as one part of another life story within myself.

In the years before I resigned from the hospital, I came to feel increasingly like Cinderella—dirty, poorly clothed, fed on scraps, forced to toil long hours without recognition, scrubbing floors, and washing the hearth while my true station as the daughter of the master was unrecognized. My initial reaction was to work harder in the hopes that my true value would be recognized. However, the bosses and colleagues who were, unbeknownst to themselves, consigned by my psyche to the role of cruel stepmother and stepsisters ignored my long hours of work, need for respect and recognition, and pleas for better treatment. (Please note that I am describing an experience of the psyche, not an objective report on my work conditions. My actual bosses and colleagues were generally dedicated, honest, and fair-minded people who were very supportive in many ways.)

When sacrifices failed to improve my lot at the hospital, I decided that I had to try to get to the ball that I heard the prince was holding in order to choose a wife. Mentors and fairy godmothers began to appear in the form of generous professional colleagues who helped in unexpected ways. One offered office space with affordable rent so that I could begin seeing private clients outside the hospital; others talked with me in detail about how to set up a private practice. The collaboration with Susan offered the possibility of continuing intellectually stimulating work, an aspect of university-affiliated hospital work that I had greatly enjoyed. So I made the move into community practice, where I felt much happier and more connected to my true self. However, I had made a move that was incomprehensible to myself and many professional colleagues. For healthcare professionals, the most prestigious positions are those as a senior leader at a university-affiliated hospital; I had progressed steadily on such a career path for fourteen years, so struggled with a sense of failure when I resigned from the hospital, thus effectively abandoning power and status. In a way, I had returned to the stepmother's house after the ball, glad that the prince had noticed me, but unable to make a lasting connection with him just yet.

I should be clear: my longed-for prince was no flesh-and-blood person, either male or female. What I sought was to find a meaningful purpose that was worthy to become the partner of my caring and hard work; such a marriage would be a true royal union.

Work with Susan on writing this book was, as I mentioned earlier, a way of healing, a crucial part of this search for my own story and for the prince. I felt a great need to reconcile my feminist beliefs with my professional career, to understand what impelled me to resign my hospital position and to author a new life story. Fairy godmothers continued to appear, enabling me to continue with renewed energy at times when I felt discouraged. The more I talked, read, wrote, and understood, the more I sensed the prince approaching, holding the exquisite and magical glass slipper.

ROSEMARY
The Garden Path

I met artist Paul Hogan briefly at Women's College Hospital when he exhibited his paintings with Susan in 1992 at the *Never Again* event. Paul's paintings were bold, whimsical images—mythological cartoons. In chapter 4, Susan briefly introduced Paul and his work as co-founder and director of the Spiral Garden at what is now known as the Bloorview Kids Rehab. In 1994, Paul was commissioned to be part of McMaster University's Health Reach study on the traumatizing effects of war on Sri Lankan children, and he remained in Sri Lanka to help co-found the Butterfly Peace Garden (BPG) in Batticaloa. The BPG offers peace-oriented art, play, and care for the earth to war-traumatized Tamil, Muslim, Hindu, and Christian children and their communities; more recently this care is also offered to numbers of former child soldiers. The Butterfly Peace Garden has since been listed in the US Congressional Records as a "Best Peace Practice." Paul also received an Ashoka Fellowship for his work with Sri Lankan children. Paul was very familiar with Susan's art, and able to read a preliminary version of her written story before our discussion.

Paul, Susan, and I met in my professional office on 18 January 1996, just two weeks before Paul left Toronto for Sri Lanka. Paul began our session by unpacking a tea box containing a special piece of cloth, a large male Kokopelli doll with a very visible penis, introduced as St. Joseph, a medium-sized female Kachina doll, introduced as Mary the earth mother, a small male Koshare doll, introduced as the wise man, a baby in a cradleboard, and freshly cut, small, green branches from cedar and pine trees. He draped the cloth over a small table in my office, and arranged the figures to make an altar displaying a nativity scene. He brought an author-published satiric book of poetry, *The Apocryphon of Mother Ralphe*,[11] from which he asked me to select a passage to read at one point during the meeting. At another point, he chanted Vajrayana mantras as he shook a rattle. Dorothy, we are not at Women's College Hospital psychiatry rounds!

ROSEMARY BARNES: Before we discuss Susan's work, tell us about your work. I was going through your articles, reproductions, and the photographs of the Spiral Garden at the Hugh MacMillan Rehabilitation Centre: I saw beautiful pictures of plants, children, masks, children in costume, totem poles. Can you tell me some more about your work there and about site-specific mythography?

PAUL HOGAN: The Spiral Garden is an integrated program involving the children from the Hugh MacMillan Rehabilitation Centre and the children from the neighbourhood who are both able-bodied and disabled: it's a mixed population. The children plant the garden in the spring and harvest in the fall. In between, in the summer, a continuous art is animated with the children and the staff. It is very much like living theatre; what's going to happen is based on what's happening and what has happened before. Ground, actuality, continuity: this is part of the principle of site-specific mythography which is one of the tools that's used to guide the process.

In the summer many different artists come and facilitate for the kids. Everything happens at once. Someone defined the garden as one thing that happens simultaneously and I would agree with that. It's not time-framed like "Now we do this" and "Now we do that" so much as it is a grand improvisation, with the exception of the few ritualistic divides in the order of the day.

RB: So it's a day-long process each time.

PH: Yes, it's a day-long process for three days each week. A fourth day is often added for staff to take account of what is happening and to make preparations for the unfolding theatre of the site. Some people might write in the accounts, for example, of different story processes that are happening. This writing takes time outside of the site for the mythographer, the "rememberer." There is also a lot of time spent in scrounging, buying, and prepping materials.

RB: What is your role?

PH: I am an animator. I am a crow sitting in a tree watching. I also squawk a lot and stir up stories. I've long done that "inside-outside" writing—regarding, reflecting, remembering. Now someone else will do that while I'm away. The structure of the garden is story. That means it is very flexible, as I've never heard a story told twice the same way by anybody. Even the person who makes up the story tells it differently the next time. We rejoice in that at the Spiral Garden. It could almost be construed as prevarication. Everything is kept on a playful, metaphorical level. It is a world of make-believe that allows both kids and adults to express different, perhaps forbidden parts of themselves in various ways.

There is also a parallel, less metaphorical, more dialogical process happening at the garden. It is very open and really is about building relationships, making a kind of family, trying to understand and make room for one another. Programming for the emergent story provides a context for exchange and dialogue. We don't always agree on how things should go. An example of this dialogical aspect would be the talking circle (or medicine circle) that Shirley Bear introduced to the Spiral Garden a few years ago.[12] These days more and more of the task is in the silence. In the talking circle, you listen much more than you talk.

For fourteen years we have been cultivating the Earth Garden. But there is also a Sky Garden which is within. In Sri Lanka, I have seriously begun to cultivate the Sky Garden. There is a Sky Garden and the Earth Garden and I feel that the Spiral Garden exists somewhere in between the two. The Sky Garden is an impelling mystery towards which we are drawn. It is entirely unspeakable. The Earth Garden is mystery too, but somehow it is much more tangible, much more strongly felt and lived in our bodies. The Spiral Garden connects those two—perhaps they are just the "the inner and the outer" aspects of our being. We cultivate the middle ground and in so doing, we—the children, the artists, the community around the garden—see who we are. The garden is an oracle for us. It shows us who we are and connects us to our deepest purpose as people.

Children are very important to creating the garden because very often their imaginations are more in touch with reality than the adult imagination. So we follow them; we follow their story leads and intuitions. But this does not usually mean that we surrender completely to the chaos of the child's whim. Kids seem to want to know everything and their imaginations are always working. They "why?" everything, test all the edges, celebrate and rejoice at their findings or else recoil in horror. What they say is very often more interesting than what we say. It is fresher, more spontaneous. So we follow and they lead us . . . back to the garden. They are the reconcilers, the peacemakers, President Clinton's comments notwithstanding when he misquoted the scripture after the Dayton accords.[13]

In the Spiral Garden and the Butterfly Garden, we learn simply by returning and re-consecrating small patches of our desacralized and debilitated earth to the children, and then follow them through its labyrinth and wonders. That is the process and it is the revelation. Sometimes we call it "rehabilitation" from the Latin *rehabilare*, coming home to ourselves, our bodies, our planet. And the children lead the way. The peacemakers show us how.

RB: This process is the site-specific mythography?

PH: Following it, charting the voyage, is the mythography. Following it is the "graphy," the writing of it. The writing is an approximation of course, because it's impossible, absolutely impossible to say definitively what goes on there at the Spiral Garden. If you want to know, you must come see. But the point of the garden is simple—it is transformation: Through expression and care to become more aware and to be, as Gandhi says, "the change you wish to make in the world." Becoming more aware helps us to realize "essence," which is the mystery of being. Just being. It has nothing to do with anything. We resist our being mightily. We resist silence, stillness, and the revelations immanent therein—the paradox and poetry. The garden is a sanctuary where we cultivate the paradox, the mystery of our being; this is poetry for us. We do this through silence, through playfulness—painting, theatre, music, and so on. We do it through gardening and through a constant dialogue of images and words among people—child and adult in a caring community.

We take our cues from the kids. Often, the children's stories are filled with wisdom. Just helping them to bring their stories forth and having them heard is healing for all. Even the jaded and weary adult soul can be replenished. Both child and adult benefit. I believe children telling their stories to be useful in many contexts, including in war-torn communities.

RB: Like Sri Lanka?

PH: Yes. This concept of community reconciliation through a child/art/earth project seems to be something perceived as feasible from the beginning. And from the outset of my early explorations in regards to gardens of peace for children in Sri Lanka, adult, even parent participation in the children's activities has been an important element to include. Sri Lankan parents seem to enjoy the process and they also want to be part of the garden and its healing processes.

There is an edge here, however. Adults everywhere, not just in Sri Lanka, have a way of dampening, if not deadening forever, spontaneity and imagination in children—it's sadly inevitable somehow. Much of the training I give facilitators has to do with letting inner worlds—one's own, others, the children's—unfold naturally as revelation, play, poetry in the fullness of time, so to speak . . . when the time is right. There's a "cultivation" aspect to this as in any garden, and also playfulness. This is very serious work, of course, making peace in war zones, but it's important not to take it too seriously or else the whole point is lost—once again we encounter the paradox, the Great Mystery, the divine teacher. Just staying alive, open, and aware, that's the big trick—especially under fire. Terror can easily highjack the imagination.

RB: I saw the paintings that you and Susan exhibited at Women's College Hospital several years ago. I understand that you also read what she wrote recently, about her experiences associated with her psychotic episode. Do you relate her experiences to what you experienced in the gardens in Toronto and Sri Lanka?

PH: As a point of entry into that question—Susan and I have communicated quite intuitively for a long time. Once we got to know each other we did some—I now jokingly call them—"medication trials." We did some medicine together, at Women's College Hospital and at Rat Plaza. We experienced more how we react intuitively in collaborative ventures. We learned something on those projects.

Whatever Susan's experiences had been in life prior to our meeting, I received many insights into her suffering, her breakdown, and recovery along the way, and was intrigued by how art played a role in her healing. There was an integrity and wholeness to Susan's view that I could relate to without even knowing more. There was also determination, humour, and a strong family/communitarian aesthetic to her life. Your healing was accomplished primarily by yourself, Susan, in communion with others which is, as James Hillman, Thomas Moore, and others point out, the only way a human being ever heals. This is one of the chief principles of the Spiral Garden—togetherness, transformation, collaboration.

I greatly admire Susan's grit, wit, and compassion, of which I see more and more as her journey unfolds. The twinkle in her eye says a lot. I am always discovering things about Susan. On the way over here today, she told me how the frustrations of her speech difficulties, caused by the psychotropic drugs, led her to begin to teach bread-and-butter English to new Canadians several years after her psychotic episode. She mentioned that these were the first people after her illness to really accept her slow language, her pauses . . .

SUSAN SCHELLENBERG: And the effect of those people accepting me as normal rather than as mentally ill was vital to my recovery at that time.

PH: That's very interesting because only now am I understanding silence as a powerful way of communicating. As you travel east, you find that silence is a valid response. You don't have to say yes or no. The absence of words will not necessarily provoke uneasiness or hostility or puzzlement. Exploring silence through meditative practices is very much a way of life in the East. Or it was in the past—it seems to be getting to be rarer and rarer a practice. Nevertheless, it still has residual influence in daily communication. There is yes, no, ... and silence.

Silence to me is a new seed to sow consciously as part of the praxis of the Spiral Garden. It is somehow the ground of everything and one can think of it as another way of knowing—like clairvoyance, or just being aware and being present. Silence seems primarily to be about being present to one's self, one's life, and others. Susan's art, her painting reflects that. Many of her images are solitary or embedded in an emotion of solitariness and perhaps dereliction. Thomas Merton talks about the contemplative as being solitary and derelict, and Susan as a contemplative artist expresses the same feeling for me. The dereliction is the falling away from one's self as well, perhaps as an initiatory movement of return, of healing.

When I think back to our engagements together in terms of artistic collaboration, they weren't necessarily peaceful. We had to do a lot of wrangling with institutions and with our own doubts and inertia. It was a fierce struggle, at times a kind of war. Maybe, though, we have the wrong idea of peace. I have a doctor friend, James, who works with Médecins Sans Frontières (MSF or Doctors Without Borders) and who experienced the mass genocide in Rwanda. He speaks of peace as "the other face of war." In certain moments in the horrendous atrocities and in certain people, peace is there in ways you can't possibly imagine when you are living in an environment of channel-surfing superficialities and commodity-oriented distraction or when you are with people who are present only for the briefest moment while in transit to some other place of distraction. We do not enter our dereliction if we can possibly avoid it. The whole culture is set up to avoid it.

Now, however, even here in Ontario, our dereliction is being forced upon us. I certainly don't applaud the Harris government, but I do feel that because of all the pain it's causing, people will get really angry and will have to start talking to one another, being present, being real to one another—and that may have some positive outcome.[14] For real healing to occur in our communities, there has to be some kind of healing crisis so that a deeper, heart-felt connection can be made between people. Some genuine empathy must be established to lead us out of our present bewilderment and narcosis.

Susan, you experienced a profound psychotic breakdown, and your art has been part of your recovery. This is a model for people: how your soul moved deeply from within and then, in a corresponding movement, compelled you to find others in community who would help to reconnect you to a more meaningful world. I too know this journey of the solitary derelict. Susan and I are soulmates. We've shared a lot. It hasn't all been grim—there has been a lot of laughter. That's part of the garden path for sure. Very often, when space opens up, there is laughter—we intuit very new possibilities: dances and harmonies emerge. Laughter is one sure sign of healing.

● ● ●

When Paul discussed entering into silence, experiencing the dereliction within oneself, opening to the mysteries revealed in being, I recalled the longing I had experienced for time to reflect. Limiting hospital work hours and responsibilities helped but did not permit the inner stillness to be with myself and others in the deeper way that I desired. Producing a steady stream of results in terms of patients seen, meetings attended, reports submitted, and projects completed seemed to require either quick, superficial responses to complex problems or exhausting hours that came to feel like drudgery.

When trying to determine how to stem my growing unhappiness, the intuitive voice within advised, "Slow down." Entering community practice created its own pressures and anxieties, but eliminated excuses that the boss or organization were to blame for my lack of control over my time and resources. Gradually, I identified beliefs that interfered with slowing down, for example, the way I prized hard work and overtime hours that I learned from my parents, the way I admired being impossibly busy as a badge of professional importance and prestige. Like Susan, I had to confront unhelpful beliefs and develop a different sense of myself while facing fears: in my case, fears of financial ruin, professional obscurity, and personal worthlessness. The more I allowed time to be quietly with myself as Paul described, the greater my sense of well-being became.

● ● ●

Talk proceeded with discussion of the Chong artists and the Rat Plaza street theatre event. I brought cookies and a vacuum bottle of tea that we shared as we talked.

SS: Paul and I share a similar understanding of the word *healing*. Healing and cure in the medical sense means that illness has disappeared. Where art and essence are located, I understand healing to mean a strengthening of regard and compassion for self and others, a strengthening of one's ability to cope, a deepened sense of wholeness and well-being. This kind of healing shapes life into a cycle of deaths and rebirths, and has for me and for many I've encountered been the catalyst which led us in the direction of wholeness and away from our addictions.

I was approaching a crossroad just before Paul asked me if I wanted to take part in the 1992 Chong street event. Up to that time, I lived in two worlds. I had one life as a mother and newly ex-corporate wife and another as a highly anxious artist always on the cusp of bolting from her art. Near endgame within this psychological split, I was being forced to face that my soul wasn't committed to anything definite and to own how I had chosen to remain stuck in this floating back and forth. That is who I was when Paul asked if I would like to take part in—What was the full title of it, Paul?

PH: "Rat Plaza Reunion: Shake a Snake Awake." It was a formal de-obsession of Chong cults.

SS: Paul collaborated with "The Chong" artists for a number of years. Mother Ralphe whose book Paul brought today, is patron saint of the Chong. When Paul asked if I would like to be part of this festival, I really felt like the odd man. These were all inner-city artists, and I still had a very suburban persona. But I also felt strongly about the fact that Paul was offering an opportunity. I knew that if I didn't take it, I might never have another like it. It wasn't that I did anything spectacular at the event. It was more the fact that I got in, did it, and got through it.

PH: You survived. We all survived. [All laugh]

SS: Of course. In hindsight, Rat Plaza was an almost perfect set-up for everything the unconscious was trying to get me to change at that time. The Chong became the mirror for the unresolved conflicts that were keeping me from being fully present to myself as an artist. It was uncomfortable. But I did commit and brought hidden parts of myself to the process. And some of those parts were stubborn as well as an embarrassment. My conforming, suburban, convent-raised part was particularly critical and rebellious of what I was doing at Rat Plaza. Yet, a meltdown of that part began to occur when I took to the streets with a bunch of people dressed as sardines, a rat, and various other Chong illusions.

As with dream, it took time to understand everything that happened to me during that event and I am still learning from it. I know that the poultice wasn't putting on a costume and walking in the parade. The poultice was my intention to be open with myself and with others who were also committed to "being" in this non-judgmental playful way. Everyone became a witness or mirror in that setting. The event was an essentially safe environment where old demons could relax and inner learning and change could occur. And I did make changes because of my experience. So, even though more talented ones than I were chosen to be the sardines, a little more order came out of the Rat Plaza's back alleys for me. I felt great and still do about the fact that I got in and did it.

PH: All I have to say about the Chong experience, if I may just add a little bit to what Susan's saying, is this. A Chong experience such as Rat Plaza is like suddenly finding yourself in a river—a torrent you've jumped into. There were sixty-four people in procession through the alleys in downtown Toronto on June 21, 1992 for about four hours. There were six months of preparation, so you just flow along with this mysterious event, working hard to make it happen, and suddenly you're in the parade. You are in the river. This is a connection of an initiatory kind. It takes people to completely different places in their lives. Susan, I don't quite recall what happened to you, but I do remember that afterwards, you felt totally isolated from the Chong, and very isolated in general, didn't you?

SS: Yes. As a group, the Chong were kind and welcoming, so my feelings did not originate with them. I had just been burnt for stepping outside a twenty-seven-year suburban, corporate wife life and was coming to terms with the friendship, lifestyle, and material losses this change involved. The Chong artists' grounded comfort in their bodies and casual ways of dressing emphasized how rigid and lacking I was in that type of musicality in my own body. The Nancy Regan casualness of my leftover suburban clothes further nailed the contrast. Then there was also the element of public clowning involved at Rat Plaza, and I was always used to being dressed as the culture said I should be dressed—you know, as a fashion plate.

PH: And you had done modelling too.

SS: Yes, I had done fashion modelling. Paul had everybody in ankle-high black running shoes, and it just got worse from there. [Laughter] So being dressed like this out on the street ...

PH: Which is a runway, in the fashion sense, and also in the airport sense ... preparing for liftoff.

SS: So it was. Part of me warred with, "I hope to God nobody sees me" [all laugh], and the other part of me thought "This is good, just keep doing it." I persevered, did it, and survived. Anyway, a year or so ago I had a dream where I was just about to deliver a baby. Paul, you were the midwife and were wearing your pink scarf around your neck. Rat Plaza was a turning point, a time of giving birth to myself. I feel the Chong event helped me to further commit to my art. I think we can only commit in increments, but since that time I find that the more I do commit, the saner I become.

PH: That's a true sign of insanity. [All laugh] Keep on, Susan.

SS: Right. But, now I feel more able to live with that paradox. My feeling alienated following the Chong event was about learning to let go. Though visiting the Chong was exciting, I knew I didn't really belong there. I'd also done a lot of work at Women's College for the merger fight, but knew that I didn't belong there either. I became a member of the Arts and Letters Club when my marriage ended and although its artists were welcoming, I felt a stranger there as well. Added to this, the minute our marriage ended, I lost the large group of people we had been close to through my husband's business. So I came to a point where I thought, "I don't belong anywhere." I think that was when I started belonging to myself.

PH: That had a very lasting effect on me because you asked me to do these ceremonies with your family, and that shows a lot of trust. I play with children at the garden, and I play with adults in the foolish Chong sort of way. But I had not done much family ritual. I must say I consider funerals more my specialty. Some day, I may open a funeral parlour. But Susan got me doing all these births and weddings! I thought, "Why do people get married anyway?" It's part of my dereliction: not understanding this, being a solitary, a wandering idiot, et cetera. I didn't really understand but I was going to get a good lesson. I didn't understand weddings as a sacrament or anything. So this was a real learning for me. I came to understand the meaning of marriage simply as "relatedness," acknowledging our relativity and interdependence and the passing away of all things in love. I'm still meditating on this lesson…. It is the lesson of "seeing through" each other and "seeing each other through."

Susan, her daughter Carolyn, and her son-in-law Ervin had challenged me already to bring my ritual "playfulness" into a family context with the welcoming and naming ceremony of Susan's granddaughter Julia Rose. Then her son, David, picked up on it a couple of years later when he and his partner Chris included me in the planning and animation of their very special three-day wedding on an island in Georgian Bay in the late summer of 1995. That was a stretch for me given all the variables of Irish, German, and Chinese coming together—and me being, as I say, a funeral specialist, a Saturnian, a snake priest, a wanderer, et cetera.

SS: And Paul, in showing my family how to take priesthood into their own hands when important life events needed "making sacred in the post-divorce period," allowed us to discover new ways of celebrating as a family. The family story of brokenness transformed through these events into a story of us beginning to recover our ability to share laughter, closeness, and pleasure.

The atmosphere was hilarious and serious by turns. Paul transformed conversation into improv performance. The altar, Paul's unexpected twists such as asking me to select a reading from *The Apocryphon of Mother Ralphe* and our laughter gave an immediate experience of artistic creation as healing.

PH: Now, I think it must be time to . . . [Paul hands Rosemary *The Apocryphon of Mother Ralphe.* The cover of this small book shows a photograph of the face of a male with a very full dark beard, dressed in a nun's habit.] Rosemary, do you want to pick a word from the book? [To Susan] She's dying to say something. [Laughter]

RB: Is there a ritual?

PH: Well, any way you want. Every word in the book is in the index. So, you can stick a finger in or look at . . .

RB: I see. I wait for the words to speak to me. [Rosemary scans words in the book's index] How about *blackberries*?

PH: Blackberries.

SS: [solemnly] That sounds very auspicious. [All laugh]

PH: It probably is. We'll see. [Paul searches the book for the page where the word *blackberries* is mentioned] The blackness of blackberries, okay. Mother Ralphe is very black. That's her walking down beside the Clarke Institute of Psychiatry. You know I have thirty-six or so pictures of her posed with that building . . . [Reads from book] "Mulberries are ripe, blackberries black, why should I care for the bread of my wretched husband." [Laughter] That applies to you sort of, doesn't it, Susan?

SS: Why should I care for the bread of my wretched husband? Oh, well . . . [laughs]

PH: That's it. That's sort of what happened to Susan in a way. The mulberries ripened and the blackberries blackened and she realized that she didn't care for the bread of her wretched husband any more and took to the streets.

SS: With the Chong.

PH: With the Chong.

SS: There is always a temptation to concretize the oracle, but as a dream, Mother Ralphe is bang on. The old demon lover part of myself was the part that locked the bride—the artist—part of me in the closet, and deprived her of decent spiritual food. The demon lover was also the part that got metaphorically toasted in the company of the Chong. Mother Ralphe has come to affirm that when all things were ripe, when I was no longer willing to settle for crumbs, I went into the fire, burned off that cheap patriarch, and then rose anew out of the blackened bits of her Chong people's bread. I ask Karmic absolution and forgiveness for any slight I may have previously shown to Mother Ralphe. [Laughter]

The conversation turned to the healing possibilities of the gardens that Paul has helped to create in Toronto and Sri Lanka.

SS: Paul, do you feel gardens could hold healing possibilities for adults who have experienced mental illness? Could garden work be integrated into the total healing package, where persons could go back to adult types of play and ritual in a garden for the purpose of finding themselves again?

PH: I am of the Garden Path School, and I see great possibilities for the cultivation of gardens by all kinds of people, not so much as a cure for anything but simply as a means of showing care. *Colare,* the Latin root for "culture" means "to care for." I see gardens such as the Butterfly Garden and the Spiral Garden as enjoyable places, beautiful places, inclusive of everyone where we can all practise some of the lost arts, like caring for the earth and for each other. We can establish communities of transformation where people bring change into the world by changing themselves—but in a playful way, in a round way, slowly, gracefully, with kindness, space, and good humour. But make no mistake: There is a lot of careful and hard work in this and it takes a long time. When asked the purpose of the Chong, Bishop Chong [a street theatre character played by a man with a history of mental illness] answered "to civilize North America." When further queried about how long it would take, he replied, "310,000 years." But we have plenty of time in the garden. Gardens are timeless places.

RB: There's a whole literature in psychiatry about madness, creativity, and the relationship between the two. Entering into the creative process involves going within, which has similarities to going mad. How does one do art safely? I was reminded of that when we were talking earlier about that entering the mystery and crossing the river. I was thinking, "When one enters the mystery and crosses the river, is there something important to remember about how one makes that trip, so that it's not a process of no return or of disintegration?"

PH: Yes. You must have a boat to cross the river or you must know where the stepping stones are. It helps to have a vehicle, that is, a tradition you follow whether in music or painting or prayer. And the intention behind your practice is very important. Is it to bring a sense of beauty back into the soulless world? Is it to bring balance? Harmony? Peace? Is it to deepen the human sense of belonging to one and other and to the earth? Our art and our lives have been given to us. Ultimately, we must make a gift of them to someone else. All we do can be an offering in good will, for the well-being of all. There is no madness unless it be divine when we create out of this method.

RB: You mention over and over the importance of working together. It happens to some degree now, but how much more collaboration is needed to support something new emerging?

PH: Gardens like the Butterfly Garden and the Spiral Garden, which cultivate both inner and outer realms, bring together many people—from young to old and from many walks of life. They are ostensibly about particular dimensions of healing. In Canada, it is focused on children living with physical disabilities, and in Sri Lanka, it is for children affected by war. But more and more, I hear myself say, "We are not here to make a garden. We are here to make peace with ourselves, with the world. This peace is growing from within." Ultimately, that is what the garden conspiracy is about: creating inclusive communities where we can practise peace, using gardening and art as a vehicle. Of course, in today's world, much more of this type of collaboration is needed: Safe havens for imagination, little Pure Lands, as Thich Nhat Hanh calls them.[15]

● ● ●

The performance that Paul created and his explanation of what lies behind his work at the Spiral Garden and the Butterfly Garden appealed to me in complex ways. I could see how the gardens allowed children to explore, to care for themselves and others, to develop trust in the ability to heal, to sustain hope through observation of the cycles of life, death, and rebirth, to experience the continuity needed to overcome fragmentation and alienation, and to engage the imagination in ongoing creation.

Paul described a garden path that offered to awaken and support the curious, hopeful, trusting parts of children. He listened carefully, recorded the children's stories, and then assisted them in transforming the stories into painting, sculptures, costumes, and performances. These steps ensured that what emerged in the quiet and playfulness of the garden was recorded in some more or less permanent way so that the experiences could be examined and considered from fresh perspectives.

Conversation, writing, painting, and other such activities function to ground inner experience in the outer, physical world of object, image, and action. When inner experience does not receive serious attention and grounding in the physical world, it takes on the ghostly impermanence of dreams which are vivid on waking, forgotten in minutes, then return uninvited to haunt and torment. Inner experience that is grounded in physical productions can be examined to deepen and reconstruct understandings of oneself and one's relation to the world.

Attending to what is within, expressing inner experience in the outer world, then reflecting on the meaning and impact of these expressions is the core process in many forms of psychotherapy. Paul's gardens facilitate this powerful process at a group level within an environment that is likely far more playful and creative than most therapists' offices. The art of the garden and its activities thus creates conditions for transformation and healing.

Talking with Paul led me to think of Susan as having engaged in a garden process when she recorded her dreams in writing, painting, and through conversations, whether with a therapist or trusted friend. Looking back, I thought that I had engaged in a garden process when I left the hospital, slowed down, faced my fears, worked with Susan, and began to develop a new sense of myself. Like Susan, I have used psychotherapy, meditative practices, yoga, and dream journalling and been grateful for the help of mentors, including Susan and the people to whom she has introduced me.

Paul described story as the structure of the garden experience, echoing Helen Porter's explanation of story as reflecting the deep structure of psychological processes. Story as the central structure for organizing human experience is likewise the focus for narrative therapy,[16] the innovative psychotherapeutic approach I described in chapter 5. Citing advances in social sciences and the work of Michel Foucault, proponents of narrative therapy point out that story is the basic organizing structure of human thought and action: "Persons generally ascribe meaning to their lives by plotting their experience onto stories, and … these stories shape their lives and relationships."[17] These theorists repeat Paul's observation that no story is ever told twice in the same way. Further, narrative therapists argue that we are constantly enacting in our own lives the process which Paul orchestrates consciously in the garden; that is, we continually turn our stories into performances through our activities and relationships.

For narrative therapists, not surprisingly, the construction and reconstruction of personal story is central to human change. The desire to change, to reorganize stories and life performances, is understood to arise when the person is enacting a story that fails to accommodate vital aspects of his or her lived experience. Take, for example, the experience of Susan and her husband as her emotional distress progressively heightened to the point of breakdown. In the face of increasing emotional distress, Susan struggled strenuously to continue to perform within the scripts of her dominant life stories: devoted wife and mother, good daughter, observant Catholic woman, normal person. As none of these stories were adequate to incorporate her deepest feelings or to resolve dilemmas from arising within these scripts, her distress and exhaustion steadily intensified and her ways of behaving became increasingly off-script and of concern to others. As her difficulty became more visible in her speech and actions, her husband joined her in efforts to restore her ability to adhere to their mutually understood and preferred scripts. When his efforts also failed, he accepted Susan's hospital admission.

While Susan was in hospital, mental health staff listened carefully to her account of her experiences and offered a new story that was accepted by Susan and her husband because it accommodated some of her previously neglected experiences and actions. Using information provided by authoritative professional staff, Susan reconstructed her story of herself as follows. She understood herself to suffer from schizophrenia, a serious mental illness, for which she should take mediation in order to prevent serious consequences such as the inability to parent her children or even the risk that she might harm her children. Her husband's role was to provide surveillance and direction in the face of her questionable capacity to perform other major script responsibilities, such as devoted wife and mother, good Catholic. Her role was to comply with the direction of the doctor and her husband, to take medication, and to continue to perform in all other major life scripts including that of "normal person." This reconstructed story was decisive in determining how Susan and her husband responded to her difficulties for many years, until Susan again reached a point where enacting this story neglected so much of her vital experience that she could no longer sustain its performance.

Narrative therapy provides a helpful alternative to the medical model account of the profound changes associated with Susan's emotional breakdown, hospital admission, and period of apparently successful recovery. The narrative perspective underscores the centrality of story to human change and offers approaches to help the individual troubled by problems to explore their experiences in open and creative ways, to locate vital and previously neglected aspects of themselves, and to use these elements to construct new stories and life performances. In important ways, the narrative therapy approach seems roughly parallel to the process that Paul facilitates in the garden through artistic activities.

Part of what facilitates healing in Paul's artistic work, in narrative therapy, and in other mentored healing experiences is that the healer gives emphasis to bearing witness, guiding, facilitating, and coaching individuals in the process of creating new stories. The new story emerges from the process of attending to what is within, giving the inner experience some form of outer expression, and then working with these expressions to construct a new story. The healer facilitates this process but the individual remains the prime story author. In contrast, staff in medical-model mental health settings of the kind described by Susan take the role of prime authors of a new story; *they* supply a diagnosis and recommend the treatment that the patient and family are expected to accept on the doctor's authority.

Paul's artistic work in the gardens and Susan's healing through her painting and participation in street theatre with the Chong artists were consistent with the transformative change processes familiar to me in the psychotherapy framework. Paul's work demonstrated how art can extend the playfulness and creativity that the individual is able to bring to the healing process of attending within, expressing, and then reorganizing story.

Where Paul's work departed most dramatically from psychotherapy is in its engagement of community in healing. The Spiral Garden is open to both children with disabilities and children in the local community; by creating together in the garden, artists, children with disabilities and their families, and children and families in the neighbourhood become linked to one another in meaningful and loving ways. Healing at the Spiral Garden is both individual and collective. In the Butterfly Garden in Bratticaloa, Sri Lanka, Paul describes how his work engages not only children, but also communities torn by war and trauma.[18] The children's work in the Butterfly Garden is used to create stories which are then dramatically enacted as a performance in which their families and the broader community are invited to participate. The stories of healing from the children offer a cultural experience of healing and peace for the entire community.

Many of the problems likely faced by children with physical disabilities or living in the midst of war are also faced by children and adults with mental disorders—a daunting life challenge to overcome, ways of functioning that are viewed as "abnormal," a perception of abnormal individuals as frightening and deficient, a wish to suppress and avoid the "abnormal," and a tendency to exclude the abnormal individuals and experiences from the stream of "normal" life. Relying on the medical model as the exclusive response to illness, injury, disturbance, and disability not only limits potential healing but also reinforces beliefs that a person should be visible in the community only when functioning "normally"—that distress or disability should be concealed from public view. Such beliefs and practices reinforce the stigma associated with disorders both physical and mental—that "illness" or emotional disturbance is a personal shame and healing is private business. After medical treatment, one returns to the community to function as if the injury or illness never occurred; if one has a visible disability, the expectation is that one will either stay out of sight, or approximate "normal" functioning as closely as possible when in community view. The extent of stigmatization tends to be directly related to one's ability to present "normal" appearance and function.

Paul's art, however, views individual distress, injury, and disability not as a matter for pity, shame, or secrecy but as an occasion for both individual and community healing, growth, and deepening interconnection. Susan produces the same kind of socially engaged art by exhibiting her dream paintings that document her healing from mental illness at a location where they can be viewed by others whose lives are deeply affected by mental illness—the staff, patients, and families of patients associated with a major psychiatric hospital. Susan describes the healing she has experienced through producing such art, and her art offers the wider community the potential to heal, as does Paul's art in the Spiral and Butterfly Gardens. Socially engaged art allows the community to become richer and more whole as the culture enlarges to include increasingly diverse individual stories. The art provides the larger culture images and stories that can teach about illness, disability, and healing and that offer both inspiration and a vehicle for the healing of communal disorder and injury. Paul's approach provides a beautiful vision of how, as a society, we might grow and heal both individually and collectively from incorporating the experiences of those with severe emotional disturbance. In his art, I find the stuff of a new story for my own work.

Notes

1 Albert Camus, *Notebooks 1935–1942*, Vol. 3. (New York: Knopf, 1963), 141.
2 Betsy Hearne, *Beauty and the Beast: Visions and Revisions of an Old Tale* (Chicago: University of Chicago Press, 1991).
3 American educators and psychotherapists John and Joyce Weir and Alexandra Merrill teach an experiential technique called "percept language," which requires the person to speak as if every aspect of conscious experience is a projection of self; this way of speaking and thinking can be a powerful means of developing fresh perspectives on self. In chapter 4 (pp. 82–83), Susan gives an example of interpreting a dream using percept language.
4 The Myers Briggs is a personality test that classifies individuals in terms of perceptual/thinking/feeling styles.
5 Bruno Bettelheim, *The Uses of Enchantment: The Meaning and Importance of Fairy Tales* (New York: Knopf, 1976).
6 R.D. Laing and Aaron Esterson, *Sanity, Madness and the Family* (London: Tavistock, 1964).
7 Ignac Fülöp Semmelweis (1818–1865) was a German Hungarian physician who discovered that puerperal ("childbed") fever was transmittted by physicians' poor sanitation practices and introduced antisepsis into medical practice.
8 Clarissa Pinkola Estés, *Women Who Run with the Wolves* (New York: Ballantine, 1992).
9 John Bunyan, *The Pilgrim's Progress* (New York: Washington Square, 1961).
10 Estés, *Women Who Run with the Wolves*.

11 Mother Ralphe, *The Apocryphon of Mother Ralphe* (Toronto: Internity, 1979).

12 Shirley Bear is a political activist, artist, and healer from the Tobique Reserve in New Brunswick.

13 Around the time of international talks, held in Dayton, Ohio, which led to peace agreements in Bosnia, Clinton said, "Blessed are the peacemakers, for they shall inherit the earth." But Jesus said, "Blessed are the peacemakers, for they are the children of God."

14 In 1996, the Ontario government headed by Premier Mike Harris was implementing a series of major funding cutbacks and reforms that emphasized improved efficiency, increased personal accountability, and reduced government role in society.

15 Thich Nhat Hanh is a Buddhist monk who is internationally know for his teachings about peace and consciousness.

16 Narrative therapy is well described in Michael White and David Epston, *Narrative Means to Therapeutic Ends* (New York: W.W. Norton, 1990); Jill Freedman and Gene Combs, *Narrative Therapy: The Social Construction of Preferred Realities* (New York: W.W. Norton, 1996); Michael White, *Narrative Practice and Exotic Lives: Resurrecting Diversity in Everyday Life* (Adelaide, South Australia: Dulwich Centre, 2004); and Michael White, *Maps of Narrative Practice* (New York: W.W. Norton, 2007).

17 Brook, 1984, qtd. in White and Epston, *Narrative Means to Therapeutic Ends*.

18 Patricia Lawrence, *The Ocean of Stories: Children's Imagination, Creativity, and Reconciliation in Eastern Sri Lanka* (Columbo, Sri Lanka: International Centre for Ethnic Studies, 2003).

7 War and Peace

On September 11th the enemies of freedom committed an act of war against our country.... Americans have known casualties of war—but not at the center of a great city on a peaceful morning. Americans have known surprise attacks—but never before on thousands of civilians.... Our war on terror begins with al Qaeda, but it does not end there. It does not end until every terrorist group with global reach has been found, stopped, and defeated.

—George W. Bush, speech to the United States Congress, 20 September 2001[1]

Susan
Opening the Door to Making Sense

TERROR, THE BLIND TYRANT THAT had held me captive since childhood, has also prompted me to go for control, to send troops to foreign lands, and to suppress dissent at home. My initial attack on my badness was aimed at living in better accord with the feminine ideals of parents, religion, and culture but in its time the approach created greater inner chaos. The second offensive taught me to feel but with caution. At every journey point, my body's ecology, like the globe's, threatened to rebel and collapse if I resisted the needed resolution of my trauma story that would allow my life to thrive. Alice Miller, the Swiss psychologist who has written about childhood's relationship to the adult body, has an apt description for the kind of conditions I faced:

> The truth about our childhood is stored up in our body, and although we can repress it, we can never alter it. Our intellect can be deceived, our feelings manipulated, our perceptions confused, and our body tricked with medication. But, someday the body will present its bill, for it is as incorruptible as a child who, still whole in spirit, will accept no compromise or excuses, and it will not stop tormenting us until we stop evading the truth.[2]

Each resting point I reached along the journey offered hard-won insights and the physical and psychological relief that was necessary to my holding on until the end's least bearable and most frightening truths could be faced. As the nature of outer wars and the struggle to control were changing globally, I entered the door that led to the resolution of my own psychosis core. The door, recovered memories of sexual abuses, opened in 1998.

The Recall

My recall of sexual abuse by a priest occurred several weeks following the 1998 permanent installation of my *Shedding Skins* exhibit at the Clarke Institute of Psychiatry (now the Centre for Addiction and Mental Health [CAMH]). I was conscious at the time that my work with the Clarke Institute made me feel heard by psychiatrists—a feeling that was missing from my initial psychiatric hospital experience—but I had no idea that the respectful listening and validation I received from the psychiatrists, psychologists, and other Clarke Institute staff on the *Shedding Skins* planning committee was shaping in me the additional and needed psychic strength to recover the priest's abuse memory.

It was after a morning of art making and following a sitting meditation that my recall of the priest's abuse occurred. I was not in therapy at the time. Although eight or more dreams of a "faceless priest" in various disguises were attempting to reveal the abuse from the mid-1990s onward, my lack of concrete memory or suspicion of any particular priest only allowed me to interpret the dreams as warnings that I was holding on to outworn Catholic attitudes on women's inferiority and that I needed to build a more whole sense of self.

Before speaking of the abuse to anyone, multiple dreams occurred containing images that included the actual priest sodomizing me as a child, another dream where a dream voice said, "the curate raped you," and a dream with a voice saying, "He was a pedophile." In another dream, the voice said, "She [meaning me] has a hard time believing a priest could be sick." The day following the abuse recall, dreams that related to another forgotten sexual abuse also appeared. Though the recall and its multiple accompanying dreams put me in a highly frightened and anxious state, I believe my psyche worked with who I was able to be at the time.

Finding a Therapist

While my friendship with Rosemary and our collaboration on this book barred me from working in psychotherapy with her, I briefly outlined the nature of the recall for Rosemary to ask her advice on obtaining a therapist trained in treating abuse. I also stated how I wanted to resolve the abuse issue in therapy before continuing with the book. In addition to offering care, listening, and recommendations for several trauma specialists, Rosemary cautioned me that trauma therapy was in its infancy. She said that because it has received serious professional attention only since around 1990, few skilled therapists worked in this field.

Rosemary's Note

Susan had related to me her memory of her father's sexual abuse (see chapter 3) and sexual abuse by a priest. I expressed my sadness and anger that she was exposed to something so hurtful and asked a little about what she recalled— how old she was and the situation in which the abuse had occurred. As Susan talked further of the influence of these experiences on her life, I was sad, but not surprised to learn that their impact had been great.

Susan's psychotic episode and subsequent treatment for schizophrenia took place between 1969 and the early 1980s, a period when mental health professionals were unaware of the relatively high prevalence of childhood sexual abuse and of the serious psychological harms that could be associated with such experiences. Unsurprisingly, the professionals providing care to her during those years did not ask Susan about childhood sexual abuse, know of her abuse experiences, or initiate any interventions to assist with such issues.

The relationship between serious mental illness and exposure to childhood maltreatment, in particular childhood sexual abuse, is now well established. When an adult engages a child in adult sexual activities, even if the involvement occurs in a non-violent way, such developmentally inappropriate sexual contact constitutes exposure to trauma for the child.[3] Previous stresses, including exposure to trauma, increase the risk for developing a serious mental illness such as schizophrenia among those who are susceptible to such a condition. Among individuals in hospital for mental health care, 50 to 60 percent report a history of childhood sexual abuse; among those seeing a mental health professional for office appointments, 40 to 60 percent report a history of childhood sexual abuse; among adult women seeking emergency mental health care, as many as 70 percent report childhood sexual abuse.[4]

Individuals who have been sexually abused are at increased risk for anxiety, depression, a broad range of other psychological difficulties, and stress-related

medical problems. Certain psychological reactions, such as flashbacks, dissociation, and dissociative states, are common among survivors of severe or repeated
childhood trauma, but highly unusual among individuals not exposed to such
trauma.[5] Individuals experiencing flashbacks or dissociation may not understand what is happening to them and are often fearful of being perceived as
"crazy." Individuals who have experienced childhood sexual abuse are often
reluctant to disclose such abuse for many reasons: fear of not being believed,
shame about what occurred, unwillingness to think about a deeply painful experience. Knowing about a person's abuse experiences is important to understanding emotional disturbance. Nevertheless, mental health professionals sometimes
fail to ask about past trauma or maltreatment, and it is not uncommon for a
mental health professional to be unaware of an individual's exposure to childhood sexual abuse.[6]

A variety of medications and therapeutic interventions can help to alleviate the distress and harms caused by childhood sexual abuse. However, in the
absence of knowledge about a patient's past trauma or its impact, mental health
professionals may interpret flashbacks, dissociation, or dissociative states as
indication of hallucinations or thought disorders and make treatment recommendations that give little or no attention to steps that might assist in allevi-
ating traumatic distress.[7] Susan had to work out for herself how to proceed in
order to resolve the traumatic memories that stood in the way of progressing
with what was important to her in life.

Susan

When convinced that post-abuse-recall anxieties would allow me to uncover
the abuse story only under hypnosis, I asked Rosemary if she could also recommend a hypnotherapist. Hypnotherapy was initially helpful for getting my
abuse story witnessed and told in the way I was able to understand it at the
time. But I did not consciously advance in making sense of the abuse. My constant lateness and forgetting of hypnotherapy appointments and feeling the
therapist was scolding me for accusing a priest of abuse had more to do with
my inner projections and turmoil than with the therapist. My instincts to enter
and to also leave hypnotherapy were both valid at the time and for the distress
I was in.

Following hypnotherapy and prior to finding the therapist I would eventually work with, Rosemary offered to arrange and hold an abuse-related conversation with psychiatrist Cheryl Rowe. Dr. Rowe was Assistant Professor in
the Department of Psychiatry at the University of Toronto; she had headed
the psychiatric consultation/liaison service, the adult psychiatry division, and
the psychiatric postgraduate teaching program at Sunnybrook Health Sciences

Centre in Toronto and was widely known for her expertise in women's health and trauma, including childhood sexual abuse and professional sexual misconduct. At the time of our conversation on 9 February 1999, Dr. Rowe was practising in the community and providing psychiatric consultation at Alternatives East York Mental Health Services Agency, an organization working with those affected by serious mental illness.

The distress and shame I was holding at the time of our meeting with Dr. Rowe caused me to want to isolate myself more than converse. My memory of the discussion was that I warred my way through it with mixed feelings of being cared for and nurtured while wildly projecting my scolding self onto Rosemary and Dr. Rowe—"Come on, Susan, you are a non-coping failure and have dreamed up this priest's abuse to make more excuses for yourself." However, when later in our conversation both concurred that some type of abuse had taken place, I experienced a profound sense of relief. This first official confirmation that an actual abuse had occurred was vital to my going forward with my search for meaning.

Roundabout Path to a Therapist

When the therapists Rosemary recommended were unavailable for one reason or another, I approached the work from other angles. The longer my search for the right therapist took, the more suicidal thoughts, urges to destroy my art, bouts of nausea, and increasing paranoia occurred. Newly certain that my friends were stealing from me when they visited my home, I was also forced to stop entertaining for fear of wrongly accusing or losing friendships.

The fear of being caught in a false memory syndrome was constant. Research that explained how trauma memories often release in increments over time, as well as how abuses tend to remain buried longer if a trusted person inflicted them, helped me become more able to face the abuses and their effects. Added awareness on how it also takes time to form accurate narratives of what occurred better prepared me for analysis as well.

During the non-therapy interim, I enrolled in a nine-month series of courses and lectures at the Jung Foundation. Where this study approach did not deal with my or others' sexual abuse issues in any direct way, the process supported a dream analysis mindset as well as a distancing from my own dilemma that allowed me to become less anxious and more familiar with it. The Jung courses involved discussion on numerous psychological case studies and the dreams that helped to resolve each case. Compassion elicited for the principals in these case studies greatly lessened my abuse-related shame and anxiety. The Jung study functioned like a container that supported my improving instincts, which would shortly after direct me towards an analyst skilled in trauma work. I entered a three-year period of working with Jungian analyst Sylvia Shaindel Senensky, author of *Healing and Empowering the Feminine: A Labyrinth Journey.*[8]

Analysis Begins

I am in no way expert in Jungian theory or able to give an exact Jungian understanding of my dreams or healing process. My ability to heal through dream, initiated by my commitment to keep a painted record of my dreams, formed my uniquely personal dialogue with my psyche. From the 1980s onward that dialogue expanded in rhythm with the commitment that drove it.

My three-year course of Jungian analysis greatly accelerated this process. My best sense is that my psyche accepts my intention to heal and offers dream images that relate to my history and how I learn best. When interpretations and actions to resolve a dream or series of dreams are in sync with what the psyche is attempting to teach me and I get it right, I grow away from complexes; when I fail to correctly interpret or to act to bring about the required growth and change, I remain stuck.

Learning from Dreams

Analysis suited my preference for dream as well as my analytical/visual ways of learning. Although Sylvia was the opposite of controlling, the deeply personal aspect of dream helped to ensure that I did not give my power to the analyst as I had done with authority figures in my past.

To prepare for analysis sessions, I journalled my dreams and dream interpretations through the week. Prior to our weekly sessions, I typed, then emailed my past week's journal contents to the analyst. Sylvia would mainly listen and confirm whether she thought my dream interpretations made sense. If I were too off the mark in my interpretations, she would wait without giving me clues to a dream's meaning. Whatever else Sylvia did, it was her magic that I am unable to explain; I only know that analysis allowed me more growth than I thought possible. Sylvia moved out west before the entire psychosis core was cleared, but I could never have cleared it fully without her help.

I call the following my Churchill dream. The dream was of particular importance to my gaining clarity on how my depression worked and how I could lessen its effects. The dream occurred while I was in analysis and took me two months or longer to work out.

Churchill Dream

I am standing in a large formal gathering in a grand ballroom that feels part of a Viennese palace. I am in my late thirties or forties and am wearing a beautiful, slim, white satin gown. I am in the front line of guests near the ballroom's ceremonial double doors waiting with others for the guest of honour to appear.

When the doors open a midget Winston Churchill enters and walks toward me. As Churchill takes my hand, bows, and tells me I am exquisite and lovely, I become stressed and anxious that the crowd in back of me is watching a menstrual soil on the hip area of my dress. Churchill then leaves the room and the ballroom doors close.

In a short time, the doors open again and a giant Churchill who almost reaches the ceiling enters. But this time he walks past and ignores me. I feel intensely rejected. The giant Churchill exits and the doors close again. The door opens next for a normal size Churchill. He again comes toward me and takes my hand, but I choose to ignore him.[9]

Background to My Churchill Dream

The three Churchill figures immediately recalled a fairy tale that was discussed in a Jungian lecture, the Brothers Grimm fairytale, "One Eye, Two Eyes, Three Eyes." The story tells of three sisters who are so named due to the numbers of eyes they possess.

One Eye and Three Eyes cruelly withhold food and kindness from Two Eyes and ridicule her for being like common folk. One day as the hungry Two Eyes is tending her goat in the field, she is aided by an old woman who teaches her a magic rhyme to say to her goat whenever she wishes to eat. The more Two Eyes eats meals provided by the goat and ignores the scraps of food given to her at home, the more suspicious her sisters become.

In a moment of forgetfulness, Two Eyes reveals the rhyme and her sisters, spying the delicious food she has enjoyed, kill her goat in a fit of rage. The old woman reappears to instruct the bereft Two Eyes to ask her sisters for the goat's entrails and to then plant the entrails by the front of their house. Overnight the entrails grow into a magnificent tree with gold and silver branches and fruit. The two mean sisters, on failing to pluck any of the tree's fruit, become even more jealous when the tree freely gives of its treasure to Two Eyes. A prince who rides by their home notices and makes inquiries about the tree. One Eye and Three Eyes, in an effort to trick the prince into believing they are the tree's owners, hide Two Eyes under a bushel. However, Two Eyes gains the Prince's attention with her cunning and beauty and rides off with him to his palace. As soon as she is gone the gold and silver tree disappears from her sisters' home only to reappear at the palace. Many years later, her by-now old and beggared sisters repent and the happily married Two Eyes shows them forgiveness and mercy.

The Grimms' tale in a Jungian context shows how the child whose mother devalues, abuses, persecutes, and rejects their "two eye" or natural essence will develop depressive outlooks that alternate between inflated, grandiose depressed "three eye" states and narrow, limited, and depressed "one eye" states. In place of the fairytale's three separate eye symbols, my dream offered three differently sized Winston Churchills to symbolize my depression patterns. I learned of the historical Winston Churchill's lifelong battle with depression in the mid-1980s through reading *Stranger on the Earth, A Psychological Biography on Vincent Van Gogh.*[10] The Van Gogh book used Churchill's depression to reinforce how psychological wounds can be the catalyst of greatness rather than its "in-spite-of" footnote. The name "Churchill" additionally linked to how I was made ill by the church.

Active imagination and psychodrama techniques shared with my analyst allowed me to explore the meaning of the three Winston Churchills. As I enacted my encounter with the giant-sized Churchill (my inflated "Three Eye" thinking) who had walked past and ignored me in the dream, I felt rejected and diminished. When the midget Churchill (depressed "One Eye" thinking) bowed, kissed my hand, and told me I was charming and exquisite, I became highly anxious about a menstrual soil at the hip areas of my dress and felt a strong need to inflate myself in order to survive the humiliation.

As I enacted my rejection of the normal-size Churchill, I saw more clearly how my essence had been rejected as a child and how I was still hooked on behaviours that repeated this rejection of my own essence as well as that of others. The three Churchill figures' repetitious ballroom entrances gave me a clearer vision of how I perpetuated self-rejection by repeatedly flip-flopping between the one-eye and three-eye depressive states rather than enjoying a balanced two-eye perspective.

The real Churchill's battle against Hitler during the Second World War mirrored the internal healing force that was trying to help me overcome the self-destructive Nazi terrorist parts within myself. The Viennese palace recalled Austrian acts of denial and complicity with the Nazis that echoed my denial and complicity with my own self-destructive Nazi part. My late thirties and forties were the time of my psychosis and drugging. But those ages could also mean my girlhood that spanned the late 1930s and early 1940s when the sexual abuses took place. The largeness of the ballroom and slim beauty of the white satin dress showed the fragile sense of worth I held compared to the size of the abuse complex. The opening ballroom doors showed how I was becoming more open to bringing my depression and related abuse issues to consciousness. My work on this dream resulted in an improved ability to hold a "two-eye" or balanced outlook and to better monitor and manage my depression from that dream forward.

Parent and Priest Abuse

My parents' and the priest's abuse occurred close together when I was between the ages of eleven and fourteen. My sexuality by that age was already harmed from frequent punishment like spankings and enemas. During the same period, my mother forced me to confess to priests that I masturbated and said I would become schizophrenic like her sister, my aunt (mentioned in chapter 5, p. 90), if I did not obey her.

My father's abuse, which I described earlier (see chapter 3), happened when I was around the age of twelve. As I was recalling the memories of priest abuse, I also recovered the additional abuse that had occurred prior to my menses. That trauma involved my mother forcing me to strip and lie spread-legged on a bed so she and my father could see if I was menstruating. The pain of this experience was compounded by my mother's intentions to titillate my father. The conflict was further anchored by my parents' pretense of concern and the fact that once my menses did begin, my mother rationed me to twelve sanitary pads a month. Numerous public humiliations due to menstrual accidents added to the abuse and its resulting depression.

The abusing priest was the parish curate. My parents developed close ties with the curate, treating him as a family member to the degree my older brother was permitted to accompany the priest on his vacations. When I was around eleven years old, the priest announced he thought I had a vocation to be a nun. To prepare me for this vocation, he encouraged me to confess to him every week and to announce my presence in the confessional with "Bless me father, this is Susan." The loss of anonymity that resulted from this ritual was stressful. The curate later became the chaplain at St. Michael's Hospital close to the time I entered nursing.

To this day, I have no memory of the priest ever abusing me physically. The best sense I was able to make of his abuse in analysis was that it took the form of psychosexual acting out in the confessional and in his hospital apartment. Without concrete evidence, I was hesitant about wrongly accusing him. However, I became more willing to hold to the truth of the priest's abuse over the three years of dream analysis. Observations of my body's releases of energy with the working out of priest-related dreams and the corresponding disappearance of my suicidal urges and other symptoms over that time convinced me that the priest did indeed abuse his authority or worse.

It was physically and emotionally difficult to write about the priest abuse. My hips locked as I began writing one of the later drafts on these experiences. But my mind also went silent when the writing was completed. The inner chatter stopped. The only past times I have enjoyed this kind of quiet was while waking from general anaesthesia.

After several days of this silence, but still with locked hips, I tried using psychodrama techniques to see if I could discover what my hips were trying to tell me. What occurred when I confessed to the priest as a child? To prepare for this work I did a half-hour sitting meditation. Then with the question, "What was

I seeing as a child when I went to confession with Father X?" I knelt down beside an armchair to simulate the physical action in the confessional. I crossed myself and said out loud, "Bless me, father, for I have sinned. This is Susan, it has been a week since my last confession." Breathing meditatively and with an attitude that I would accept whatever the exercise revealed, even if it showed I had been wrong about the priest, I let myself be the child again in the confessional.

A blank wait followed by sensations of gagging and choking on a penis occurred first. Unable to stay calm with the process I went to my desk to journal. My writing led to questions like, "Is this sensation mirroring Catholic patriarchal values being shoved down my throat rather than psychosexual violation?" "Was this the only way the priest abused me or do I have other memories to release?" I repeated the confessional ritual again. A montage of images occurred, showing me as a young girl being raped and sodomized in different positions in and just outside the confessional. As I wrote down details of these images, I also felt an eroticism that went against my disgust and wanting to rid myself of priest memories.

I meditated next on the erotic feeling to see if it signalled that I was sexually attracted to the priest. I saw an image of the upper half of a former Ontario politician who especially repelled me but to whom I was, at times and to my shame, sexually attracted. The politician in the dream was wearing a dapper Victorian straw hat, striped blazer, and bow tie. The dream's half image of the politician and my sometime attractions to him signalled my attraction/repulsion toward the priest and how abuses had shaped a split-off and brutish aspect of my inner masculine.

While writing about this psychodrama experience, I felt a momentary urge to jump out my window, a feeling that echoed my pre-analysis suicidal urges. I next became extremely agitated, wanting to bathe one minute and get away to a movie the next. Not knowing what to do, I began to write and as I did, I felt a surge of rage and wanting to jump up and scratch out the eyes of a tall, almost shadow presence I sensed was next to me. The more I wrote and made sense of the priest's abuse, the more rage energies moved up my spine and released from my shoulders.

To aid this release of the abuse, I next made a rough sketch of a single cell and of me inside the cell kneeling at a confessional. Using this sketch as a holograph of every cell in my body and to remind myself of how each cell contained memories of the priest abuse, I imagined all my cells being cleansed of the abuses and the abuses' potential to generate illness-producing effects. Lastly, I visualized the abuses leaving my body and going into the earth to be healed. I then slept fourteen hours.

The next day I repeated the process, this time imaging myself in the priest's hospital apartment. As I imagined myself as a student nurse sitting opposite the priest, I saw myself bolting and running out of the apartment. At the time of the psychodrama exercise I recalled solely how, as a student nurse, my visits to the priest's apartment were prompted by his standing invitation and about every six months by my anxious "I must" duty feelings rather than wanting to go there. Later, I understood how the confined apartment space along with my repressed knowledge of the priest's abuse, my unacknowledged attraction/repulsion, and my anxieties over the scandal potential of a young woman being in a priest's apartment would have formed the near unbearable pressures that triggered my wanting to bolt.

Even though I cleared myself of prejudice for the meditative enactment of my visits to the priest's apartment, I did not expect the feelings of sadness and shame that radiated off the image of the priest. As I wrote in my journal about the priest's shame, I asked if the priest, by the time I entered nursing, had cleared his abuse of me as a child and/or if he felt sorrow for his past actions but the answer was no. I then asked if it was my shame I was projecting onto the priest—again the answer was no. Nor did it appear that his shame was connected to my being in his apartment or to any feelings he felt toward me at the time either. Exhausted of questions, I let the matter go.

Later that night, at what I thought was an unrelated meeting, someone told the story of a man who had been shamed for life after having been raped as a child. When I returned home and journalled the question, "Did the priest's shame come from abuses that occurred in his childhood?" the answer was yes.

As the question of the priest's shame became answered, I had a feeling that an inner authority was expressing an enormous compassion and protectiveness towards the priest as well as for me. I also felt I was being told that I had received everything I needed to heal and that my priest abuse exploration was at an end. The graphic delicacy of how the priest's shame was revealed to me, and the enormous compassion extended towards the priest as well as myself, gave me hope that there was integrity to my abuse work and that it was resolved. My determination to release all memories connected with the priest from my body and to leave all judgment of the priest to the Universe is the act of letting go I now understand forgiveness to be.

Abuse, Depression, Rage

The actual sexual abuses I experienced and the fact they did not compare in physical severity to many other people's accounts of sexual abuse made it difficult to think of them as serious. But because my mother, father, and the priest were also my key nurturers, role models of responsible living, and forceful teachers of "purity," their conflicting roles played havoc with my mind and sexuality. Unable as a child to confront the three main providers of my survival needs, I buried their abuses and assumed blame for their harmful actions and, as a result, my ability to feel was buried as well.

While I worked to unravel the effects of childhood sexual abuses, I was also drawn to question the matter of trust and the trust-related harms that had grown from maternal deprivation in childhood. My mother's inability to trust herself or her children, coupled with her rejection/nurture split from the time of my conception onward, caused me to miss key areas of trust development during childhood. Early loss of the trust instinct resulted in my tendency to mistrust the trustworthy and trust those less worthy instead. Conditioned as well to place absolute trust in the Church and in priests, the resulting self-loathing bent toward being good ensured my being an easy mark for a deviant priest. The priest needed my "see no evil" presence in the confessional to maintain his chaste exterior persona while carrying out his abusive acts. My need of my father's, the priest's, and God the Father's paternal love due to the loss of maternal love also increased my chances of being targeted by the priest.

I am convinced my father knew his actions were wrong when he and my mother jointly abused me prior to my time of menses. I recall no evidence that suggests he intended to be sexual when he came to my bed when I was a child. But the fact he did not leave my bed after he became aroused in my pre-teen years suggests a different story. The realization that I carried his sexual projections in my body and psyche for the greater part of my life allowed me to further clear the abuse. Prone for the larger part of my life to paranoia and fears of someone attacking me from behind, the abuse work allowed me to shed this reaction as well.

Naming the Abuse Puzzle

The priest's and my father's sexual violations during my adolescence, a peak period of hormonal change, eroticized my hip area and caused psychological harm similar to physical rape. Alice Miller's writing in *Thou Shalt Not Be Aware: Society's Betrayal of the Child* reinforced how as a child I would have seen and absolutely known at one level of my psyche the real truths about the priest and my father that contradicted my everyday knowledge of them.[11]

Simultaneous to my child mind's absorbing the priest's sexual violations, I was schooled to believe that priests took God's place in the confessional. To be the cause of a priest having impure thoughts was named among the gravest of mortal sins. Being trapped in a priest/god message that admonished rigorous adherence to "purity" formed an insidious torturing god within my psyche. That is, I was taught to value and embody the absence of sexual desire or expression while being eroticized through and conflicted by the priest/god's message that "I can be sexual with you, but you must never be sexual with me or anyone else."

From my early childhood onward the church that systematically and repeatedly instructed me to avoid sexual desire and expression also exposed me to heroic tales of violent deaths in the name of purity. The church encouraged my veneration of numerous young women saints who, like the twentieth century's Saint Maria Goretti, underwent torture and death rather than commit the so-called sin of being raped. Rather than using the example of Maria Goretti and other raped women saints to decry the fact that a rape occurs every two minutes in our culture, the church named rape as women's sin and responsibility to avoid. My need to please God feasted on this schizophrenic purity diet. Contrary to the infinitesimal numbers of sermons, encyclicals, and media-reported church announcements in my lifetime that have focused on women's responsibility concerning purity, birth control, and abortion, I have never once heard any church condemnation of rape. I cannot say this was every Catholic woman's experience but it was mine.

Once able to divide and conquer the priest and father entities that had formed in my mind, I was next able to name the god of this dynamic a tyrant bastard and rid myself of him. To name the god entity was an easy-to-overlook healing step when an actual cleric had shown himself to be the carrier of the betrayal energies and my culture's invisible god stood as the omnipotent container of society's highest values. But the "Thou shalt honour the Lord thy God" commandment imbedded in my psyche by abusive authority figures needed destroying for me to heal my abuse story fully. The Catholic god I had internalized was the fourth of my abusers.

Oppositely pulled due to inheriting my mother's unlived issues around being abandoned by her own father, I was needy and fearful of being abandoned by men as well. My mother's split injunctions to be "pure and good" while encouraging me to "be seductive" were not conducive to my understanding seductiveness as a beautiful feminine energy. My mother's statement, "You upset your father last night," the morning following my father's abuse likely held some truth, but I experienced her words as meaning I had done something bad to my father and assumed blame for my father's death and all negative experiences with men after that time. These split-off injunctions nailed down the virgin/whore split I brought into marriage.

If my mother, my father, or the priest had been out-and-out rotters rather than the traumatized people they were, their impact might have been easier to uncover. Long-term, their abuses forced my psychic energies to be spent on maintaining mental balance and sanity rather than on pursing more creative purposes. Forever juggling diverse opposing childhood messages and forceful moral injunctions from each abuser that I pay the highest honour and respect to the other members of the abuse trio led me to extremes in either/or, black/white ways of thinking and judging and in scrupulous negating of my feelings in all subsequent relationships.

I liken the mental effects of my abusers' double-sided messages to the mythical push-me/pull-you animal in *Doctor Dolittle* or to the maddening quality of a "make haste slowly" directive. When faced with finding the energy to live the no-escape "caged" nature of the complex, I often chose paralysis and became a proverbial Lazy Susan. As an alternative to paralysis, I coped in workaholic fashion, holding fast to many projects and relationships long after I possessed any feelings to do so. When outer life stressors led me to the same "no way out" of the inner complex, psychosis resulted. The payoff for my years of holding on to my sanity was the gift of tenacity—the same tenacity allowed me to persist on my healing journey.

Depression, a paralyzing black hole during crisis times, and otherwise an enveloping dull haze, was systemic in my parental and marital homes. If any family member spoke at a feelings level, we could be laughed at or put down. I recall with particular sadness how my older brother's teen passion for jazz was ridiculed and put down until his silence on this love was secured.

Abuse Effects on the Marriage

My first serious opening to feeling began with marriage and motherhood, closely followed by wrench and loss with the death of my father. If at the time of my father's death I had been able to fully feel and grieve his loss, that opening to feeling might have brought the abuses and my rage to consciousness sooner. But the need to keep my father's memory alive for a mother made rudderless by the loss of her husband and for myself to avoid associating my marriage with that of my in-laws caused me to continue repressing his abuse. In addition to other religious and cultural messages that valued women's stifling their feelings, the more I conformed to these messages as a corporate wife, the more my husband's seniors regarded me a suitable executive partner and company asset when they considered his advancement.

While giving energy to burying childhood trauma, I was also juggling the negation of my sexuality in the marriage. Continually reminded after the fact that what I felt was nothing as compared to what my former husband felt, I worked first at feeding his myth and then at mentally separating from his put-downs. Conditioned by abuses to negotiate splits and to consider my feelings less important than the feelings of others, I inwardly acknowledged my own pleasure and outwardly accepted my husband's view of our unequal pleasure. Mental gymnastics such as these filtered into most aspects of the marriage except cooking. My unconscious grief and trauma remained in a festering state until exhaustion combined with the retreat experience brought on the psychosis.

As I withdrew from the drugs and my long-buried traumas began surfacing in never-before-experienced levels of rage, my husband began tying the return of his love to my going back on the drugs. With only primitive understanding and means to preserve my sanity, I targeted my husband's behaviour as the sole reason for my inexplicable rage and projected it onto him.

Later unravelling of the abuses and their effects showed that my rage against my husband mirrored my conflicted "priest/father" rage against men who aroused me sexually outside the structure of marriage. My unconscious by that time knew our marriage was no longer true. Couple therapists suggested we both needed to learn our childhood stories to save the marriage but linked this recommendation to our communications difficulties rather than to any mention or questioning of us about the possibility of childhood trauma.

My rage against men was dramatically mirrored in the transference experiences that I briefly touch on in chapter 4. Both transferences involved one-sided attractions, one toward the speech therapist in the early 1980s and the other toward a tai chi master in the mid-1990s. Each transference reflected my priest/father issue but in ways that were emotionally intolerable to me. My inability to cope with my feelings in each of these situations triggered overwhelming psychological disruption to the point of near psychosis, including a vision of seeing my speech therapist while skiing at Whistler (see chapter 3).

Today I interpret this vision as a waking dream that was telling me how the addictive distractions of the corporate-wife life I was living at that time kept me from resolving my abuse issues and freeing my ability to practise art. But at the time, I was only able to hang onto my sanity in a disintegrating marriage and wait until the transference receded during my busy year of art studies with Angela Greig.

Years later, after the priest abuse surfaced, I determined to clear my 1980s transference with the speech therapist. Several unsuccessful exchanges of phone messages with the therapist occurred before I left Toronto for Whistler to attend a nephew's wedding. It seemed ironic that I was able to connect with the therapist from Whistler only where I had experienced the 1980s vision of him. Our conversation on the transference allowed me to clear the shame I carried from that time, but I never thought to speak to him about the vision, nor have I given much thought to it since.

During my transference to the tai chi master, and despite the fact that I was open with him about my feelings almost from the time it began, unusual dreams and physical symptoms occurred. In one dream, my bed turned into an operating table and an overhead surgical light shone from the ceiling. While two stern surgeons spent what seemed like an entire night pulling stuff out of my belly, they asked questions about my life and I answered. The room was filled with the smell of burning sage and I could hear the voices of my various mentors talking in the background. The dream felt more like real life than any other in my experience.

The following day as I sat on my bed recording the dream, I paused to look out my apartment window, which overlooked Lake Ontario. As I looked out,

I saw the Four Horsemen of the Apocalypse come thundering out of the clouds over the lake. I was terrified, but as has been the case throughout my journey, it was not long after that I heard about and read Edward Edinger's *Archetype of the Apocalypse: A Jungian Study of the Book of Revelation*.[12] Edinger's work allowed me to understand the Four Horsemen image as a waking dream that foretold how my present inner world was disintegrating to make room for a new inner world to come into being.

A book called *Farther Shores: Exploring How Near-Death, Kundalini and Mystical Experiences Can Transform Ordinary Lives*, by Dr. Yvonne Kason, helped me to better understand some of these psychic occurrences.[13] The *Farther Shores* book, in spite of its title and content, is a very meat-and-potatoes practical work in which the author outlines a number of psychic experiences including near-death ones that can occur but do not necessarily signify or need to develop into mental illnesses. The book was also helpful in explaining how, for some people, psychic phenomena can occur more frequently once their body's Kundalini energy centre has been opened. Kundalini energy as I understand it is a life force that lies at the base of our spines. The awakening of this energy's flow upward along the body's energy paths can occur in varying degrees at any age but is usually activated when an individual attempts to live a mind/body/spirit-connected life. Kason discusses how people affected by such occurrences can take precautions to lead normal lives and to ensure these occurrences do not cross over into mental illness. She also cautions that psychiatrists and clerics are often the least skilled in differentiating between spiritual experience and mental illness or in advising and helping persons who face these challenges.

Added awareness on abuse and its effects allowed me to understand how my abuse symptoms were mirrored in both transferences. In both cases, I was convinced each man had the power to enter my soul, a belief that echoed my deep childhood knowing that the priest was violating my boundaries. My refusal to feel my sexual feelings for each man, even though psychosis threatened to return, reflected my conditioned obedience to the god/priest's and my father's "I can be sexual with you, but you must never be sexual with me" messages. To fully feel my attractions towards these men also meant reaching a feelings level that would have exposed my buried abuse stories. It was only later through the strengthening of self-love that I was able to risk the loss of my father's and God's love in order to complete the work on abuse.

Making Sense of Psychosis Onset

As I went deeper into analysis, the onset of my psychosis at a Catholic retreat seemed less an accident. The retreat was 90 percent filled with priests and nuns with only a few laypersons like myself. The retreat-master, a Catholic layman and psychologist who lectured from a table at the foot of the chapel altar, opened the retreat late on the first evening with the reading of a highly erotic passage from the Song of Songs. As he read, I experienced an orgasm. Rather than feeling pleasure, I felt distress and certain that the clergy sitting around me knew about and disapproved of my orgasm.

I was in a state of physical exhaustion when I was listening to the priestly layman retreat master. His choice of Mother Teresa and her "higher calling" as a nun for the centrepiece of each of his sermons was a close-enough approximation of my childhood confessional experience to trigger emotional stress. My isolation as a married woman at the retreat was compounded as well by the number of nuns there who reinforced the Mother Teresa effect. My inability to see my orgasm as either a private or as healthy response to the Song of Songs poetry, let alone my lack of the sense of self to enjoy it as a pleasurable rebellious act against an asexual religion, further emphasized contradictions in my early confessional experiences. As a desperate worn-out young mother, I could not question obedience to the Church's birth control rules in this setting. With more pressure than I could bear on my unresolved childhood issues and birth control issues and no prior experience of a psychosis, I got pulled in by an insidious build-up of psychotic thinking and was unable to return once it started.

During analysis, when meditating with the question "What did I become when I repressed my sexual energies?" I was given an image of a giant devouring Victorian ghost woman. When my addictive, devouring, repressive energies were turned inward my mind/body health became increasingly compromised. When I turned these negative energies outward, my creative abilities were lessened and my relationships failed. I was greatly helped through this difficult stage of my analysis work by a book called *Witness to the Fire: Creativity and the Veil of Addiction*.[14]

The task of owning and forgiving my own worst offences and abuses towards others began to occur next. Like Scrooge in Dickens's "A Christmas Carol," I experienced a unique grace leading me through and giving me the strength to face past events where my dereliction had dishonoured others' lives and stories. Although I loved my children and intended to be a good mother, I saw more clearly how my addictive controlling behaviours, my layering of repressed rage with "sweetness," and my abandonment of the children through escape into mental illness and marital separation may have influenced their lives in ways that I did not intend or want.

The painful weight of self-examination gradually lightened with an infusion of new awareness on self-forgiveness. With the coming of forgiveness, I entered next into a dormant state of grief, observing the dying of my old life and unfolding of a new one. A new sense of trust in myself, others, and the world flowered into an opportunity to do a mutually and deeply felt clearing and forgiveness ritual with my former husband. At the same time, as parents we took each of our children aside to express our sorrow at the pain we caused them and for their pain at having to witness their siblings go through similar suffering. Some time following these clearings, I explained to my former husband about my work on this book and the graphic portrait of our marriage it contained. Once he became clear about my intention to create awareness through our story on how whole families can be adversely affected by over-drugging and gender-biased diagnoses and treatments, his initial resistance dissolved. These changes gave new dignity to our divorce and helped free the lost memories that now mark our celebrations when important rites of passage in our children and grandchildren's lives occur.

Old fears that my art would lead me into another psychosis lifted. My dreams and psyche began inviting me to take more risks, become more confident and passionate in my art making, and to trust that I was ready and supported.

Prompted by strong feelings that I would be culpable if I did not report the abuse to the Catholic authorities. I sent a letter outlining my experiences with the priest to the Monsignor who handled priest abuse complaints for the Toronto diocese. Although receipt of my letter was confirmed by the Monsignor's secretary when I phoned his office, the letter remains unanswered to this day.

Final Painful Steps

In late 2006 as we made final revisions to the manuscript of the present book, Rosemary asked if I had an interest in including some account of my reactions to the conversation with Dr. Rowe in early 1999. Shocked that I had blocked this conversation from my writing on the abuse, I was not eager to revisit it. The sole inducement to revisit and work on that conversation was my knowledge of past benefits I'd gained from walking into my worst fears.

As I reviewed the discussion tape and transcript, I was surprised to find that I was a far more coherent participant in the discussion than I had recalled being at the time Cheryl, Rosemary, and I met. The following part of the conversation, heard at this stage of my abuse clearing, made a significant difference to my ability to probe deeper.

ROSEMARY BARNES: *[To Dr. Rowe]* I know that you've had a chance to read over Susan's recent writing and clinical records. I thought I would start with some of the realizations that Susan has come to in the last year in terms of the relationship with the priest. There seemed to be a sexualized relationship that was very problematic. What's damaging about a person in authority such as a priest expressing sexual feelings in some way towards a young person?

DR. CHERYL ROWE: There's a lot damaging when an authority figure expresses sexual feelings. It's also very complicated because it depends on *how* those feelings are expressed. There is physical and emotional direct trauma from someone who reaches out and becomes sexual in a shocking and surprising way. There's often a different level of trauma that occurs when the lead-up to it [sexual content] is implicit or suggestive. The person becomes confused, maybe takes much more responsibility when the sexual feelings or innuendos are being expressed; they may begin to doubt themselves and their own judgment about what's happening. So, there are different levels and different means of impact.

Almost always though, there is a trusted authority figure who is behaving in a way that is totally outside the expectations of the recipient of these feelings. The recipient is then left to make sense of it. Depending on where they're at in their own developmental stage and what's going on in their background, how they make sense of it can be extremely damaging and detrimental to their personality.

● ● ●

While earlier parts of this chapter contain insights that grew from reviewing our conversation with Dr. Rowe, it is important to specify how my last reading of this conversation enabled me to absolve the guilt and the sense of responsibility I took as a child for the priest's actions. Once able to admit to the erotic feelings I both fought against and felt toward the priest in his apartment and in the confessional, the final clearing of the psychosis occurred.

Previous attempts to address my struggles with erotic feelings towards the priest were limited by question such as "Did I have a crush on the priest?" or "Was I in love with the priest?" As memory and dream told me that neither was the case and I had no memory of physical violation, I could understand how his psychosexual acts could bleed onto my psyche but I missed how I, as a child, could take responsibility for the unseen psychosexual energies the priest was directing at me. It was only in revisiting Dr. Rowe's explanation of the responsibility factor that I was able to admit to such (hugely forbidden) erotic feelings I had as a child towards the priest in confession. In the case of my transferences to the speech therapist and tai chi instructor, I repeated this pattern to the point of near-repeat psychosis because I could and would not own or act on these erotic feelings.

The night following this insight and clearing, I entered a semi-dream, semi-out-of-body state where I began to consciously witness and experience past psychotic auditory and physical effects release from my body. The power of the experience was unsettling to the degree I needed the added help of visualizing with my hibiscus image to remain centred for its duration. The dream was a noise-filled replication of my psychosis at its peak. It included a cacophonous chorus of raging voices, dogs barking, and car horns honking except that this time I had the additional feeling of the priest's presence and myself choking on a penis. As I was in no way psychotic while this experience was taking place, I took the dream to signal that I had at last reached and resolved the core of the psychosis and abuse.

After journalling and owning my erotic feeling experiences and the psychosis-like dream, I dreamed the face of a woman patient from my first year of nursing training. The patient was sad but her Korsakoff's syndrome, rapidly clenching and unclenching overbite jaw, foul language, chloral hydrate [a type of sedative medication] breath, and rage made it hard for nurses to go near her or, as it appears from the dream, to forget her either. I understood without a doubt how the dream was telling me that the patient was manifesting the true face of sexual abuse and how that same patient's fate might have been mine but for my commitment to heal.

A recent Internet search on Saint Maria Goretti confirmed that the Catholic Church continues to this day to teach that prevention of rape is exclusively the woman's responsibility. Had I continued to adhere to such a religion, I would have followed teachings that left me no option but to sink deeper into a belief in my badness. If it were not for mentors and my commitment to heal, I can see how like my long-ago patient, my only way of coping with my trauma dilemma could have been psychosis reoccurrence, addiction, chronic decline, and psychiatric medications.

Because psychiatrists failed in 1969 to imagine my story might involve trauma-related depression or to prescribe therapies that would aid in the resolution of my psychosis, my family and I suffered years of further distress when trauma memories were forced even deeper into my unconscious with drugs. Unresolved, my psychosis core presented in my later adult life as rage, depression, paranoia, lack of focus, urges to isolate, and to seek life energy through addictive behaviours.

Notes

1 George Bush, speech to the United States Congress, 20 September 2001. Available at http://www.white-house.gov/news/releases/2001/09/20010920-8.html.
2 Alice Miller, *Thou Shalt Not Be Aware: Society's Betrayal of the Child,* American ed. (New York: Farrar Straus Giroux, 1984), 318.
3 American Psychiatric Association, *Diagnostic and Statistical Manual of Mental Disorders,* 4th ed. (Washington, DC: American Psychiatric Press, 2000).
4 Judith Herman, *Trauma and Recovery* (New York: Basic Books, 1992).
5 American Psychiatric Association, *Diagnostic and Statistical Manual.*

6 See, for example, Catherine J. Wurr and Ian M. Partridge, "The Prevalence of a History of Childhood Sexual Abuse in an Acute Adult Inpatient Population," *Child Abuse and Neglect* 20 (1996): 867–72; and John Read, "To Ask, or Not to Ask, about Abuse—New Zealand Research," *American Psychologist* 62 (2007): 325–26.

7 Colin A. Ross, *Schizophrenia: Innovations in Diagnosis and Treatment* (Binghamton, NY: Haworth, 2004).

8 Sylvia Shaindel Senensky, *Healing and Empowering the Feminine: A Labyrinth Journey* (New York: Chiron, 2003).

9 The Churchill painting, which is part of the *Casting a Vessel* series, is reproduced in plate 30 in the colour section, which follows page 230.

10 A.J. Lubin, *Stranger on the Earth: A Psychological Biography of Vincent Van Gogh* (New York: Holt, Rinehart and Winston, 1972).

11 Miller, *Thou Shalt Not Be Aware.*

12 Edward F. Edinger, *Archetype of the Apocalypse: A Jungian Study of the Book of Revelation*, ed. G.R. Elder (Peru, IL: Open Court, 1999).

13 Yvonne Kason, *Farther Shores: Exploring How Near-Death, Kundalini and Mystical Experiences Can Transform Ordinary Lives* (Toronto: HarperCollins, 2000).

14 Linda Schierse Leonard, *Witness to the Fire: Creativity and the Veil of Addiction* (Boston: Shambhala, 1989).

8 An Eye
     to Delight

Life is always balanced on the edge of annihilation. Within the
tension of the moment, we must learn to relax, breathe, open.
Whatever happens now on earth—as always—happens either
out of fear or love. Our response to it, likewise, will be either one
of fear or love. I don't think we can deny all of the portents and
manifestations of extinction we see arising all around us. But
too, I don't think we should fear them. Life in the beginning, as
now and in the end, is the Great Mystery. Why does the Mona
Lisa smile? Why do the Buddhas smile? They must know
something we don't know. We must keep love alive in the ragged
manger of our own hearts—in the grim details of the daily
struggle, in the disappointment, the injustice, the atrocity. There
the eternal child is born. We must tend to this reality with the gift
of our hearts. And it helps to remember the paradoxical, the
poetic, the possibility of any thing—and to smile with the
accomplished ones.

> —Paul Hogan, conversation, 18 January 1996

Rosemary

WORLD WAR II ENDED BEFORE I WAS BORN, and I never fought on the front
lines of the Cold War, the Vietnam War, or the present "war against terror,"
yet my psychic struggles have mirrored the complexities, contradictions, and
protests that have accompanied these great world events. Most recently, my
attachment to professional prestige battled inner promptings towards more
meaningful life purposes. My passion for this book arose from my desire to

end the war and to heal its wounds within myself, including the splits, disappointment, anger, and the sense of failure associated with my earlier career. As Susan suggested various readings and conversations, new possibilities opened up.

I thought for a time that Susan and I were working out how to end the world's wars, if not for ourselves then for our children and grandchildren. Then Susan reminded me of Paul Hogan's story about his physician friend in Rwanda during the time of the genocide. This man described peace as "the other face of war" and pointed out how peace was present in certain moments and people even in the midst of horrendous atrocities. In a similar vein, Paul speaks of the opportunity in each moment to choose to live in love rather than fear. I realize now that peace is not some hoped-for future state, but rather the peace of the heart present even in the midst of war. Though wars continue as they have for millennia, I have reached some understandings that bring peace and that I would like to share.

Bringing Forth a World

"The truth is out there" was the signature statement of *The X Files,* an American television program in which government investigative agents combat threatening situations. Agent Mulder was certain that acceptance of paranormal phenomena was essential to understanding and overcoming threats while Agent Scully adhered to scientific understandings of tangible reality. Both agreed, however, that the truth "is out there" and could be ascertained in even the most bizarre of circumstances. The views of agents Mulder and Scully are securely grounded in the intellectual tradition of modern thought. Modernists hold that a single, stable reality exists and is known to humans, more or less accurately, through our senses and capacities for reason and reflection.[1] Words and images in the mind are presumed to correspond to this external reality, much as a rug in a photograph is recognizable as the rug in the hall. Our understandings may be imperfect but one can be confident that "the truth is out there" and a rug is a rug.

In a modernist perspective, scientific theories are understood as approximations of the truth that are constantly being refined to reflect more accurately the reality "out there." In practical situations, theories are treated as true and used as the basis for action. Psychiatric diagnoses such as "schizophrenia," and other clinical concepts, like "anxiety," are theoretical constructs subject to testing, criticism, and refinement through science, but they are treated as realities by the practising clinician. Antipsychiatry critics argue that the limitations of the medical model and problems related to its theoretical constructs (e.g., "schizophrenia"), indicate that these concepts inaccurately approximate the reality of mental illness; some argue that such conceptualizations should be improved while others argue that they should be abandoned.[2] Such critiques agree that, one way or another, "The truth is out there."

However, well-developed intellectual streams in both the humanities and science argue for something stranger than anything that Agents Mulder or Scully would believe, namely that reality is not "out there" but is instead the product of our own inner processes and communications with one another. Although we ordinarily treat what we perceive and remember as a more or less accurate recording of an external reality, psychological science has demonstrated a myriad of ways in which the brain and mind actively construct reality through various learned and innate perceptual, attentional, conceptual, and memory mechanisms. The active role of the brain in constructing reality is revealed when one sees, for example, visual illusions or considers the vagaries of memory. The theoretical work of Chilean neuroscientists Humberto Maturana and Francisco Varela goes even further.[3] These scientists argue that sensations and thoughts do not represent an external world, but rather create a world within the brain and mind in accordance with the individual's biological makeup and history. Capra explains this scientific understanding as follows:

> According to the Santiago theory, cognition is not a representation of an independent, pregiven world, but rather a bringing forth of a world. What is brought forth by a particular organism in the process of living is not *the* world but *a* world, one that is always dependent on the organism's structure.... We humans, moreover, share an abstract world of language and thought through which we bring forth our world together. (italics in original)[4]

Within the humanities, a parallel stream of thought is postmodernism. Postmodernists note that rather than living in a universal external reality, we humans create the realities in which we live through language and other symbolic exchanges.[5] In this view, a rug exists because human beings with common sensory systems, similar histories, and shared language agree that certain experiences constitute the reality of a rug. People with different sensory systems, for example, those who are blind, will construct a different reality of a rug. People with different histories construct experiences differently; what North Americans constitute as a rug might, for example, be constituted elsewhere as a door covering. In this view, a human matrix of meaning is understood not to mirror an independently existing external reality but rather to bring forth a world, to constitute a reality for those humans who share the matrix.[6]

From a postmodern view, then, reality is not "out there," but rather created in every moment by human understandings and actions. We are continually engaged individually and collectively in organizing lived experiences into meanings that we treat as reality. Society organizes itself around systems such as the mental health care system and the legal system, through widely accepted statements, practices, and institutional structures. These systems of meaning and values are regarded by narrative therapists as critical to each individual's construction of a personal story. An individual's personal story in turn organizes and generates lived experience—it creates reality, brings forth a world.[7] We are continually engaged in bringing forth a world and multiple realities co-exist. No reality has any greater claim to "truth" than any other. We direct more attention to some socially constructed systems than to others, and are surrounded by vital lived experiences that have not been incorporated into social systems or personal stories. As well, we can find subjugated knowledges or systems of meaning, that are not readily accessible as a result of being ignored in the dominant society or known only to a limited number of people (see chapter 5 for examples in relation to feminism).

Socially constructed systems profoundly influence us all. As an example, several socially constructed systems were highly influential in Susan's life. The structural-functional conception of marriage supported her in the creation and performance of a preferred story of herself as a good wife and mother in the early years of her marriage. Family and friends, religious and school instruction, law, media presentations, and health care all spoke and acted in ways directed to creating and valuing the structural-functional organization of marriage where the husband was the financially successful breadwinner and household head while the wife was the financially dependent homemaker and helpmate. This system guided Susan's choice of preferred story—her bringing forth a world where she was a devoted wife and mother.

The constructs of mental illness and medical-model care were and are products of similar socially constructed systems. When Susan experienced overwhelming emotional distress, family and friends, religious and school instruction, law, media presentations, and health-care structures all spoke and acted in ways that created and sustained the authority of physicians and other professional staff to name her experience a disease condition and to direct a response. Susan's decision to accept and perform the story of herself as mentally ill patient was influenced by this larger system as well as by what she learned in nursing training and was told by her husband and hospital staff.

Since reality is not "out there," postmodernists understand "mental illness" and "medical-model care" as constructs arising out of society's efforts to bring meaning to vital experiences and not as independently existing truths. In this view, even extensive research findings or sophisticated taxonomies such as the *DSM-IV* do not and cannot "prove" the presence or absence of mental illnesses or effective treatment. For example, describing certain behaviours as indicative of schizophrenia, doing scientific studies on schizophrenia, and evaluating how medications or other interventions alter schizophrenic behaviours do not and cannot prove the presence or absence of schizophrenia. From this perspective, constructs such as "mental illness" and the "medical model" are problematic not because such ideas exist or are incorrect but because they often function to suppress other possibilities, other understandings, other stories of human distress and healing. Postmodernists "discourage foreclosing meaning making experience through the pre-emptive adoption of only one construction of disorder" in order to explore other possibilities and to encourage richer understandings of emotional disturbance and possible responses.[8]

Postmodern thought implies that we possess extraordinary creative power. We have the power to bring forth a world, indeed *are* bringing forth a world at every moment by what we choose to think, say, and do. Given this extraordinary power, what world do we choose to bring forth?

Familiar Values: Power to Transcend Nature, Social Control, and Normality

Susan's stories of herself as devoted wife and mother, observant Catholic, and mentally ill patient and my story of myself as a successful professional can be understood in light of core values which we humans have maintained through beliefs, practices, and institutions for hundreds of years. Within this framework, what is prized as giving meaning to human existence is the power to transcend our human condition by dominating nature and inferiors in the outer world and subduing the bodily sensations and emotional impulses in inner experience. *Beyond Power* by author and scholar Marilyn French provides a meticulously researched and detailed analysis of beliefs and practices through which we maintain this core valuing of power to transcend and thereby bring forth our present world.[9] Although other scholars provide similar perspectives, I will refer to French's writing to sketch out how the valuing of power to dominate and transcend forms social structures and practices relating to mental health care; French is also useful to explore the destructive consequences of valuing power as well as alternatives to such values.

Considering several millennia of history, French concludes that we humans have created and sustained forms of government, business, science, religion, law, and health care that are based on the belief that people are superior to animals and nature by virtue of some superior knowledge or quality such as being chosen by God, possessing reason, or being capable of controlling our destiny. The purpose of human existence is to become godlike by transcending our earthly body through dominating and controlling both the external world of nature and the inner world of feeling and frailty. We honour as leaders, heroes, and exemplary persons those humans who appear victorious over such outer and inner forces, which are perceived as threatening or evil, such as aggressive beasts or shameful laziness.

Though exceptions exist, French describes a myriad of examples where this prizing of power has been enacted in the world's great military, religious, political, and corporate empires. Military conquests, for example, are understood as victories because they demonstrate an emperor's power to dominate people and the earth; these military victories are also of deep psychic importance because they symbolize the transcendence of ideals like "justice" by defeat of an enemy and transcendence over time and mortality, especially when the fame of the emperor is spread over large areas of land among many people and prolonged through the emperor's heirs.

The valuing of power to transcend and dominate found new expressions during the Industrial Revolution when modes of work changed to require the separation of producer from product, people from land, home from workplace, and families from one another. According to French,

> For the few, the Industrial Revolution established a new language of values, one suited to the power-seeking men who were suited to thrive in such an atmosphere. It is difficult to describe this new vision without offering a bookful of biographies, because it subtly infiltrates most of our culture. It is a vision of control without end, control for its own sake, boundless ambition; home is superseded by a state of permanent exile, the pursuit of power; the excitement of the chase is substituted for the affections of the heart. The vision has been made into an image of "modernity" and glamour, of a man who controls technology and is invulnerable to emotional need. Power in its many manifestations is not just the greatest but the *only* good. (italics in original)[10]

What we say, the practices we enact, and the institutions we sustain are guided by an understanding, usually implicit, that dominance and transcendence are of prime importance in every realm of contemporary society, including mental health care. Susan and I both participated in such arrangements. When Susan learned as a girl and young woman to subdue, for example, her artistic interests and sexual passions for the sake of being an observant Catholic and good daughter, she was learning with the assistance of her parents, religious authorities, and others to transcend by conquering and dominating her inner nature. When I learned as a girl and young woman to set aside fun and games for the sake of earning good grades, achieving an advanced education, and establishing a career, I was learning with the assistance of parents, educational authorities, and others to transcend by suppressing personal desires and interests for the sake of professional prestige and power.

Learning self-control is an aspect of maturing and not inherently problematic. However, when self-control is prized over all else, an individual risks losing awareness of body, feelings, and relationships and thus failing to recognize and integrate vital experiences into one's personal story. For example, Susan describes neglecting exhaustion and illness in the time prior to her psychotic break and adding volunteer work to already-heavy family responsibilities for the sake of being a good Catholic. I found it difficult to care for my body and heart as a hospital psychologist, in part because I and many of my colleagues shared the belief that bearing fatigue, illness, or emotional adversity without allowing these to affect work performance indicated admirable good character. We were prizing self-control and personal power to transcend bodily nature, in extreme cases over life itself, when we dismissed health or safety problems for the sake of work performance.

Familiar Values: The Exercise of Power in Mental Health Care

In relation to emotional disturbance and mental health care, French describes the prizing of power that is enacted when professional leaders, loyal staff, and compliant patients engage in subduing passions, illness, and frailty for the sake of "normality." French, like many feminist and antipsychiatry critics, points out that medical-model care imposes control on a large and unruly part of the population by ensuring that people maintain, insofar as possible, the appearances and performances of "normal" stories, such as good wife, dutiful husband, productive worker, and so on.[11] As French puts it, such approaches "try to produce humans fit for this world rather than a world fit for humans."[12]

Susan describes how she, her family, and health professionals worked for years to shoehorn her life into "normality." Everyone took part in performances within the disease-based medical model where the authoritative doctor prescribed treatment to an obedient patient who was deemed cured so long as she appeared normal—free from overt emotional distress and able to perform socially approved roles as attractive, obedient wife and selfless mother. Part of this enactment went well; hospital interventions pulled Susan out of the water when she was drowning. Over succeeding years, however, Susan felt increasing emptiness and despair as she, her family, and mental health professionals neglected her dissatisfactions with her marriage, memories of childhood sexual abuse, and interests in art. The conquest-of-illness and normality approaches did not help to identify or accommodate vital aspects of her experience. They did not take her into the garden.

French's analysis helped me to understand my successful career in university-affiliated hospitals. As my resumé gleamed ever brighter with the gold coin of the professional realm—positions at prestigious institutions, appointment as a department head, academic titles, and research publications—my work satisfaction steadily diminished. As my knowledge grew, I became increasingly confused and distressed over the contradictions between the stated purposes and the *realpolitik* of organizational life. I eventually realized that my personal values were at odds with what I and others in the hospital said and did.

Hospitals publicly commit to transcendent ideals such as "health" and "excellence," just as the courts are devoted to "justice" and governments are devoted to "life, liberty, and the pursuit of happiness" or "peace, order, and good government" or "liberté, egalité, fraternité." I found the hospital ideals meaningful and felt confident of my connection to the larger community as a professional dedicated to these ideals. But I was shocked and bewildered when I noticed irregularities such as the poorly skilled clinician selected to head a new program, the researcher whose shoddy work was promoted through a significant grant, and the general lack of interest in community initiatives. Then there were the systemic errors described in earlier chapters of this book and elsewhere: narrow focus on symptoms, diagnosis, and medication; bias in respect to gender, race, religion, or sexual orientation; prescribed treatments causing serious, sometimes irreversible damage; failure to nurture the patient's desire to heal; and failure to recognize the importance of creative expression.[13] I could see that such errors, at best, limited the effectiveness of clinical interventions and, at worst, harmed individuals who were already emotionally vulnerable.

Initially, I took these occurrences to be regrettable but inadvertent mistakes. However, I gradually realized that clinical practices, hiring, promotion, funding, programs, and awards were regularly at odds with stated hospital ideals and rarely of great concern to senior hospital leaders. I decided that the hospital where I worked was dysfunctional. After I moved to a different hospital and talked with colleagues elsewhere, I realized that these occurrences were common. I then decided that hospitals are peculiar and disappointing institutions.

After my father died and my mother remarried, I listened to my stepfather's stories about being an airplane navigator in World War II and a chemical engineer who designed, built, and operated oil and gas refineries all over the world. I was startled to recognize in his stories the same puzzling anomalies that I noticed at hospitals and realized that my experiences were common to most, if not all, large organizations. The near-universal nature of such experiences was further underscored by *Dilbert*, the widely popular cartoon whose humour satirizes corporate environments and echoed many of my hospital experiences. I became convinced that power to dominate is the highest value in organizational culture and that it routinely undermines the organization's ability to attain its stated ideals.

Individuals within institutions learn to pay their "dues," to accommodate and support the valuing of power by adopting attitudes deferential to superiors, professing loyalty to the institution, and conforming to the appearances, whether dress, manners, or speech, required of a good employee.[14] In return employees expect that good work and loyalty will be rewarded by advancement and security. However, these promises are routinely betrayed; job performance is loosely if at all related to promotion, pay, or security of tenure. We cannot rely even on securing the larger goods to which the organizations are ostensibly dedicated. As Marilyn French sees it,

> The betrayals made by institutions are not limited to exploitive treatment of individuals or failure to fulfill their promises to individuals and groups. Institutions and the men [and women] who govern them betray even themselves and their own reason for being. Political and religious groups, and even states, all claiming to exist for the sake of the people who are their adherents, often destroy their entire following.[15]

The corporate scandals of the 1990s are examples of such betrayals. Think of Enron, where senior management encouraged employees to invest their retirement savings in the company even when it became apparent that the company was on the cusp of financial collapse. Although French attributes such problems to men, women can be as committed as men to social systems organized to bring about domination and transcendence; both men and women can and do choose different commitments.

At hospitals where I worked, "excellence" often served as code for a commitment to dominate the professional terrain by means of amassing the biggest hospitals, most influential scientific publications, and largest research grants. Such commitments allowed mental health professional leaders to impress peers, government, or funding bodies while giving little or no attention to the voices of those seeking help or to broader public concerns. Excellence came at the expense of poor accountability to the larger community. Paradoxically, when excellence and competitive advantage were pursued to the exclusion of other interests, scientific quality suffered when considerable resources were expended on projects that aimed to enhance individual or institutional prestige with little regard to community concerns or priorities. Despite the fact that I never worked in a managed care setting, what I have learned about this approach indicates the same problems I experienced in hospitals: profits and shareholder returns take the place of scientific or administrative prestige as trophies to be secured by the practices of power.[16] Both hospital and managed care environments can suffer from the same disparities between stated purposes and organizational *realpolitik*, the same de facto disregard for individuals seeking help or for the larger community.

Work with Susan, *Dilbert* cartoons, talks with my stepfather, and reading all helped me to realize that my work experiences mirrored those of many people in a society where we know little else but to enact statements and practices that bring forth a world where power is prized as the greatest good. My good intentions and high ideals could not change the fact that my daily work supported beliefs and practices that I believed to be wrong and harmful to myself, to the individuals who came to the hospital for care, and to the community as a whole. This disconnection became increasingly disturbing. French offers an analysis so clearly describing what I experienced that she could have been writing me a personal letter:

> What one must be on the job has an effect on what one is off the job. Young people who enter large institutions may at first find them intimidating, oppressive and even immoral. They may try to behave as they must on the job and be themselves—"let it all hang out"—in their private lives. But to keep this up they must either become hypocrites or schizophrenics.... [In] actuality, few people are hypocrites; indeed, sustained hypocrisy would seem to lead to madness. People who find their work too dehumanizing eventually leave the workplace; others embrace the values and the role and persuade themselves that both are worthwhile.
>
> It is impossible to condemn people for doing this. The values of the workplace are the values of the public world, and most people are neither arrogant nor foolhardy enough to challenge that world single-handedly.[17]

In the end, this was indeed the choice that I faced, either to leave hospitals or stay. Staying would require that I embrace the power-oriented culture and my career as worthy and thus risk loss of connection to my life purposes as well as madness, which for me would likely have taken the form of depletion and despair. I left.

I worked towards bringing forth a different world within my own life. Some years later, I realized that my choices freed me to bury my hospital commitments with respect, just as Susan had buried with respect the worn and untenable aspects in her own life.

EMERGING VALUES
Bringing Forth a World with an Eye to Delight

Many people are concerned that practices of power are failing to generate systems that incorporate experiences vital to the survival and flourishing of human life. Thinkers in a wide range of disciplines have been inspired by the difficulties facing humanity and the earth's natural systems to describe the need to transform our relationships to ourselves, one another, and our planet.[18] French warns that as long as we continue to speak and act in ways that value transcendence and domination as our highest social priorities, we will have difficulty in imagining alternatives to the bleak scenarios that haunt our present lives: global war, global totalitarianism, desiccation of the planet.[19]

At a personal level, when we place the greatest value on control, appearances, and normality, we engage in efforts to transcend and thereby deny the drama inherent in our human experience. We all have good and evil, strengths and flaws in our character. We all have moments of triumph and moments of shame, anger, sorrow, and helplessness. Our lives are continuously unfolding stories. To strive to be "normal," successful, always in control, is to aspire to an unattainable and banal transcendence over the complex realities of our own nature and our interconnection with human and natural systems.[20] Susan experienced increasing emptiness and despair as long as she confined herself to "normal" appearances and the enacting of stories as a devoted wife and mother, observant Catholic, or mentally ill patient. She reached a point where she felt that her well-being had to have priority over the expectations most familiar to her and others around her. When she committed to healing, Susan gradually learned of the profoundly meaningful drama unfolding in her life.

Just as Susan shifted to a different way of living in the face of despair, so humanity appears to be struggling with overwhelming and desperate problems. Our current ways of living seem inadequate to the challenges we face. What is the alternative? Creating something different cannot be achieved through revolution, though revolutions, violent and otherwise, are historically familiar approaches to change. French points out that revolutions are simply arguments about which persons, practices, or transcendent ideals will be accorded respect as most powerful but they fail to challenge domination as the central value.[21]

French also observes that we cannot expect to discover new values because all possible values are known already. Instead she suggests a new ordering of values to give the highest priority to well-being and life purposes, in short, to pleasure:

> The great end is pleasure…. It includes all the values we currently entertain; it excludes nothing. While there are parts of human experience we would like to exclude—cruelty, death—we cannot accomplish this. To pretend that we can, to create symbols that suggest that some people live forever, is to implant in human experience a falsehood so profound as to distort it utterly. Life carries sorrows for all creatures; sorrow and deprivation are not escapable. But it is possible to live with an eye to delight rather than to domination.[22]

Just as Susan turned within to discover what she needed when the old approach was failing, so French suggests turning within to identify what makes living desirable and satisfying. She suggests that we accept with grace that we are all dependent on the earth and on other people for our existence. While we will continue to value transcendence and domination at times, priority should be given to the deep pleasures associated with the beauty of the earth, the company of other people, and the freedom to chose commitments and means of self-expression. "The qualities on which we have depended for several millennia, which we have imagined have kept us afloat—power-in-the-world, possession, status, hierarchy, tradition—are in fact sweeping us to ruin; what is necessary to prevent that ruin are the very qualities we have feared to trust – the flexible, fluid, transient elements of affection and communality."[23]

Many scholars and scientists are exploring the transition to a different way of being on the earth and recent scholarly writing outlines new possibilities. Fritjof Capra in *The Web of Life* argues that the philosophy of deep ecology and current scientific knowledge both imply that mental and physical experiences are differing aspects of a single web of life.[24] Jane Jacobs in *The Nature of Economies* calls for a reorganization of economic activity to recognize the intimate connection between sustainable economies and the earth's natural living systems.[25] Rosemary Radford Ruether in *Gaia and God* describes the need for a new consciousness, symbolic culture, and spirituality which supports communities that care for the earth on which they are located, justice for individuals, and ways to establish compassionate solidarity in place of competitive alienation and domination.[26] Thomas Berry in *The Dream of the Earth* calls for a "new story" of the earth to heal the split between religions preoccupied with spiritual fall and redemption and sciences disconnected from humanity.[27] Martin Seligman and Mihaly Csikszentmihalyi argue for psychological research focused on "positive subjective experience, positive individual traits and positive institutions to improve the quality of life and prevent the pathologies that arise when life is barren and meaningless."[28] In daily life, Thomas Moore in *Care of the Soul* comments that overcoming the "loss of soul" requires giving primacy to "life in all its particulars – good food, satisfying conversation, genuine friends, and experiences that stay in the memory and touch the heart."[29]

Susan introduced me to how a shift in values is being articulated within art. Art historian Suzi Gablik notes a historic shift as a growing number of artists break from the observer-recorder role and move to roles as partners in their communities.[30] Like French, she argues that such change is a necessity in the face of the urgent human and psychological problems facing the planet at the beginning of a new millennium:

> The mode of distanced, objective knowing, removed from moral and social responsibility, has been the animating motif of both science and art in the modern world. As a form of thinking, it is now proving to be something of an evolutionary dead-end.... We are in transitional times.... It is a good moment to attend to the delineation of goals, as more and more people now imagine that

our present system can be replaced by something better: closeness, instead of distancing; cultivation of ecocentric values; whole-systems thinking; a developed
discipline of caring; an individualism that is not purely individual but is grounded
in social relationships and also promotes community and the welfare of the
whole; an expanded vision of art as a social practice and not just a disembod-
ied eye.[31]

Susan's emotional disturbance, personal turning point, and step-by-step reorganization of her life reflect a struggle with the valuing of power-in-the-world,
possession, status, hierarchy, and tradition. Her story serves as a metaphor for
the larger struggle facing us individually and as a society.

Emerging Values: Healing from Emotional Disturbance

To live with an eye to delight is to hold dear the earth that is our home, the
relationships that sustain us, and the opportunities for self-expression that
emerge within the flow of experience. We attend to our lives as unfolding
within a great web that extends from the earth systems described in the Gaia
hypothesis down to the intricacies within single cells.[32] From this perspective,
serious emotional disturbance is an eruption of vital experience that over-
whelms the familiar and forces the reorganization of self and relationships
within the web of life.

Emotional disturbance can be like a hurricane going through a settled
area—powerful sensation, feeling, thought, action, and relational changes shat-
ter existing structures, both within and without. First, one struggles simply to
survive in the awesome intensity of the elements. Then, people cope with the
immediate devastation, provide rescue and care to the injured, secure temporary shelter and emergency supplies, salvage belongings, cordon off and clear
away unsafe structures, and find and bury the bodies of those who have per-
ished. When the worst seems past, sometimes the calm turns out to be only
the eye of the storm passing over and a further storm must be endured and
emergency measures renewed. Eventually, the time comes for mourning what
has been lost and then for longer-term reconstruction where buildings are
cleaned and repaired, fields replanted, and daily living re-established, likely
with provisions that allow a future storm to be weathered with more safety
and confidence.

Responding to emotional disturbance is a complex undertaking. At every
stage, many things need attention and not everything can be done at once. The
medical model explains emotional disturbance as a biochemical imbalance in
the brain that can be righted through accurate diagnosis and correct medication. For some individuals, this approach provides an entirely satisfactory
account of vital experience and an acceptable basis for reorganizing their sense

of self, relationships, and place in the community. Indeed this approach was acceptable to Susan for several years after her psychotic break when she and her husband were able to relate well with a mutual unspoken accommodation of their individual woundedness. However, for many people, the medical model is not fully satisfactory—something more is necessary to understand and respond to what has transpired.

To speak of *healing* offers another possibility. We think of healing as growth in ability to love and forgive self and other, to cope, to feel pleasure, to engage in meaningful activity, and to follow the psyche's inner direction away from addiction and towards greater wholeness. Healing involves recreating and reorganizing so as to accommodate the raw experience of emotional disturbance into the web of life, both in the inner realm of thought, feeling, and dream and in the outer world of family, friends, work, and community. Healing opens the way to new stories of self, relationships, and place in the larger world. The richer and more compassionate the new story, the more stable and skilful the individual's relationships to self, family, friends, community, and the natural world is likely to become.

For some, as Susan describes and Helen Porter elaborates, the snaky "Aaaagh!!!" of emotional disturbance may indicate the emergence of profound personal growth, the beginning of a vital new life story—an emphasis on well-being and healing can help the individual and his or her family to give birth to this new story. For many, even those with serious mental illness, a period of suffering will likely be followed sooner or later by some degree of recovery; an emphasis on well-being and healing will help to alleviate distress and improve the speed and extent of such recovery. For some, emotional disturbance will stretch throughout their lives with no lasting improvement, as permanent as the loss of a limb or a sense. Yet even where cure is impossible, healing is always possible and desirable; life can always be lived with an eye to delight, with an emphasis on meaning, creativity, caring, and connection to the earth and one another. The first step is to decide to make a better life, to live with an eye to delight, to value one's own well-being and life purposes above all else.

The Garden Path

Finding healing activities that advance one's own life purposes can feel overwhelming, even impossible at the beginning. Healing can feel like putting together a jigsaw puzzle where there is no picture on the front of the box and one is confronted by a large pile of pieces with no order or meaning. The person who decides to assemble the puzzle often starts by sorting pieces into piles by colour or straight edges or some other principle and searches by trial and error for pieces that connect easily to one another. It is a gradual, often frustrating process, particularly in the beginning, and one often moves restlessly from one organizing strategy to another, takes breaks, or seeks others' help to search for patterns.

Thinking of Helen Porter's advice in fairy tales, I realized the Grimms' tale "The Queen Bee" is a story instructing about healing. In this story, three royal princes set off to seek their fortunes. The eldest two are proud, clever, sophisticated, and unsuccessful. The youngest, Witling, is a simple man who is ridiculed by his older brothers for insisting on protecting from harm even nature's smallest creatures—ants, ducks, and bees. The brothers face the task of freeing a castle from an evil enchantment by performing three tasks. Those who fail are turned to stone. The first task is to collect by sunset every one of the princess's thousand pearls strewn in the moss of the wood. Each of the proud elder brothers tries and fails to collect the pearls; they are duly turned to stone. The younger brother tries, is equally overwhelmed and weeps bitterly. However, the ants he had earlier befriended take pity on him and gather every one of the pearls so that the task is completed by sunset.

The second task is to obtain the key to the princess's bedroom from the bottom of the lake, another task not humanly possible. However, the ducks whose lives Witling had saved dive to the bottom of the lake and retrieve the key for him. The final task is to choose from among three sleeping princesses, each with a different sweet in her mouth, the youngest and loveliest, whose mouth holds a spoonful of honey. In this task, the bees whom Witling had protected come to direct him to the princess holding the honey. So Witling is able to break the spell of the enchanted castle, free all who had been turned to stone, and marry the princess.

To find fortune is to find the inner treasures of peace, love, and wisdom, in other words, to heal. To secure these treasures, it is necessary to perform a series of tasks in order to break the evil spell guarding the enchanted castle. The story tells us that when pursuing treasures, it is important to keep trying, to do all that we are able on our own, and to be open to help from unexpected sources. Heeding the childlike inclination to befriend instinctual parts of the self—body, intuition, emotions—can enable us to receive help in healing when faced with tasks that cause our rational adult selves to become overwhelmed and turn to stone.

The literal garden path described by Paul Hogan (see chapter 6) gives a further account of how to locate the inner treasures that assist with overwhelming tasks. The physical garden enclosures at the Spiral and Butterfly gardens in Toronto and Sri Lanka each provide a setting of unhurried calm where play is possible. In the garden, Paul listened carefully to the children, then assisted them in expressing themselves in painting, sculpture, costume, and performance. Art expressions ensured that the children could examine what emerged— their own feelings, intuitions, or dreams—in the quiet and playfulness of the garden and opened the possibility for unexpected insights.

With or without an actual garden, anyone can take such a garden path, that is, we can attend to thoughts, feelings, intuitions, or dreams, express these vital experiences, and reflect on what has been expressed with friendly curiosity. One needs first, a garden, a kind of refuge, or "sane asylum," a setting of unhurried calm where one can notice and play with thoughts, feelings, intuitions, dreams. Talking, writing, painting, and other activities ground such inner awarenesses in the outer, physical world of object, image, and action. Like assembling a jigsaw puzzle, the garden process allows the individual to survey and name the inner world, to sort pieces, and gradually to notice promising combinations. Engaging in this process in a sustained way provides openings for the emergence of previously unknown stories of self and others.

Having in mind that she wanted a better life, Susan created a garden for herself, first within the guidance and reassurances offered by mentors such as the psychiatrist and then the art teacher Angela Greig, then later within the understanding that developed as she attended with more openness to her inner life. She began with simple tasks such as exploring her body, attending to the textures of what she touched during her day-to-day life. She talked of her wretchedness to an understanding physician. She learned practices of yoga, tai chi, and drama as means of attending to bodily experiences while learning how to relax and breathe into the physical and emotional discomforts that accompanied the release of buried feelings. She learned ways to hold dream images in mind while observing where her body was responding. She learned the Percept approach to analyzing dreams (see chapter 7). She recorded and painted her dreams. Gradually, she accumulated insights that opened up new possibilities.

Confidence, Relationships, and an Ecology of Healing

First, decide to make a better life. Then, take the garden path. Along the way cultivate three fields: confidence in life's healing capacity, supportive relationships, and an ecology of healing—activities of the mind, body, heart, and spirit that advance one's own life purposes and preferred stories. Here are things to consider about these aspects of healing:

CONFIDENCE IN LIFE'S HEALING CAPACITY. We humans share with other living creatures remarkable capacities to heal. Unfortunately, everyday statements and practices may obscure the healing powers of the body and psyche through stories that emphasize externals, as in "I saw the doctor to get a broken bone fixed," "an infection cured by antibiotics," or "a cancer eliminated by surgery." These stories are unhelpful when they diminish confidence in the healing capacities of one's own body and psyche.

Medical procedures such as diagnosis, laboratory tests, scans, X-rays, surgery, and medication can be very helpful and even necessary but none of these practices actually create healing. The body heals through its own natural processes. A physician or other clinician facilitates healing by investigating injury, disease, or imbalance and offering treatments intended to support the body's regenerative and regulatory functions. When the body's healing systems fail, medical treatments alone cannot produce healing. The doctor sets a broken bone, for example, while the body initiates and governs the processes by which the bone ends knit together and become stronger than before the break occurred. The doctor does not have the power to knit the bones together.

The doctor selects an antibiotic suitable to kill a particular infectious agent, but the body's own immune defences are responsible for overcoming infection and healing. This fact became tragically clear to me when I worked in hospital in the early years of the AIDS epidemic. Antibiotics were helpful in controlling life-threatening infections such as *pneumocystis carinii* pneumonia so long as the person with AIDS was able to sustain overall immune system function above a certain level. When the immune system was critically weakened by HIV infection, antibiotics ceased to be effective and the person died of the secondary infections. The situation with surgical removal of cancerous tissue is the same: the surgeon aims to tip the balance towards recovery, but is relying on the body's own capacity to effect healing following surgery. The surgeon does not have the power to cause bones, organs, blood vessels, connective tissue, muscle, and skin to repair, knit together, and resume functioning. When the individual's own body is unable to complete these tasks, the person dies even if the surgeon successfully removed all diseased tissue.

The psyche has enormous healing capacity in the form of creative imagination and persistent initiatives to engage with the world. Indeed, psychotherapies such as narrative and solution-focused therapies assume that all individuals possess such capacities.[33] Psychoactive medications and psychotherapy, like casts, antibiotics, or surgery, must be understood as providing conditions that facilitate the psyche's natural healing processes. For example, hospital admission and medication alleviated Susan's delusions, terror, and disorganization. The story that she was suffering from schizophrenia, needed extra help, and should continue medication relieved her distress for some time. However, Susan still lived her life and brought forth her world. Moment to moment, day to day, week to week, and year to year, decisions about what she said and did remained her own. Her life was not and could not be created by medication, by health care professionals, by any other person, or by outside intervention.

Vital aspects of Susan's experience were not addressed following her psychotic break, including her inability to reconcile birth control with her Catholic beliefs, difficulties in her marriage, lack of attention to her personal needs, and her interests in art. Neglect of these matters by Susan, her family, and health care professionals, together with the debilitating side effects of medication, eventually led Susan to experience despair and thoughts of suicide. When Susan decided to make her life better, she began to attend to these neglected aspects of her experience. This attention allowed her gradually to set for herself and learn from others the practices that allowed her innate healing capacities to flourish. Physicians, psychotherapists, naturopaths, tai chi instructors, and speech therapists assisted. But the healing capacities of Susan's own psyche—her creativity, her ability to bring forth a world, her initiatives as author and performer of her own story—were critical in enabling their interventions to be effective.

Much can be done to nurture confidence in healing in the midst of emotional disturbance. Susan nurtured her healing capacity by committing to feeling better, becoming aware of her feelings and needs and taking responsibility for her life rather than relying solely on others' advice. Taking more personal responsibility is usually gradual and involves unexpected turns and obstacles. An individual with emotional disturbance who is taking this approach will ask over and over, "What is important to me? What do I know? What can I do? What step can I take right now?" then act on the basis of answers to these questions. Family members, friends, and health professionals will ask themselves similar questions.

Family, friends, and health professionals can nurture the capacity to heal by expressing belief that the person with emotional disturbance has vital knowledge and powers. Words count. Actions speak even louder. Helpful actions include listening carefully, asking the person to make life decisions to the full extent of his or her ability, respecting the person's wishes, and looking for ways in which the person's interests, creativity, skills, temperament, and knowledge may be used as part of the recovery process. The psychiatrist who helped with discontinuing medication nurtured Susan's confidence by listening, encouraging her involvement (e.g., giving her a book on Jungian analysis), affirming that medication was not the answer, and explaining how to discontinue medications safely.

Friends, family, and health professionals must take care that respecting personal self-determination and nurturing a desire to heal does not deteriorate into abandoning the person in distress or into blaming and burdening him or her. Capabilities, vulnerabilities, and circumstances must be considered carefully. In crisis, heightened feelings along with the practical limits to one's ability to help can make it easy to lose a sense of balance. When an individual is highly disorganized, others may need to make decisions on his or her behalf, as was the case for Susan at the time of her psychotic break. However, even in this situation, confidence in the person's capacity to heal can be expressed by treating the person with tact and respect, explaining what steps are being taken and why, and involving the person in decision making as soon as possible. Mutual respect, good judgment, compassion, and cooperation are essential; each individual's needs, wishes, and goals must be reconciled with others' similar claims. However, the potential for benefit more than justifies taking on the challenges inherent in nurturing the distressed individual's desire to have a better life and in helping him or her to exercise personal responsibility and self-determination. Realistic encouragement helps to affirm that we each bring forth a world, and healing flourishes when each individual is respected as the prime author of his or her own story.

SUPPORTIVE RELATIONSHIPS. Because all life is interconnected, healing always occurs in relationship. Relationships make possible exchanges of information, ideas, caring, assistance, and material goods, and by these means form the basis for creating and sustaining a sense of self in the world.[34] Relationships enable us to bring forth a world by giving expression to the story of our lives through what we say and do with one another. Supportive relationships use words and practices that demonstrate mutual respect, open and honest communication, and shared responsibilities and pleasures. Like Susan, many people with emotional disturbance describe caring relationships with individuals who had faith in them as critical to their recovery.[35] An honest and open relationship with a supportive therapist has long been known to be essential to the effectiveness of psychotherapy.[36] Sustained collaborative relationships among individuals and organizations with diverse commitments and expertise —whether it's art, business, fitness, health care, or communications—foster healing for both individuals and community.[37]

The structure and culture of conventional mental health care invited Susan, as it often invites professionals and patients, to accept a story in which relationships are hierarchical and power oriented. Susan's hospital experience illustrates how this occurs. The doctor (or nurse, psychologist, social worker, occupational therapist) is seen by themself and patients as the confident, powerful, infallible expert responsible for maintaining order by making quick, accurate diagnoses and providing effective treatment. Patients are seen by themselves and others as weak, foolish, distressed, and sometimes threatening dependents responsible for "getting well" by following the doctor's orders. Sometimes, the healing potential of the doctor/patient relationship is subverted by administrative procedures that transfer patients from one doctor to another as if people could be sorted like door hinges without regard for human connection.[38]

Both doctors and patients come to disown parts of themselves. Professional staff have difficulty accepting or showing compassion for their own or colleagues' feelings, mistakes, shortcomings, and times of personal vulnerability; staff may have equal difficulty in accepting wisdom, concerns, creativity, strength, confidence, or independence in patients. Patients can become either "good patients" who disown their own knowledge, originality, power, confidence, and autonomy and rely unquestioningly on professional staff for direction, or "bad patients" who rebel unthinkingly against the doctor's orders or become intensely angry or despairing when the doctor makes mistakes or otherwise displays shortcomings. Such relationships undermine healing.

As she healed, Susan continued to use the services of experts in mental health and other fields, but she formed relationships quite differently. She remained clear that she was responsible for her own life and in charge of decisions about what was helpful and what was not. She found health professionals who were able to accept and nurture her healing through mutually respectful and cooperative relationships. She established caring relationships with individuals who were not mental health professionals such as her art teacher and various other mentors. For Susan, as for most individuals with serious emotional disturbance, healing was a series of stages with shifting needs and approaches to nurturing her mind, body, heart, spirit, family life, friendships, and community involvement.

AN ECOLOGY OF HEALING. Because all living systems are interrelated and interdependent, a crisis such as serious emotional disturbance disrupts every sphere of experience—sensation, feeling, thought, action, relationships, and life involvements such as work. The cultivation of activities that incorporate vital experiences and enhance well-being in mind, body, heart, and spirit is essential to healing.

Attending to all realms of life can be described as "holistic." Holistic approaches are widely popular, and the complex interrelations of mind and body have attracted scientific interest and stimulated entire new areas of study, such as psychoneuroimmunology.[39] Years of research on mental illnesses like schizophrenia indicate clearly that such conditions have no single cause and must be understood to result from complex genetic, neurophysiological, psychological, interpersonal, and social interactions; treatments that address multiple spheres are most effective.[40] For just about as many years, mental health professionals have emphasized using a biopsychosocial model to formulate how a particular crisis has developed in any given individual with a particular genetic and physical makeup, unique life experiences, and temperament, unfolding in a specific social, political, economic, cultural, religious, and environmental context.[41] Unfortunately, this conceptual stance is often more aspiration than practice in actual clinics or treatment programs.[42] Symptom investigation, diagnosis, and biological treatments often greatly overshadow all other aspects of mental health assessment and intervention, as Dr. Toner noted in chapter 5 and others have also lamented.[43]

The idea of "holistic" fails, however, to convey the constant interplay that is characteristic of living systems, including personal lives. Scholar and physicist Fritjof Capra suggests the term *ecological* to highlight this dynamic aspect of life:

> "Holistic" is somewhat less appropriate to describe the new paradigm. A holistic view of, say, a bicycle means to see the bicycle as a functional whole and to understand the interdependence of its parts accordingly. An ecological view of the bicycle includes that, but it adds to it the perception of how the bicycle is embedded in its natural and social environment—where the raw materials that went into it came from, how it was manufactured, how its use affects the natural environment and the community by which it is used and so on.[44]

In an ecology of healing, we think not only of body, mind, heart, and spirit functioning within a complex socio-political environment, but also of where we came from prior to serious emotional disturbance, and where we will go after—our life purposes and stories.

Susan had a home, family, and important work to take up on leaving hospital. For those with serious mental illness who lack the basic structures of daily life, that is, a reasonably safe and clean home, food, caring relationships, and meaningful daily activities, establishing these basics is central to healing. Pat Capponi describes eloquently how stigma and poverty dehumanize and torment those struggling to cope with serious, chronic emotional disturbance.[45] In some communities, psychiatric consumer-survivors own and operate businesses that offer work opportunities to those affected by serious emotional disturbance. Spiritual support, community programs, housing, education, and a justice system that seeks to maximize respect for human rights and to minimize interpersonal violence could all contribute to healing from emotional disturbance by constituting an ecology of healing within the broader community.

Susan involved herself in conventional health care, alternative health care, and activities not typically associated with health in any direct way. She saw physicians, speech therapists, and naturopaths and learned the practices of meditation, shiatsu dream work, and tai chi. She entered into conversations of the heart, spent time in nature, taught English as a second language, volunteered in community television, formed new friendships, and studied art, drama, Jungian concepts, and stories. What is important is not what activities Susan undertook (others will make different choices) but rather that personally meaningful activities in varied spheres of life form a personal context—a personal ecology that nurtures healing.

Simmie and Nunes refer to conventional mental health care and alternative sources of help as parallel systems and outline steps that a person coping with emotional disturbance can take to make use of all that both systems have to offer.[46] For example, a wide range of self-help organizations are active in many communities and provide free or low-cost sources of support and knowledge that may be relatively unknown to staff in mental health hospitals or clinics. Many conditions and activities which support healing—for example, gym workouts, continuing learning courses, or volunteer activities—are outside the domain of the mental health system. Indeed, the realms where healing takes place are so vast that it is unrealistic to expect mental health professionals ever to be a sole source of knowledge or guidance. Each individual needs to scout out his or her own potentially helpful activities.

Fortunately, because of the interconnection and interdependence of all aspects of life, steps in one area often lead to positive changes in other areas, even in areas that were not specifically a focus of change. Taking regular walks, for example, can lead to improved sleep which leads to improved energy levels and better mood which makes it easier to think through problems which leads to more enjoyment of relationships which makes it easier to feel motivated to go on walks. Susan's experience that the small step of watering her dying house plant led to the bigger step of seeking out a sympathetic physician demonstrates the principle that is a premise of solution-focused therapy—small changes are generative and lead to further helpful changes.[47] Healing flourishes when an individual forms a personal healing ecology—a system of activities that incorporates vital experiences and nurtures mind, body, heart, and spirit with a view to the individual's own life story and purposes.

A Well-Being, Healing Approach to Mental Health Care

Bodily awareness, emotions, knowledge of her own and family life experiences, dreams, painting, and new relationships were vital experiences which Susan experienced initially as fragmented and lacking in inner connection to one another. Some experiences such as rage seemed to have been long present but split off from consciousness. Other experiences, such as the stories offered by her art-teacher mentor, were new and offered possibilities for understanding self and others. Gradually over a period of years, Susan developed a fuller awareness of the scope of her inner experiences and knit these experiences together to form new webs of meaning and understanding. In time, she organized these experiences and understandings into new stories. She developed a new relationship to herself, a new presence in relationships with others, and a new sense of her place in the world. She created and performed a new story. She brought forth a new world. She healed.

Healing is supported by any and all of a vast array of people and experiences so long as emotional disturbance is approached with an eye to delight where well-being is the highest priority and attention is given to the nurturing of confidence, supportive relationships, and a healing ecology. Mental health services, conventional and otherwise, can be helpful but are not sufficient and for some people, not even necessary to heal. Vital experiences, people, practices, knowledges, and programs grounded in well-being and healing perspectives abound among us all right now. A myriad of approaches nurture healing, in conventional health services such as medication and psychotherapy, in alternative health practices such as meditation, acupuncture, and massage and in activities altogether outside of the health domain such as exercise, storytelling, conversations of the heart, sports, academic studies, business, and artistic activities. We can learn much about healing from areas other than traditional mental health disciplines, such as philosophy, literature, and cultural anthropology and from non-European peoples and cultures who have different understandings of emotional disturbance and appropriate responses.[48]

Some mental health programs embrace a philosophy and practices consistent with a well-being and healing approach and many include professionals who work this way.[49] While no service will lack shortcomings, healing-oriented health providers tend to be better able to avoid the systematic errors and thus the harms that can befall individuals receiving conventional medical-model care. Knowing what to look for and attending to one's own feelings and intuitions about a service can help in locating such programs or practitioners.

Because I am a psychologist and my own healing has led me to question the medical model and to seek alternatives, I have been thinking about how mental health services can support healing in relation to emotional disturbance. In healing-oriented programs, the statements and, more importantly, the *practices* of the staff, the physical facilities, and the program activities should demonstrate a commitment to nurturing confidence in healing, supportive relationships, and an ecology of healing. Healing-oriented services demonstrate concern for the patient's needs, for example, in hours of operation, location, assistance with attending appointments. Often individuals with emotional disturbance can receive services without a professional referral. Psychiatric diagnoses are avoided unless there is a specific need for such services. Efforts are made to encourage client involvement—listening carefully to patient concerns, educating the patient about the available services, and planning interventions with the patient. Efforts are made to consider patient preferences concerning the professionals whom they see and to ensure the continuity of relationships with treating professionals rather than transferring patients from one professional caregiver to another for administrative convenience.

Healing-oriented professionals nurture confidence in the capacity to heal by encouraging personal responsibility and self-determination. How this can be done can be explained by an example from Susan's hospital admission where staff learned something about her abilities and interests. Unfortunately, hospital professionals described Susan's interests in community involvement and art as "obsessions," naming them as indications of pathology. Pursuing these interests may not have been very realistic at a time of emotional crisis, but both Susan and the staff would have gained considerably had the staff looked at her interests with an eye to their healing possibilities. An interest in the community could be understood as a valuing of generosity and responsibility. An interest in art might suggest art therapy as a modality for creative therapeutic work. As Susan felt less overwhelmed, staff could ask more and talk with Susan about whether she wished to pursue these interests in some way as part of her recovery process.

Another way that well-being-oriented professionals encourage confidence in healing is through the clinical interview. An interview is conducted differently when the first priority is to understand and, to the extent possible, address the patient's goals and expectations as opposed to establishing a diagnosis. The doctor can do a great deal to clarify important goals to the patient and to recommend professional expertise in relation to such goals. The patient's talents, interests, and past accomplishments are also carefully investigated and considered. The psychiatrist who helped Susan to decide about medication and to discontinue medication safely is an excellent example of using professional expertise to encourage confidence in healing. If making a diagnosis will likely help to meet important patient goals, then the interview proceeds with the investigations necessary to establish a diagnosis. However, knowing a diagnosis sometimes contributes little to important patient goals, so a diagnostic interview is not the invariably appropriate clinical investigation.

Well-being-oriented practitioners will offer psychotherapy in a framework that has been adapted or developed to foster healing. Most psychotherapeutic approaches can be adapted to incorporate the valuing of well-being and the nurturing of confidence in healing, supportive relationships, and a healing ecology.[50] As well, recent new approaches to psychotherapy explicitly incorporate elements consistent with healing-oriented approaches into theory and clinical practice, emphasizing for example, the encouragement of self-determination, the positive use of power, how to avoid "power-over" relationships, how relationships influence the sense of self, the role of story in psychological change, and the premise that small changes generate larger changes. Examples are relational therapy,[51] narrative therapy,[52] and solution-focused therapy.[53]

As Helen Porter and Gail Regan pointed out, practitioners need to engage in their own healing and know their own stories in order to support others' well-being and healing. Life is such that we all have occasions for healing. Who among us has not faced loss, deceit, confusion, ugliness, betrayal, cruelty, shame, fear, and despair? When we face adversity with healing commitment it can be transformed into wisdom and compassion, the qualities essential to allow the practitioner—indeed all of us—to support the healing of individuals who experience emotional disturbance. When we know our own stories of healing, we are able to move away from the "we/they" attitudes and towards the sense of "this could be my story" that Gail Regan identifies as the basis for "all of us as a community building what the community needs."

Healing-oriented practitioners and programs nurture an ecology of healing by recognizing their services as one of many and maintaining collaborative relationships with other professionals. Practitioners assist patients in using community and professional resources, including but not restricted to psychiatric and medical services; practitioners assist each patient in deciding what best meets his or her needs and goals. Bulletin boards, libraries, internet access, or other facilities may help the patient to take an active role in finding relevant information. The valuing of activities that nurture mind, body, heart, and spirit may be evident in the information provided, the quality of conversations, or in activities such as food preparation that encourages healthy eating; sports or exercise equipment or opportunities for creative expression are also important. A healing-oriented approach will consider the individual's situation in relation to adequate food and housing, personal safety, general health, access to education, meaningful work, and adequate pay. Efforts are made to investigate and respond to potential difficulties related to social class, financial circumstances, culture, immigration experiences, language, racism, trauma, gender role, homophobia, gender identification, disability, and religious prejudices.

Well-being- and healing-oriented mental health care is distinctive also in its organizational structure, policies, practices, and relationships to the broader community because it is difficult for individual practitioners to sustain healing-oriented services without a broader organizational commitment to this approach. Well-being and healing must be given primacy at every level of planning and decision making, from statements of mission and values to strategic planning, policy development, and implementation, hiring and resource allocation; consumer/survivors and community members should be involved at all levels to assist in ensuring the programs are accountable to those whom they are intended to serve and to the larger community. Programs need to nurture confidence in healing, supportive relationships, and an ecology of healing, both among staff within the program and in links to other mental health services and broader community life—business, schools, recreational facilities, and the arts. For example, organizations and programs can, benefit enormously from engagement in visual arts, music, drama, and ritual, as Helen Porter's storytelling and Paul Hogan's gardens demonstrate. Health professionals, mental health agencies, and hospitals can support businesses run by psychiatric survivors by using the services of these businesses whenever possible.

Finally, well-being and healing practices need not be confined to mental health services. Several Toronto productions exemplify the healing potential of socially engaged art, including Susan's 1994 play *My Old Movie of Dreams* and her *Shedding Skins* paintings installed in the lobby of the Centre for Addiction and Mental Health. *Survivors in Search of a Voice*, a 1995 exhibit at the Royal Ontario Museum, consisted of works created by well-known Canadian visual artists following discussions with women who had breast cancer concerning the impact of this illness on their lives. *Not by the Book*, a 1995 video program produced by TVOntario, tells stories of schizophrenia, depression, and bi-polar disorders and was created as a collaboration among the Derosier dance company, patients, and their families. Initiatives such as these bring the vital experiences of well-being and healing from the personal to the larger community sphere. As chapter 6 discusses, such socially engaged art offers the opportunity for individual distress, injury, and disability to be experienced not as matters evoking pity, shame, or secrecy but rather as opportunities for extending the ecology of healing by furthering understanding, growth, and interconnection within both individuals and the broader community.

The Proven Benefits of the Well-Being and Healing Approach

All individuals experiencing emotional disturbance can benefit from a well-being and healing approach. However, I would like to discuss serious mental illness in greater detail because Susan's difficulties were of this type and because public and professionals alike often regard the prospects as hopeless for those who experience psychotic symptoms, severe depression, or hospital admission. Many believe, as Susan did in the years after her hospital admission, that serious mental illness is invariably chronic, irreversible, and degenerative. However, scientific findings indicate otherwise and individual experiences vary greatly even among those with the same initial problems or diagnoses.[54]

What I am describing in this approach has many similarities to psychosocial rehabilitation and competency-based approaches that have been in use to some degree for many years.[55] For example, according to Coursey, Alford, and Safarjan, a traditional approach to serious mental illness relies on a disease-based, medical model where individuals seeking help and their families are viewed as pathological, dysfunctional, helpless, uninformed, and passive; health providers are authoritarian and focused on a narrow triad of hospital, medication, and psychotherapy services for all patients.[56] The traditional approach is contrasted with an emerging perspective using a health-based, bio-psychosocial competency model with attention to multiple potentially helpful forms of assistance, including both traditional treatments and other supports such as life skills, income, housing, and self-help groups. In this perspective, individuals seeking help and their families are viewed in terms of competency, strengths, and active participation; health providers foster respectful, egalitarian, cooperative relationships where varied, flexible, and coordinated interventions are used to enhance the coping skills and abilities of clients and families. Coursey and his colleagues note that a critical aspect of moving towards the competency approach is a shift in values, attitudes, and roles among both health professionals and individuals with serious mental illness.

Competency-based, psychosocial rehabilitation or recovery approaches can lead to quite positive outcomes even for individuals seriously disabled by mental illness.[57] A well-known example is a large scale study that investigated outcomes for individuals released from state mental hospitals in Maine and Vermont. The researchers were interested in what happened to individuals diagnosed with chronic schizophrenia and residing in state hospital "back wards." Like Susan's uncle Leo Regan (see Appendix II, fig. 1, pp. 241–42), these individuals had been deemed incapable of living in the community and would likely have spent their entire lives in institutional care but for the advent of new psychoactive medications and shifts in government policy. Mental health policy mandated the "deinstitutionalization" of such patients in the 1950s and 1960s. The Vermont and Maine study groups were quite similar in terms of the length of their hospital admissions, severity of their psychiatric diagnoses, and their gender and age. Upon hospital release, individuals in both groups received access to government financial assistance and psychoactive medication. No further services were offered to the Maine group. However, individuals in the Vermont group were also provided with a biopsychosocial rehabilitation program that was in place for ten years (1955–1965) with a multidisciplinary professional team. The Vermont rehabilitation program focused on patient well-being and competencies as a basis for providing individualized treatment planning and follow-up; staff assisted former hospital patients with housing, vocational training, educational programs, social skills training, and social supports.

In the 1980s, researchers located and interviewed these former Maine and Vermont state mental hospital patients. The individuals were interviewed on average thirty-two years after their first hospital admission for mental illness. Recovery or significant improvement was defined as an individual experiencing nothing worse than "some mild symptoms (e.g., depressive mood or mild insomnia) or some difficulties in several areas of functioning, but generally functioning pretty well, has some meaningful relationships and most untrained people would not consider him sick."[58] In Maine, 48 percent of the former state hospital patients were significantly improved or fully recovered from their serious mental illness by the 1980s. This figure clearly challenges the commonly held belief that individuals with schizophrenia or other serious mental illnesses suffer from a condition that is inevitably irreversible and permanently disabling.

To evaluate the possibility that an improved diagnostic system could better identify patients with schizophrenia and thus poor prognosis, a further study carefully evaluated Vermont patients' past medical records to identify individuals who could be diagnosed with schizophrenia using *DSM-III* criteria, the most advanced system available at the time the study was conducted. However, even among the group identified as suffering from schizophrenia using this more stringent approach to diagnosis, one-half to two-thirds showed a long-term outcome characterized by "and evolution into various degrees of productivity, social involvement, wellness and competent functioning." [59]

In Vermont with its comprehensive biopsychosocial rehabilitation program, former state hospital patients showed an even more striking rate of improvement; between 62 and 68 percent of the former patients were fully recovered and showed no signs at all of mental illness in the 1980s. About half of these former patients continued to use psychoactive medications either regularly or when needed and half took no medications of this type at all. The results of these studies are consistent with those reported from several other longitudinal studies of individuals with schizophrenia.[60] With sustained, well-being- and healing-oriented help, the majority of those with serious mental illness were able to make remarkable improvement and many recovered completely.

In reflecting on what supports healing among individuals with serious mental illness, Harding, Zubin, and Strauss discuss the importance of seeing the essentially well person behind the disorder rather than allowing the disturbance and disorganization associated with times of crisis and poor functioning to define the person in his or her entirety.[61] This perspective guided the successful 1955–1965 psychosocial rehabilitation program in Vermont. George Brooks, a clinician central to that program, identified four key factors: "Drugs relieved the anguish and fevered mental activity. People were trusted and hence expected to be capable. Goals (jobs, homes, companions) were an experience of new hope for many. People were allowed, even encouraged, to show compassion (aide to patient, patient to patient, patient to aide)."[62]

What was healing for chronically disabled psychiatric patients in Vermont was the same as what was healing for Susan following her psychotic break, namely, giving priority to well-being and the nurturing of healing capacity, supportive relationships, and a healing ecology.

Of course, some individuals are unable to overcome serious mental illness and many simply learn to live with certain recurring difficulties. In the Vermont study group, those who were functioning well included individuals who continued to experience hallucinations or delusions but had learned to control these experiences or not to tell others.[63'] Such accommodation is comparable to learning to live with chronic medical conditions such as arthritis or diabetes. Even in favourable circumstances, healing is, as Susan's story demonstrates, a long and gradual process requiring persistent effort over some years. At times, we choose the difficult process of healing because the only alternative, unremitting hopelessness and disability, is worse. Yet even when emotional disturbance is chronic, attention to well-being and healing is always possible and desirable.

Despite the documented effectiveness of well-being and healing approaches, many individuals in developed countries now receive mental health services within essentially the same limited approach that characterized Susan's experiences thirty to forty years ago. Conventional medical-model care remains the basic organizational chassis. In fact, *Science*, the prestigious journal of the American Association for the Advancement of Science, reports that care emphasizing healing and well-being appears to be more available to people with mental illness who live in developing countries than to those living in countries such as Canada and the United States.[64] A recent article describes patients at the Schizophrenia Research Foundation (SCARF) program in Chennai, India, making chalk sticks, sturdy shopping bags, dolls, and candles for sale at local shops and taking part in Hindu religious observances. Despite the greater availability of psychiatrists in developed countries, "a long string of studies beginning with WHO's [World Health Organization] International Pilot Study of Schizophrenia, launched in 1967, have reported that patients in India and other developing countries are more likely to have long-term remission of symptoms and fewer relapses than patients in the developed world."[65]

The *Science* report attributes these positive outcomes to the greater availability in developing countries of mental health programs emphasizing work, family, and community, as well as providing medication. Such care is noted to be available only to a minority of individuals with mental illness in the United States. Coursey and colleagues write that, although the psychosocial competency approach is implemented in some American states, "much remains aspirational rather than operational;" the same could be said for Canada.[66]

The Recovery Movement

Although I was unaware of these developments until recently, the healing and well-being approach that I am describing is also very much in keeping with the recovery approach to emotional crisis that has emerged within the mental health consumer/survivor movement.[67] At an International Recovery Perspectives Conference held in Toronto in November 2006, Susan and I learned of a vibrant and creative international collaboration propelled by individuals who have experienced emotional crisis and the unhelpful or harmful effects of conventional medical-model care. These individuals with first-hand knowledge are essential to involve in the reorganizing of our approaches to emotional crisis.[68]

Confusion sometimes surrounds the word *recovery*. One sense of this word is restoration to a previous level of functioning. This definition, however, excludes individuals with serious mental illness who do not experience such restoration. Recovery can also be described as "living well in the presence or absence of mental illness" and understood to encourage an individual to assume increasing control over his or her own psychiatric condition, while reclaiming responsibility for his or her own life, particularly when life has been subsumed by the illness or taken over by others.[69] In this sense, recovery fits most closely a dictionary definition of "obtaining usable substances from unusable sources," and typically involves acceptance of the illness, a sense of hope, and a renewed sense of self.[70]

The tasks of recovery include renewing hope and commitment, redefining self, incorporating illness, being involved in meaningful activities, overcoming stigma, assuming control, becoming empowered, exercising citizenship, managing symptoms, and being supported by others.[71] For mental health professionals, use of a recovery approach requires an expanded vision of the nature and purpose of care, including what is considered possible for the person with emotional disturbance and the person's own role in pursuing those possibilities.[72] This expanded vision emphasizes the individual reclaiming a life in the community rather than waiting to find a treatment that eliminates symptoms.

The recovery perspective moves significantly beyond the ideas of the psychosocial competency approach. Recovery emphasizes the importance of self-determination for individuals experiencing emotional disturbance and argues for involving consumer/survivors at every organizational level in the development and administration of mental health care systems. Such participation is essential to propelling broad change and to keeping policies, funding, and programs accountable to the people they are intended to help. The recovery movement has, in many places, developed innovative programs where consumer/survivors provide support and services to one another rather than relying exclusively on services provided by credentialed professionals. Such programs can improve the scope and effectiveness of support offered to people affected by emotional disturbance. As well, the recovery movement argues for organizing social and economic environments to support the functioning of people with emotional disturbance, much as we have devoted design and construction resources to making streets, buildings, and transportation accessible to persons with physical disabilities; supportive social environments include adequate income, decent housing, and meaningful employment.[73] Such changes move our responses to emotional disturbance away from the narrow individual focus and towards more ecological and community perspectives. In Marilyn French's words, we can choose to create a world fit for humans.

Significant initiatives are under way in New Zealand, Canada, the United States, and England to ensure that a recovery model is widely understood and used at every level of mental health care from the most senior policy levels to the day-to-day.[74] In 2006, the Canadian Senate Standing Committee on Social Affairs, Science, and Technology released a comprehensive report on mental illness, government policy, and funding that provides a compelling summary of the problems faced by those suffering from emotional disturbance. It recommends the recovery model as the basis for mental health reform in Canada and describes the law, policy, and funding arrangements that could support implementation of this model.[75]

The recovery movement offers great hope for the transformation of our understanding of emotional disturbance and the organization of individual, family, professional, and community response. Susan's artistic work and this book thus join the work of others committed to bring forth a world with an emphasis on well-being and healing and with a deep respect for the healing capacity, interconnectedness, and interdependence of all life.

Working with "an Eye to Delight"

Working with an eye to power was, for me, a continual effort to perfect performances of stories that originated outside of myself, whether as successful professional or passionate activist. While my performances drew accolades, I worried about being more or less a fraud as I scrutinized the reactions of actual or imagined audiences. What I appreciate most about choosing pleasure as a central life priority is the moral authority to author a story originating from a deeper level of inner experience. I was always free to take such authority. I have, like Susan, enjoyed the great privileges conferred by middle-class status, white race, professional education, and financial security. However, like Susan, I believed that my particular inner wounds could be soothed only through excellent performances of the stories that were grounded in others' expectations rather than in the satisfactions of my own body, mind, heart, or spirit. Because others' responses are outside of my control, leaving my sense of worth in "their" hands was an inherently flawed life strategy.

Unhappiness and emotional depletion helped me to slow my pace of work and to turn within to understand what I valued most deeply. Fortunately, I practised a profession deeply meaningful to me in many ways, what Thomas Moore describes as work of the soul.[76] Independent practice was an obvious possibility. I do not believe that well-being or healing can be achieved by simple or rote solutions and what worked for me may be wrong for others. Each individual has to proceed with consideration for the requirements of his or her own inner drama. While leaving a large organization helped me to realize my power to author my own story and to heal, staying in such a work setting is just as powerful when the decision is made in the context of commitment to well-being and healing. I left hospitals with great respect for the many professionals and programs that use a well-being and healing approach when the strains of institutional *realpolitik* often pull for different values.

As I planned to leave the hospital to develop a community practice, I tried to remain aware of my power to bring forth a world by focusing on what would be my ideal work situation in terms of specifics such as location, hours, income, focus, and variety and in terms of generalities such as engagement in social change, personal growth, and intellectual engagement. Some of these matters I could influence directly and in other areas, I could only keep my goals in mind and watch for opportunities. At times, opportunities came that I could never have anticipated and that far exceeded my hopeful expectations.

Committing to a better life freed me to create a new story of my work. I deeply appreciate my hospital experiences and in my current practice I make constant use of what I learned. I am also far more certain about what values and practices I do not wish to perform or support. These are positive legacies of my years as a hospital psychologist. I now pursue work opportunities that allow me to use my professional expertise to advance social justice initiatives like the civil rights of lesbians, gay men, and their children, and legal and policy recognition of the detrimental impact of harassment, violence, and sexual violation. Such projects are positive legacies of my experiences as a lesbian and feminist.

However, by far the most significant part of my new story of work has to do with what I now know about where I stand in the world—self-knowledge that is a legacy of both hospital and lesbian-feminist experiences. Valuing well-being and healing above career advancement and prestige has helped me to slow down and enabled more depth and complexity in my work. I try to help individuals in distress to feel and function better. I listen carefully for the individual's life stories and try to locate vital experiences, the inner drama, and the new story possibilities. I encourage the bringing forth of a world based on rich and respectful human relationships, creative self-expression, and meaningful commitments. I seek out work where I believe that my time, energy, and expertise may nurture what I value in the world. My work "output" has diminished in terms of institutional measures such as number of clients seen, papers published, presentations given, committees chaired, staff supervised, and budgets administered. However, I have greater satisfaction and more confidence in what I do.

The commitments that changed my work life have also furthered my personal healing. I am not spared the usual human quota of ignorance (my own and others'), frustration, doubt, fear, shame, discouragement, and sadness; these offer daily opportunities to learn to live more deeply. I am far from feeling this particular healing adventure is concluded and struggle with many unanswered questions. Despite a rich network of friends and colleagues, I feel somewhat lonely and disconnected from more public discourses. What do I want in the way of more formal means of working with others? How do I want to engage in art and ritual in my life? What rituals are meaningful to me? The prince, you recall, has not yet arrived.

Yet despite cares and confusions, my life is on track. Susan's story of woundedness and healing parallels my own at deep psychic levels; our work together has furthered my healing because I have been able to go within, locate and describe vital experiences, reflect, and consider reorganizing relationships. Likewise, the story of each client, colleague, and project in my work life in one way or another becomes part of my own inner healing drama. Just as working with Susan to produce this book has advanced both her healing and my own, so work with each client, colleague, and project helps both myself and others to form new stories, to bring forth a new world, to heal. I feel increasingly confident in giving myself over to this process. My work feels deeply satisfying and life affirming for both myself and others.

● ● ●

Case Study
Dr. Barnes 2007

In late September 2007, Ms. Schellenberg phones my office and says she was released from hospital the week before; her psychiatrist, Dr. Medmodel, who now works at Merged Health Sciences Centre, remembered me from Women's College Hospital and suggested she contact me about psychotherapy. Her husband has workplace health benefits that cover most of the cost of psychological services. Am I a licensed psychologist? she asks. This is necessary for her to obtain reimbursement from the insurance company. Do I have appointments available? She can meet only on Wednesday or Thursday mornings, when she has care for her young children.

I see Ms. Schellenberg at 10 o'clock on a Wednesday morning in my pleasant, carpeted office, furnished with comfortable chairs upholstered in a warm gold, rose, and green floral-patterned fabric. A large window provides a view of the small shops and businesses along the street outside. I am wearing pants, a cotton knit top, a jacket, and comfortable laced shoes. I begin the appointment by explaining what we will do.

"When I meet with someone whom I have not seen before, the first couple of meetings are for me to ask in some detail about what is concerning you and to get some background information so that we can decide what will be most helpful. If we decide to continue for psychotherapy, we will make a plan that includes the goals, appointment schedule, and length of time that we will meet." I explain that information Ms. Schellenberg shares with me is confidential, but that under certain circumstances that may not apply in her situation, I am required to share information even without the permission of the person I am seeing. If necessary, I will alert appropriate authorities where I am concerned about the risk of children being abused, when I am concerned about an immediate danger to people's physical safety, where other health professionals have acted in a sexually inappropriate way, or if required by a court to disclose information. I explain that I am a member of a regulated health profession and thus subject to having my practice audited and files reviewed by the College of Psychologists of Ontario. I also explain that I meet regularly with a group of other psychologists, and sometimes discuss information about clients without names or identifying information in order to receive suggestions from my colleagues about how to improve my clinical work.

I ask if Ms. Schellenberg has any questions or concerns about any of these areas. She is looking down at her lap and says quietly, "I am not going to harm my children."

"Has there been something that has brought this to mind for you recently?" I ask.

"At the hospital," says Ms. Schellenberg, "Dr. Medmodel said he was concerned that I might harm my children."

"Do you know why Dr. Medmodel brought this up?" I am feeling a little worried as I try to recall the questions to ask to evaluate the risk for child abuse—this issue rarely comes up in my practice with adults.

"He asked about whether I thought of harming the children when I went through the bad time recently," Ms. Schellenberg says.

"Did you find yourself thinking about harming the children during that time?" I ask.

"No."

"Have you ever considered doing something to hurt one of the children? Or actually hurt one of them?"

"No."

I ask if she discussed this matter with hospital staff. "I told them that I would not harm the children," she says. I point out that I am obligated to notify child protective services only if I feel that there is a significant risk that she will harm the children, but that I cannot see that there is such a risk from what she is telling me. I say that if I feel that she is having a problem in that regard, I will try to help her to find a means to address the problem and would involve child protective services only if we can find no other means to ensure the children's safety.

Later in the interview, I talk with Ms. Schellenberg in detail about what occurred at the time of the psychotic break and how she managed the children during that time; she mentions bringing them to the retreat and the help of the nanny. Although the experience was likely puzzling to the children, they do not seem to have been placed in any danger. I ask Ms. Schellenberg if she has ever heard voices telling her to harm one of the children. She has not. I ask about how she disciplines the children when they misbehave and what she does when she feels frustrated with one of the children. She describes reprimanding the children when they have done something wrong, asking them to go to their rooms if they disregard what she is saying, or taking away toys or privileges. When she feels very frustrated, she asks the nanny to look after the children while she does something else for a time. I explain that I can see no reason to feel concerned that she will harm her children and ask her if she knows why Dr. Medmodel might have been concerned for the children's safety or if he ever mentioned notifying the Children's Aid Society.

By this point in the interview, we have a reasonably good rapport. Ms. Shellenberg says that Dr. Medmodel did not mention the Children's Aid Society. She thinks over my question, then comments, "It may have been an answer that I put on one of the psychological tests." I ask further and she explains her fear for the children's safety due to traffic on the neighbourhood street and the lack of locks on the back doors of the car. I decide that there was perhaps a misunderstanding between Dr. Medmodel and Ms. Schellenberg, but ask her permission to obtain a copy of her hospital records as a final check on the safety of the children. Ms. Schellenberg agrees and signs a release form.

At a second meeting, I spend more time asking about Ms. Schellenberg's background and symptoms. I ask if she and her husband continue the walks they began at the hospital or whether some other activity might enable her to exercise regularly. I ask Ms. Schellenberg what she sees ahead for herself and what she would like to do in her life over the next several years. She mentions how much she loves her husband and children, her concern for them given her recent hospitalization, and her wanting to be a good wife and mother. I ask if she would like for us to discuss what is involved for her in being a good mother and wife and how best to care for her husband and children. She agrees that this would be helpful, and we arrange a series of meetings.

I feel excited about our coming conversations. Ms. Schellenberg is thoughtful, interested in her life, and able to reflect on her experiences. I look forward to learning about her understanding of what it means to be a good wife and mother, how she decides what is best for her children and husband, and whether she has ever been unable to care for them as she wished when she was unable to care for herself. I am interested in whether her recent difficulties interfered with her being a wife and mother and in what steps she has found helpful in minimizing such interference. I am interested in what values and experiences have led her to devote time to volunteer work and how she makes decisions about allocating time to various commitments. I feel that discussing these matters will likely bring up other issues and lead to further helpful conversations. If I find reason to be concerned about the medications that Ms. Schellenberg takes, I will refer her for a second opinion to Dr. Relational, a community practice psychiatrist who is knowledgeable about serious mental illness and shares my outlook on well-being and healing.

I feel hopeful that our conversations can clarify what is precious to Ms. Schellenberg and thus improve her ability to live in a manner in keeping with her values and with care for her own well-being. I feel confident that she will have important and creative ideas concerning these matters, and that I will not need to be solely responsible for devising a resolution for her concerns. I look forward to asking about others in Ms. Schellenberg's life who share her values and to find out how her commitments to husband and children affect the lives of others who are important to her. I greatly enjoy such conversations, and at the end of a working day find myself tired but with a full heart.

● ● ●

The Latest Story

Psychologist Laura Brown draws on her Jewish heritage to describe concerns about contemporary professional practice that are roughly parallel to those I have described in this book.[77] She tells the story of the prophet Ezekiel being taken by God and instructed to prophesy over a valley of dry bones and stone hearts. The bones and stones, she relates, represent the people of Israel who at the time of Ezekiel were survivors of war and captivity; they had seen the destruction of all that meant most to them and been forced into a foreign land as slaves. They suffered devastating trauma and loss; they experienced emotional numbing and disconnection, extreme fear and hopelessness, loss of a sense of identity and of their place on the earth. Brown argues that psychologists, and indeed all of us, enter the valley and become dry bones and stone hearts in a foreign land when we become disconnected from the values that nurture life and healing.

Brown describes professional work that gives greatest priority to social justice, to what I call healing and well-being, as work that leads away from the valley of dry bones towards the identification of vital experiences, life-affirming interconnection, and genuine human encounters. She finds this kind of professional practice falls within the tradition of *tikkun olam*, a term from Jewish ethical thought. Tikkun olam refers to the paramount moral obligation to save one human life as the most effective step to save the entire world, "the healing of the world, through the healing of the one human life in front of them at that moment."[78] Brown points out that tikkun olam, the saving of life, involves not just the flesh-and-blood body, but also the individual's core emotional vitality, the individual's confidence in his or her own voice and place in human community on the earth. She calls for professionals to resist the statements and practices, the core valuing of power, that undermine our ability to practise tikkun olam—the healing of the individual and the world.

Like Brown, I feel that my work is tikkun olam, a sacred means of healing myself, others, and the world. Brown's paper was based on a talk given to psychologists, so it focuses heavily on professional practice. However, I feel confident that the ethical tradition in which she situates her work is not confined to professional practice but widely applicable to all. In the Biblical story, God instructs Ezekiel to speak to the dry bones and stone hearts of a hopeful and healing vision so that the bones can come together, be covered again with sinews and flesh, and filled with the spirit of life. The wounded people were to be healed, reconnected, made human, returned home. Whenever any of us nurture the human capacity to heal, to recover life in body, mind, heart, and spirit, to reconnect, we practise tikkun olam, the sacred work that restores life and furthers the healing of the world.

We are all entrenched in bringing forth a world where power to dominate inner and outer nature is often prized as the greatest human purpose; few, if any, of us can imagine a life, a world, that gives primacy to other deeply meaningful life purposes.[79] Like Susan when she began, we must turn within to find what we value most deeply, then use these values as guides to create stories of life with one another and the earth that is our home. Just as Susan did not know where such a commitment would take her, so we cannot know where we will find ourselves individually and collectively when we choose to live with an eye to delight. Still, I feel much more whole and at peace knowing that I and we have the power—and it will be a pleasure—to follow Susan along the garden path of healing.

SUSAN
The View from Here

Although past experience tells me it is unlikely that I could have properly heard or followed all the threads of Rosemary's explanations about well-being and healing at the time of my psychiatric hospital admission, I am convinced that the tone and care intended in her words would have immediately registered in more helpful and hopeful ways than what I actually experienced. My ability to say this with certainty is rooted in a writing process that involved the reliving of and healing from my psychiatric experience that access to my psychiatric hospital records allowed.

It was like striking gold to find in those records a psychological report that validated how my childhood history of sexual trauma had been projected onto me as a "cauldron of snakes"; however, the same records' multiple opinions that the snakes needed a long-term lid held down with psychoactive drugs illustrated a system divorced from healing.

The work of healing spared me the illusion that psychiatrists could have cleared the roots of my psychosis core because the essence of healing is learning how it is ultimately one's job to arrive at those roots as well as to creatively transform one's wounds. But I do believe that the non gender-biased, less belittling, more story-oriented healing approaches to mental illness crisis and aftercare that Rosemary outlines would have inspired me to act in my own best interest sooner rather than to submit passively, as I did, to my actual diagnosis and treatment.

Had a psychiatrist and I worked as a team from an ecological story perspective, our shared goal to uncover the story behind the psychosis would have empowered me and lessened my exposure to traumatic physical and psychological outcomes. These benefits in turn would have set the stage for my former husband and I to move through a less conflicted and prolonged marriage breakup and offered greater protection for our children's lives and well-being than my actual psychiatric treatment did.

My psychiatric caregivers never did encourage or empower me to commit to healing. Yet the following universal truth about the power of commitment as stated by Scottish mountaineer W.H. Murray rang like truth to me the second I committed to healing my mind and body and to painting a record of my dreams as I healed:

> Until one is committed, there is hesitancy, the chance to draw back, always ineffectiveness. Concerning all acts of initiative (and creation), there is one elementary truth that ignorance of which kills countless ideas and splendid plans: that

the moment one definitely commits oneself, then Providence moves too. All sorts of things occur to help one that would never otherwise have occurred. A whole stream of events issues from the decision, raising in one's favour all manner of unforeseen incidents and meetings and material assistance, which no man could have dreamed would have come his way.[80]

My idea of an improved mental health care system would most definitely include facilities where fostering and encouraging commitments to heal is an expectation not just for the mentally ill but for all who work in the field of psychiatry and mental health.

Conclusion

The soul's language is image. The painted dream image in my case forged missing links to trust of self and life that my mother had been unable to give me. With artistic expression, the unconscious material locked in my body's matter (Latin *mater*, meaning "mother"), slowly evolved into healing as well as an awareness that healing of self is inseparable from the healing of the planet, our Great Mother Earth.

As an artist, I see how the written and painted dream journey that helped me to reconcile the split-off parts of myself echoes the larger current needs of the world. The incidence of collective alienation, of being split off from self and others, which manifests in escalating global violence, the dishonouring of children, the lack of spirit in institutions, political corruption, and destruction of the environment speaks of our collective need to heal inner/outer partnerships and find the global will to commit to wholeness.

My hope for my story and dream art is that they contribute to contemporary meditations on what it means to heal and encourage greater trust in the power of healing commitments among mental illness sufferers and their carers. The passion and size of this hope are best expressed for me in the following Raymond Carver poem:

> And did you get what
> you wanted from this life, even so?
> I did.
> And what did you want?
> To call myself beloved, to feel myself
> beloved on the earth. [81]

Notes

1 These theories are summarized in the following sources: Jill Freedman and Gene Combs, *Narrative Therapy: The Social Construction of Preferred Realities* (New York: W.W. Norton, 1996); Robert A. Neimeyer and Jonathan D. Raskin, eds., *Constructions of Disorder* (Washington, DC: American Psychological Association, 2000).

2 See the following for examples of such critiques: Richard P. Bentall, ed., *Reconstructing Schizophrenia* (New York: Routledge, 1990); Peter R. Breggin, *Toxic Psychiatry* (New York: St. Martin's, 1991); Thomas Szasz, *The Myth of Mental Illness* (New York: Harper and Row, 1974); Thomas Szasz, *Schizophrenia: The Sacred Symbol of Psychiatry* (Syracuse University Press, 1988); and Philip Thomas, *The Dialectics of Schizophrenia* (New York: Free Association, 1997).

3 The work of these scientists is summarized in Fritjof Capra, *The Web of Life* (Toronto: Anchor, 1996).

4 Capra, *Web of Life*, 270.

5 Freedman and Combs, *Narrative Therapy*; Neimeyer and Raskin, *Constructions of Disorder*.

6 Neimeyer and Raskin, *Constructions of Disorder*.

7 For development of this argument in the mental health field, see Freedman and Combs, *Narrative Therapy*; Neimeyer and Raskin, *Constructions of Disorder*; and Michael White and David Epston, *Narrative Means to Therapeutic Ends* (New York: W.W. Norton, 1990).

8 Jonathan D. Raskin and Adam M. Lewandowski, "The Construction of Disorder as a Human Enterprise," in *Constructions of Disorder*, ed. Robert A. Neimeyer and Jonathan D. Raskin (Washington, DC: American Psychological Association, 2000), 19.

9 Marilyn French, *Beyond Power: On Women, Men and Morals* (New York: Ballantine, 1985).

10 Ibid., 342.

11 See, for example, Breggin, *Toxic Psychiatry*; Phyllis Chesler, *Women and Madness* (New York: Avon, 1972); French, *Beyond Power*; and Szasz, *Myth of Mental Illness*.

12 French, *Beyond Power*, 382.

13 See, for example, Persimmon Blackbridge and Sheila Gilhooly, *Still Sane* (Vancouver: Press Gang, 1985); Breggin, *Toxic Psychiatry*; Bonnie Burstow and Don Weitz, eds., *Shrink Resistant: The Struggle against Psychiatry in Canada* (Vancouver: New Star, 1988); Chesler, *Women and Madness*; Wendy Funk, *What Difference Does It Make? (The Journey of a Soul Survivor)* (Cranbrook, BC: Wild Flower, 1998); Courtney R. Harding, Joseph Zubin, and John S. Strauss "Chronicity in Schizophrenia: Revisited," *British Journal of Psychiatry* 161 (suppl. 18) (1992): 27–37; Irit Shimrat, ed., *Call Me Crazy: Stories from the Mad Movement* (Vancouver: Press Gang, 1997); Szasz, *Myth of Mental Illness*; and Thomas, *Dialectics of Schizophrenia*. A particularly excellent account of the historical and philosophical roots of conventional psychiatric practice is provided by Patrick Bracken and Philip Thomas, *Postpsychiatry: Mental Health in a Postmodern World* (Oxford: Oxford University Press, 2005).

14 French, *Beyond Power*.

15 Ibid., 320–21.

16 Laura S. Brown, "The Private Practice of Subversion Psychology as Tikkun Olam," *American Psychologist* 52 (1997): 449–62.

17 French, *Beyond Power*, 323.

18 See, for example, Thomas Berry, *The Dream of the Earth* (San Francisco: Sierra Club, 1988); Capra, *Web of Life*; Suzi Gablik, *The Reenchantment of Art* (New York: Thames and Hudson, 1991); Jane Jacobs, *The Nature of Economies* (Toronto: Random House, 2000); Thomas Moore, *Care of the Soul* (New York: HarperCollins, 1992); Rosemary Ruether, *Gaia and God: An Ecofeminist Theology of Earth Healing* (New York: HarperCollins, 1992); and

Martin E.P. Seligman and Mihaly Csikszentmihalyi, "Positive Psychology," *American Psychologist* 55 (2000): 5–14.

19 French, *Beyond Power.*

20 Ibid.

21 Ibid.

22 Ibid., 542.

23 Ibid.

24 Capra, *Web of Life.*

25 Jacobs, *Nature of Economies.*

26 Ruether, *Gaia and God.*

27 Berry, *Dream of the Earth.*

28 Seligman and Csikszentmihalyi, "Positive Psychology," 5.

29 Moore, *Care of the Soul*, xi.

30 Gablik, *Reenchantment of Art.*

31 Gablik, *Reenchantment of Art*, 177–78, 181.

32 Capra, *Web of Life.*

33 See, for example, Freedman and Combs, *Narrative Therapy*; John L. Walter and Jane E. Peller, *Becoming Solution-Focused in Brief Therapy* (New York: Brunner/Mazel, 1992); and White and Epston, *Narrative Means to Therapeutic Ends.*

34 Narrative therapy and relational theory are examples of accounts explaining the development of self within relationship. See, for example,White and Epston, *Narrative Means to Therapeutic Ends*; Freedman and Combs, *Narrative Therapy*; Michael White, *Narrative Practice and Exotic Lives: Resurrecting Diversity in Everyday Life* (Adelaide, South Australia: Dulwich Centre, 2004); Michael White, *Maps of Narrative Practice* (New York: W.W. Norton, 2007); Jean Baker Miller, *Toward a New Psychology of Women* (Boston: Beacon, 1976); Judith V. Jordan, Alexandra G. Kaplan, Jean Baker Miller, Irene P. Stiver, and Janet L. Surrey, *Women's Growth in Connection* (New York: Guilford, 1991); Jean Baker Miller and Irene P. Stiver, *The Healing Connection* (Boston: Beacon, 1997); Maureen Walker and Wendy Rosen, eds., *How Connections Heal* (New York: Guilford, 2004); Judith V. Jordan, Maureen Walker, and Linda M. Hartling, eds., *The Complexity of Connection* (New York: Guilford, 2004).

35 See, for example, Breggin, *Toxic Psychiatry*; Scott Simmie and Julia Nunes, *The Last Taboo: A Survival Guide to Mental Health Care in Canada* (Toronto: McClelland & Stewart, 2001); Patrick A. McGuire, "New Hope for People with Schizophrenia," *Monitor on Psychology* 31 (2000): 24–28.

36 See, for example, Sol L. Garfield, *Psychotherapy: An Eclectic-Integrative Approach* (Toronto: John Wiley and Sons, 1995).

37 See, for example, Breggin, *Toxic Psychiatry*; Robert D. Coursey, Joseph Alford and Bill Safarjan, "Significant Advances in Understanding and Treating Serious Mental Illness," *Professional Psychology: Research and Practice* 28 (1997): 205–16; and Diane T. Marsh and Dale L. Johnson, "The Family Experience of Mental Illness: Implications for Intervention," *Professional Psychology: Research and Practice* 28 (1997): 229–37.

38 Brown, "The Private Practice of Subversion Psychology."

39 Kathryn P. White, "Psychology and Complementary and Alternative Medicine," *Professional Psychology: Research and Practice* 31 (2000): 671–81. See, for example, Janice K. Kiecolt-Glaser et al., "Psychological Influences on Surgical Recovery: Perspectives from Psychoneuroimmunology," *American Psychologist* 53 (1998): 1209–18; and Gregory E. Miller and Sheldon Cohen, "Psychological Interventions and the Immune System: A Meta Analytic Review and Critique," *Health Psychology* 20 (2001): 47–63.

40 See, for example, Bentall, *Reconstructing Schizophrenia*; Coursey et al., "Significant Advances"; Harding et al., "Chronicity in Schizophrenia"; and Thomas, *Dialectics of Schizophrenia*.

41 Coursey et al., "Significant Advances."

42 See, for example, Coursey et al., "Significant Advances"; and Simmie and Nunes, *Last Taboo*.

43 See, for example, Breggin, *Toxic Psychiatry*; Coursey et al., "Significant Advances"; Simmie and Nunes, *Last Taboo*; and Thomas, *Dialectics of Schizophrenia*.

44 Capra, *Web of Life*, 6–7.

45 Pat Capponi, *Upstairs in the Crazy House* (Toronto: Penguin, 1992).

46 Simmie and Nunes, *Last Taboo*.

47 Walter and Peller, *Becoming Solution-Focused*.

48 See for example, Bracken and Thomas, *Postpsychiatry*; Rupert Ross, *Returning to the Teachings: Exploring Aboriginal Justice* (Toronto: Penguin, 1996);Michael White, *Narrative Practice and Exotic Lives*; and White and Epston, *Narrative Means to Therapeutic Ends*.

49 Examples of such programs familiar to me in Toronto are the Brief Psychotherapy Centre for Women at Sunnybrook and Women's Health Care Centre, the Alternatives East York Mental Health Services Agency, the Gerstein Centre, and Sheena's Place. The Brief Psychotherapy Centre approach is described in the following: M. Anne Oakley, "Short-Term Women's Groups as Spaces for Integration," in *Women and Group Psychotherapy: Theory and Practice*, ed. Betsy DeChant (New York: Guilford Press, 1996), 263–83; and Shirley Addison, Shelley Glazer, and Eimear O'Neill, "A Feminist Approach to Psychotherapy," *Canadian Women's Studies Journal* 14 (1994): 69–73.

50 For ideas about how this can be done, see, for example, Judith Worell and Pam Remer, *Feminist Perspectives in Therapy: An Empowerment Model for Women* (Toronto: John Wiley and Sons, 1992).

51 For example, Miller, *Toward a New Psychology of Women*; Jordan, Kaplan, Miller, Stiver, and Surrey, *Women's Growth in Connection*; Miller and Stiver, *The Healing Connection*; Walker and Rosen, *How Connections Heal*; and Jordan, Walker, and Hartling, *The Complexity of Connection*.

52 For example, White and Epston, *Narrative Means to Therapeutic Ends*; Freedman and Combs, *Narrative Therapy*; White, *Narrative Practice and Exotic Lives*; and White, *Maps of Narrative Practice*.

53 Walter and Peller, *Becoming Solution-Focused*.

54 See, for example, Bentall, *Reconstructing Schizophrenia*; Coursey et al., "Significant Advances"; Courtenay M. Harding et al., "The Vermont Longitudinal Study of Persons with Severe Mental Illness, I: Methodology, Study Sample, and Overall Status 32 Years Later," *American Journal of Psychiatry* 144 (1987): 718–26; Courtenay M. Harding et al., "The Vermont Longitudinal Study of Persons with Severe Mental Illness, II: Long-Term Outcome of Subjects Who Retrospectively Met *DSM-III* Criteria for Schizophrenia," *American Journal of Psychiatry* 144 (1987): 727–35; Courtenay M. Harding and James H. Zahniser, "Empirical Correction of Seven Myths about Schizophrenia with Implications for Treatment," *Acta Psychiatrica Scandinavica* 90 (suppl. 384) (1994): 140–46; Harding et al., "Chronicity in Schizophrenia"; and McGuire, "New Hope."

55 See, for example, Coursey et al., "Significant Advances"; Harding et al., "Chronicity in Schizophrenia"; Harding and Zahniser, "Empirical Correction"; Marsh and Johnson, "The Family Experience"; and McGuire, "New Hope."

56 Coursey et al., "Significant Advances."

57 See, for example, Coursey et al., "Significant Advances"; Larry Davidson et al., "Recovery in Serious Mental Illness: A New Wine or Just a New Bottle?" *Professional Psychology: Research and Practice* 36 (2005): 480–87; Larry Davidson, Courtenay M. Harding, and LeRoy Spaniol, eds., *Recovery from Serious Mental Illness: Research Evidence and Implications for Practice*, Vol. 1 (Boston: Center for Psychiatric Rehabilitation, Boston University, 2005); Larry Davidson, Courtenay M. Harding, and LeRoy Spaniol, eds., *Recovery from Serious Mental Illness: Research Evidence and Implications for Practice*, Vol. 2 (Boston: Center of Psychiatric Rehabilitation, Boston University, 2005); Harding et al., "The Vermont Longitudinal Study of Persons with Severe Mental Illness, I: Methodology, Study Sample, and Overall Status 32 Years Later"; Harding et al., "The Vermont Longitudinal Study of Persons with Severe Mental Illness, II: Long-Term Outcome of Subjects who Retrospectively Met *DSM-III* Criteria for Schizophrenia"; and McGuire, "New Hope."

58 Harding et al., "The Vermont Longitudinal Study of Persons with Severe Mental Illness, I," 722–23; and Harding et al., "The Vermont Longitudinal Study of Persons with Severe Mental Illness, II," 730.

59 Harding et al., "The Vermont Longitudinal Study of Persons with Severe Mental Illness, II," 730.

60 Scientific studies of outcomes for people diagnosed with schizophrenia are summarized in Harding et al., "Chronicity in Schizophrenia"; Harding and Zahniser, "Empirical Correction"; and Richard Warner, *Recovery from Schizophrenia: Psychiatry and Political Economy* (London: Routledge, 1994).

61 Harding et al., "Chronicity in Schizophrenia."

62 Brooks quoted in Harding et al., "Chronicity in Schizophrenia," 33.

63 Harding et al., "The Vermont Longitudinal Study of Persons with Severe Mental Illness, II."

64 These articles together make this point: Greg Miller, "The Unseen: Mental Illness's Global Toll," *Science* 311 (2006b): 458–61 and Greg Miller, "A Spoonful of Medicine—and a Steady Diet of Normality," *Science* 311 (2006a): 464–65.

65 Miller, "A Spoonful of Medicine," 464.

66 Coursey et al., "Significant Advances," 207.

67 See, for example, Bracken and Thomas, *Postpsychiatry*; Davidson et al., "Recovery in Serious Mental Illness"; Davidson, Harding, and Spaniol, *Recovery from Serious Mental Illness*, Vols. 1 and Vol. 2; Nora Jacobson, *In Recovery, the Making of Mental Health Policy* (Nashville: Vanderbilt University Press, 2004); Mary O'Hagan, "Recovery in New Zealand: Lessons for Australia?" *Australian e-Journal for the Advancement of Mental Health* 3 (1) (2004) www.auseinet.com/journal/vol3iss1/ohaganeditorial.pdf ; and Ann Thompson, compiler, *A Mental Health Recovery Reader for Providers, Survivors and Families* (Toronto: Canadian Scholars' Press, 2006).

68 Authors who emphasize this point include McGuire, "New Hope"; O'Hagan, "Recovery in New Zealand"; Simmie and Nunes, *Last Taboo*; and Thompson, *A Mental Health Recovery Reader*.

69 O'Hagan, "Recovery in New Zealand."

70 Davidson et al., "Recovery in Serious Mental Illness."

71 Ibid.

72 Ibid.

73 See, for example, Davidson et al., "Recovery in Serious Mental Illness"; O'Hagan, "Recovery in New Zealand"; and Thompson, *A Mental Health Recovery Reader*.

74 See, for example, Bracken and Thomas, *Postpsychiatry*; Davidson et al., "Recovery in Serious Mental Illness"; Jacobson, *In Recovery*; O'Hagan, "Recovery in New Zealand"; and Thompson, *A Mental Health Recovery Reader*.

75 The Standing Senate Committee on Social Affairs, Science and Technology, *Out of the Shadows at Last, Transforming Mental Health, Mental Illness and Addiction Services in Canada* (2006). Retrieved 19 March 2008 from www.parl.gc.ca/39/1/parlbus/commbus/senate/com-e/soci-e/rep-e/pdf/rep02may06part1-e.pdf.

76 Moore, *Care of the Soul*.

77 Brown, "Private Practice of Subversion Psychology."

78 Ibid.

79 French, *Beyond Power*.

80 William H. Murray, *The Scottish Himalayan Expedition* (London: J.M. Dent & Sons, 1951), 6–7.

81 Raymond Carver, "Late Fragment," *A New Path to the Waterfall* (New York: Atlantic Monthly, 1989).

I Appendix

Susan Schellenberg's
Art and Text

Shedding Skins, 1983–1991

Most of the dream paintings in the *Shedding Skins* series were first exhibited in December 1992 at the Women's College Hospital event called *Never Again: Women and Men Against Violence.* The text that accompanies the art was rewritten close to the time the art became permanently installed in the main lobby at the Centre for Addiction and Mental Health (CAMH), a psychiatric teaching hospital in Toronto, Canada.

The images are reproduced in this volume as plates 1–16 in the colour section following page 230.

Apotheosis (Plate 1, oil on canvas, 20 × 23.5 in.)

I become ill; I abandon art. Ten years later, I withdraw from drugs and resume artmaking. Art stirs feelings of chaos and terror.

A passionate teacher keeps my fragile mind busily structured for a year. Anatomical drawing and studies on Rembrandt bridge my Catholic past to a new perspective. The teacher's finely honed consciousness in body and mind imparts my first awareness of the feminine. My health strengthens, my art terrors lessen.

I paint Beethoven in the hope of learning the secret of creativity. Beethoven teaches that my ability to create is lessened by belief that art and goodness are outside myself.

The Clown (Plate 2, oil on canvas, 24 × 39.5 in.)

After I commit to healing, I enter what the nineteenth-century poet Matthew Arnold called a "wandering between two worlds, One dead, the other powerless to be born."[1]

My slate of old beliefs becomes blank. Animals become important to my story. Nature rather than familiar religious images offer a new sense of mystery. Wakened by respect and justice in the natural world, I learn how essential these same qualities are to mental and physical health.

The white unicorn colt with a red horn appears in a dream. Synchronous to the dream, I learn how the unicorn was a Christ figure symbol during the Middle Ages. Trust in my dreams and in the possibilities of healing expand.

The clown is a deliberate invention, an antidote for my depression and brooding seriousness. As I paint the clown's balloons, I see the inflated, prideful, flip side of my low self-worth.

I saw and sketched the flautist on a recent trip to Paris. He was playing his flute outside the Jeu de Paume.

Bury It with Respect (Plate 3, mixed media, 27.5 × 38.25 in.)

Prior to leaving my marriage, I dream that Andy Warhol and I are standing at the top of my crescent-shaped rock garden. To my left at the bottom of the garden stands a bishop. As I watch, the bishop disintegrates into a pile of dead leaves. A dream voice says, "Bury it with respect."

Leaving my marriage, religion, home, and garden is painful but I come to accept that the price for my staying in the relationship is my agreeing to remain ill and drugged.

I interpret the dream bishop's leaves as my leaving or returning to the Mother Earth or feeling part of me that will fertilize the next period of my life. Years of growth are necessary before I understand that my need to hold onto and to possess others originates in my not being in possession of myself. I must learn to let go, and to bury the past with respect.

Image from the Desert (Plate 4, mixed media, 27 × 38.5 in.)

It is 1988. Cancer and surgery force me to work on my rage. A wilderness/dream workshop in the New Mexico desert offers needed spiritual courage to face how I turn loss and emotional pain into physical illnesses. My concept of self-awareness shifts from a product to a never-ending process. To complement dream work, I utilize yoga, tai chi, and movement, and begin to write my story.

The blue on the face remains a mystery for several years. Then, my teacher during a tai chi class shows me a narrow black-and-silver martial arts wand, sometimes called a flute, and directs his full attention toward showing me how to hold the flute close to my face. That night, I dream a buried childhood memory of my mother hitting me full force on the side of my face with a steel black-and-silver hairbrush. This memory, coupled with those of my mother frequently saying "I have never been able to stand the sight of your face, not since the day you were born" helps me uncover the origins of my "Who could love this face?" attitude. I must research the story of my mother's life and understand her pain before I feel compassion and forgiveness for her. As this occurs, I also learn how I in turn projected this unconscious mother onto women authority figures, my former husband, as well as my other relationships.

Joan of Arc (Plate 5, mixed media, 27.5 × 39 in.)

Joan appears when I need to fight feelings of powerlessness.

With a hand on her horse Joan tells me to connect to the animal or instinctive feeling part of myself. Joan says, "Live in and with your feelings." Her haircuts and suits of armour have always charmed me. Her fashion messages: "You mask your sense of being evil with a fashionable appearance," "You armour yourself against rejection," "You settle for approval and admiration rather than love." I attempt to change my style, my fear of love.

Joan, as my warrior part, finds added expression in tai chi sword forms. Internal as well as external attitudes of self-defence build.

The Duenna (The Chaperone) (Plate 6, mixed media, 27 × 37.75 in.)

In the New Mexico desert, I dream I am speaking to a beautiful young Pueblo nun; her large brown eyes are filled with love. She sits gazing at the young man across from her. A loving Mother Superior chaperones the couple's courtship. I say to the young nun, "Don't I know you? Are you Thérèse?" My sole Thérèse memories are of St. Thérèse Lisieux and St. Teresa of Avila, but these Catholic saints have not been in my conscious mind since primary school.

Vita Sackville West's *The Eagle and the Dove* advances my understanding of the Lisieux and Avila stories.[2] Where I honour and find their stories heroic, I gain added support for my own decision to leave a patriarchal religion in order to become whole as a woman.

Both women were left motherless at an early age. My mother's inability to nurture me psychologically and my unfinished work on that issue means that my children, former partnership, and I existed in a state of spiritual motherlessness. Learning how both women's loss of their mothers fuelled their desire to do something heroic for God made added sense of how I am pulled towards doing the heroic rather than what I love to do in order to feel worthy of love.

My mother, like the Pueblo dream nun, had brown eyes. Duty love for my mother begins to transform into authentic love for her as both a flawed and creative human being. I also begin to mother myself in more positive ways.

The young couple echoes how my masculine and feminine parts, though coming together, are still young and not yet fully integrated.

The Eagle and the Dove (Plate 7, mixed media, 28.75 × 40.75 in.)

I paint Lisieux and Avila. I see Thérèse as coltish and express her contemplative nature by placing her in the ocean. Teresa of Avila is more difficult. Though I have an idea of their physical portraits from reading Vita Sackville West's account of both women, I am unable to feel Avila in my body as I must if I want to draw her.[3] My shiatsu/dream therapist suggests that I try to dance Avila. Dance allows me to know in my torso that just as history records, Avila was like a sumo wrestler, a big, strong but not sloppy body. Then a strange thing happens. I develop an ache over my left eye and my legs refuse more dancing.

The therapist waits and then says, "Can you name the feeling in your legs?" "It is 'don't come near me' energy," I eventually say, and shortly after remember a buried sexual trauma from my past. The ache over my eye that was my not wanting to see or examine this hurtful issue begins to lessen. I go home and place Avila into the picture.

The Blue Nuns (Plate 8, mixed media, 27.5 × 40.75 in.)

This work tells the story of the rage at the heart of my addictive behaviour. The blue nun's half-dressed figure echoes my mind–body split. She reminds me of a mermaid, a woman who is unable to bear life or to create. The nun in the cloister on the right is sewing, the other reading. I used these figures to symbolize the mind–body connection I desire. The grille of the cloister represents my goal to achieve a positive self that can create and keep personal boundaries but still be open to the world.

The meaning for me of the white neck area on the nun becomes apparent one day as I notice two elderly women animated in passionate chatter. These women remind me of the inner chatter, located in my throat. It becomes clearer that my constant self-talk is also an addiction aimed at keeping painful feelings and rage pushed down. This addiction keeps me in my head, prevents me from connecting to life, the feelings in my body, and to my creativity.

Abe and the Bear (Plate 9, mixed media, 26.5 × 38 in.)

The parked car, the prostitutes, the theatre, the blue, the bear, and the Abraham Lincoln are all parts of myself that I am working on at the time of this painting: the stalled part, the part I dishonour, my journey, the true-to-myself part, the instinctive animal part, and the masculine part.

The meaning of each dream symbol is personal. The more I record my dreams and learn what my symbols mean, the more they recur and become part of my dream language. My fear that each dream will show that I am evil constantly prods me to find more courage for the work. Childhood conditioning about good and evil has shaped my intention to be perfect rather than human. As I grow in self-love, I learn to embrace all my parts, including my dereliction.

The Faceless Priest (Plate 10, mixed media, 28.75 × 40.75 in.)

I stand at the back of the dream cathedral. I am locked in this building and cannot escape. Nazi soldiers surround the building. They carry machine guns. I think I know the priest in the pulpit, but his words are all garbled and his face featureless.

Where my strict religious training was rich in ritual and story, the low self-worth/terrorist parts of me were shaped by religious myths of the feminine that implied the inferiority of women. I do not presume to say that this is every Catholic woman's experience. It was mine.

The inner dream Nazi symbolizes the ways I put myself down. My willingness to think I deserve put-downs and take responsibility for the actions of others if they put me down causes me in turn to put others down. My Nazi part kills inner and outer relationships and creativity.

The faceless priest motif recurred in eight or more other dreams. My eventual recall of a psychosexual abuse by a priest during my childhood convinces me that my becoming psychotic at a retreat that was heavily attended by priests was not an accident.

The Pinto and the Nun (Plate 11, oil on masonite, 36 × 44 in.)

After leaving New Mexico, I have dreams in which a nun rides horses in the desert. The horse varies from dream to dream. I research horses and am pulled against all other preferences to the pinto. Though discouraged, I honour the impulse and am later thrilled when I discover that the name pinto means "painting."

Good Grief (Plate 12, mixed media, 26.75 × 38.25 in.)

The figure in this painting contains a coded record of my various life encounters with pain and a similar record of the good that ultimately resulted from that pain.

As the meaning of my illness becomes clearer, I am less controlled by and more able to let go of outworn behaviours. The alternating love–reject, charm–betray, tyrant–victim, and abuse patterns that I bring to and seek in relationship become a one-day-at-a-time challenge to change. Rather than needing to act on the extreme side of any of these behaviours while burying its opposite or becoming split off because of them, I learn to forgive and to accept other peoples' total selves more and to enjoy more authentic relationships with others.

Lot's Wife Redeemed (Plate 13, mixed media, 28.75 × 40.75 in.)

Prior to this painting, I am drawn to the biblical story of Lot's wife, the woman who is warned that she will turn to a pillar of salt if she looks back while on her desert journey.

Later, when I sit on the banks of the Rio Puerco in New Mexico, I see my shadow cast upon the water. I perceive this as a metaphor for the redemption of the Lot's wife part of me.

Where I do not turn into a pillar of salt as Lot's wife did, my difficulties with processing feelings makes me recycle rather than let go of the past. The more I block feelings, the more rigid (pillar of salt) my body becomes in its movement and the more prone I become to illness.

The Naming of Julia Rose (Plate 14, mixed media, 28.75 × 40.75 in.)

My daughter gives birth to Julia Rose. Julia is respectfully welcomed into the community of a healing, caring Mother Earth. Her naming ritual suits our changed sensibilities and connects us to the story of baptism in a profound new way.

Artist/healer Paul Hogan teaches our family how to take priesthood into our own hands. This occurs at a time when, as a family, we are numbed by the pain of divorce and lack meaningful sources of ritual to mark the sacredness of Julia's birth. Julia's naming is healing in that it tells a story of us having fun and celebrating rather than being depressed. We are no longer as bound to our old story.

The Crone (Plate 15, mixed media, 28.75 × 23.75 in.)

The old woman, or crone, in a dream signifies wisdom. I had this dream after some painful work examining and owning one of my negative mother issues.

I had recently failed to honour a young person's pain or to trust in his ability to solve a problem; instead, I had become a rescuer.

Once, when I was very frustrated, I confessed to a wise mentor that I never seemed to learn except the hard way. She laughed and said, "Yes, that is how we learn!"

Hawk (Plate 16, mixed media, 28.75 × 40.75 in.)

It is early morning in High Park. I hear a powerful rustle of feathers. A few feet away a majestic hawk lands atop a white cruciform post. I stand still. The bird appears to want my attention—our eyes meet. The hawk's capacity for intimacy is greater than mine. Its eyes offer a strong, clear, non-intrusive love. After a while, the hawk lifts into the air, disappears, and I go home to paint it.

This artwork is affirming to me as it suggests that my past and present theologies, rather than being ruptured, are knitting into a new whole. I've learned many life lessons from the hawk during my walks through the park.

Viv Moore and Dave Wilson Gestures, 1995–1997

From the mid-1990s until 2003, "connection" as an expression of the inner masculine/feminine became uniquely alive for me through artistic collaborations with Toronto dancers Viv Moore and Dave Wilson. To see Viv and Dave express some of my dreams in dance and to intimately feel the dance as I rendered nudes of their gestures allowed a rare exploration of my dreams and an ongoing meditation on the meaning of wholeness. To enter myself through executing Viv and Dave's dream gestures enriched beyond the place of words or tears. Both sets of nudes were an integral part of my 2005 *Casting a Vessel* show.

Viv has been a dancer, choreographer, and actor since 1979, in Sweden, Australia, England, and Canada. A much-sought-after movement coach for plays, Viv has since gone on to obtain her master's in dance. We met when Viv was chosen to play Ann, the character based on my life story in the workshop production of my play, *My Old Movie of Dreams*. To learn the story and role, Viv danced and created interpretive gestures for my *Shedding Skins* dream works. Viv went on to play me while I rendered her gestures in a mixed media of watercolour, charcoal, and pastel. Each drawing is 27 × 39 inches. See figures 1–8 (pp. 231–34).

Dave Wilson at that time was artistic director of the McMaster Dance Company and the Parahumans Dance Theatre. He has since become artistic director of the Centre for Dance Performance, McMaster University. Dave's interests included mind/body/spirit and healing topics as well as the filming of dance. His enthusiasm for the *Moore Gestures* and the process Viv and I had undertaken led to our collaborating on a series of Faceless Priest dreams that occurred in the mid-1990s. Our initial photographing of Dave's gestures preceded my recall of priest abuse in childhood. Where I was able to work steadily on Viv's gestures, I was able to commit Dave's gestures to egg tempera only after I entered analysis and began work on the recalled abuse memories. I sometimes experienced Dave's face as the real priest's face as I was working.

Dave Wilson's gestures appear as part of the *Casting a Vessel* series, which is reproduced in this volume. See plates 23, 25, 27, 29, and 32 in the colour section, which follows.

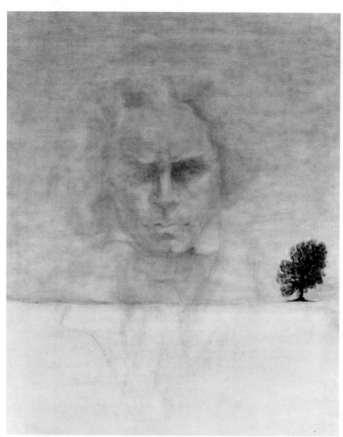

[PLATE 1] APOTHEOSIS

[PLATE 2] THE CLOWN

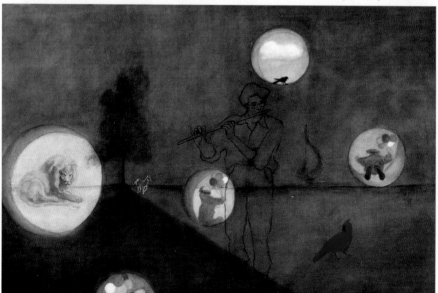

SHEDDING SKINS

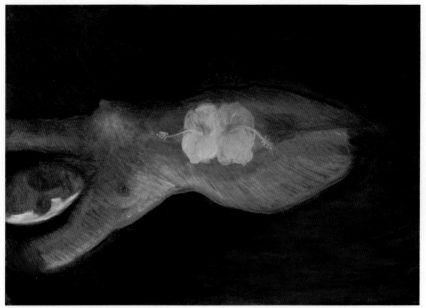

[PLATE 4] IMAGE FROM THE DESERT

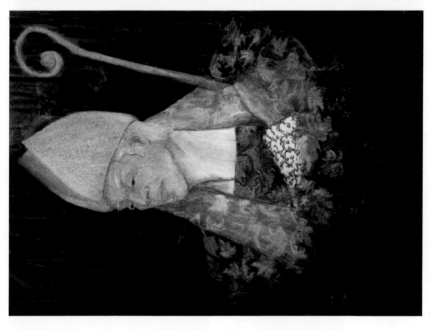

[PLATE 3] BURY IT WITH RESPECT

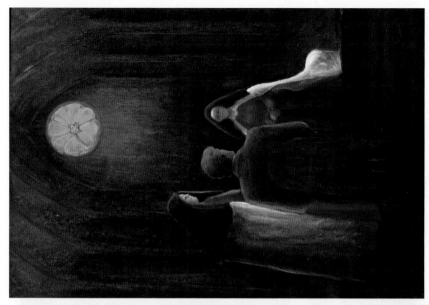

[PLATE 6] THE DUENNA (THE CHAPERONE)

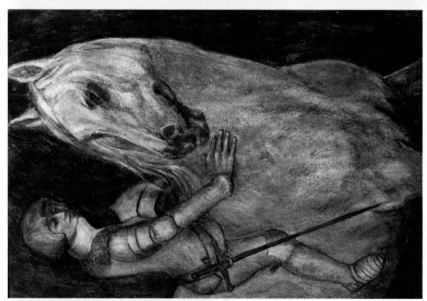

[PLATE 5] JOAN OF ARC

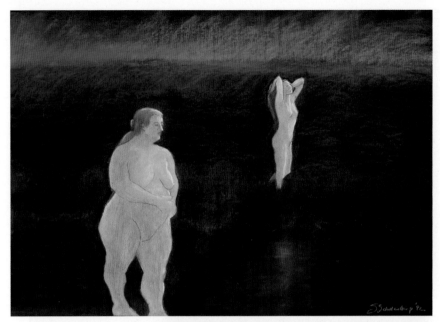

[PLATE 7] THE EAGLE AND THE DOVE

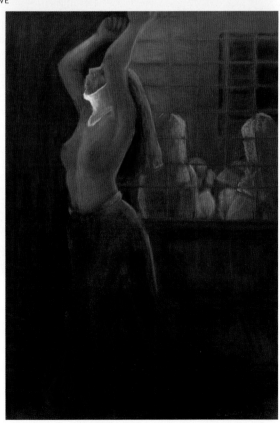

[PLATE 8] THE BLUE NUNS

SHEDDING SKINS

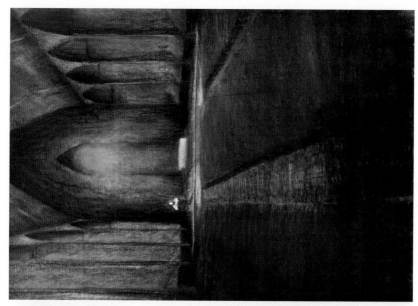

[PLATE 10] THE FACELESS PRIEST

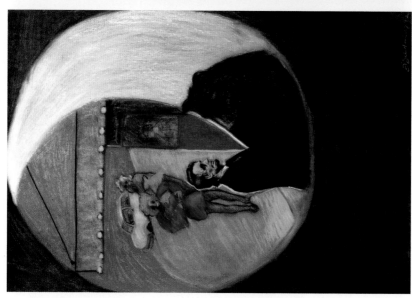

[PLATE 9] ABE AND THE BEAR

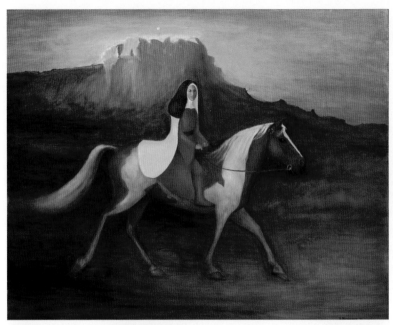

[PLATE 11]
THE PINTO AND THE
NUN

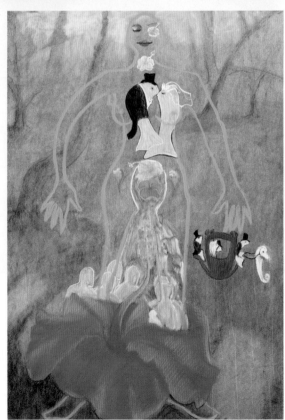

[PLATE 12]
GOOD GRIEF

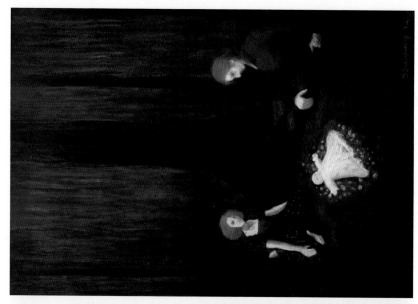

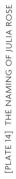

[PLATE 14] THE NAMING OF JULIA ROSE

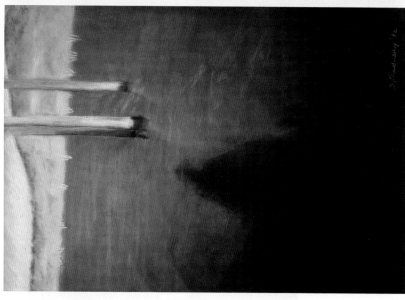

[PLATE 13] LOT'S WIFE REDEEMED

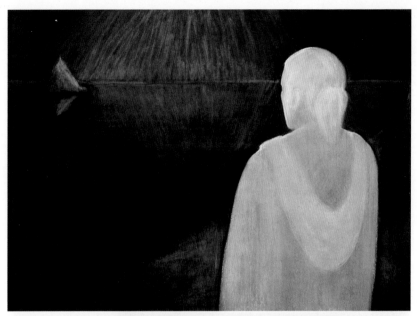

[PLATE 15] THE CRONE

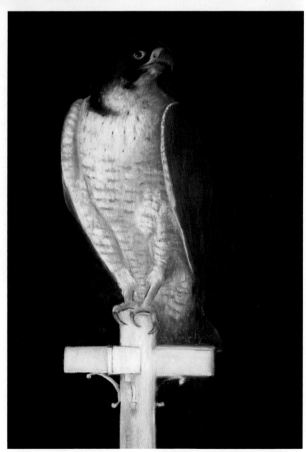

[PLATE 16] HAWK

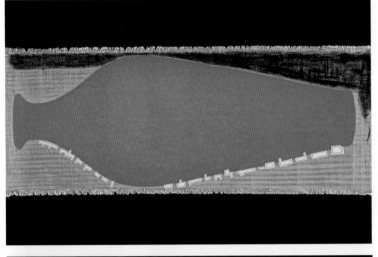

[PLATE 19] WORDLESS

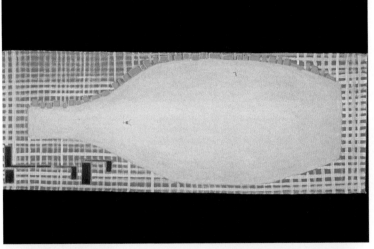

[PLATE 18] THROUGH THE GRILLE

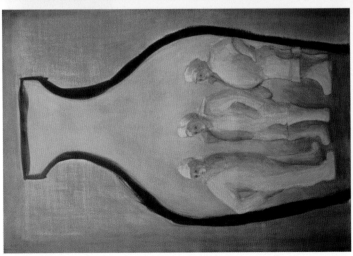

[PLATE 17] MANAN MAGI #4

CASTING A VESSEL

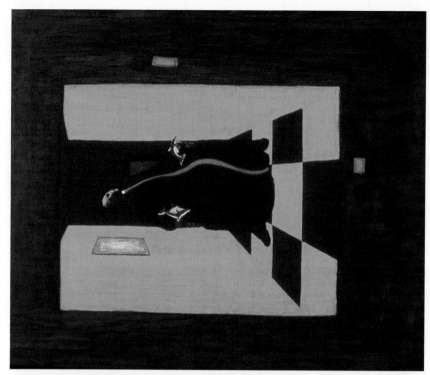

[PLATE 21] GRILLED FISH

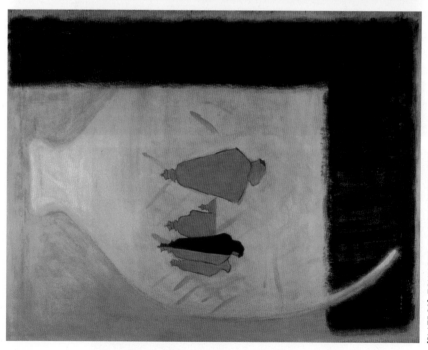

[PLATE 20] TOWARDS AN EARTH THEOLOGY

CASTING A VESSEL

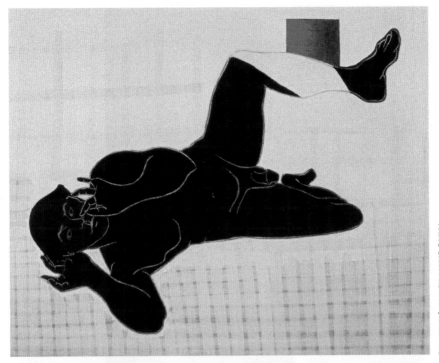

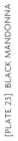

[PLATE 23] BLACK MANDONNA

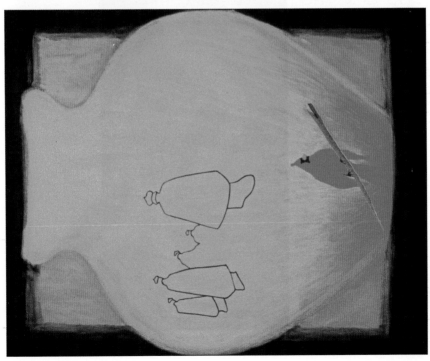

[PLATE 22] THE CARDINAL

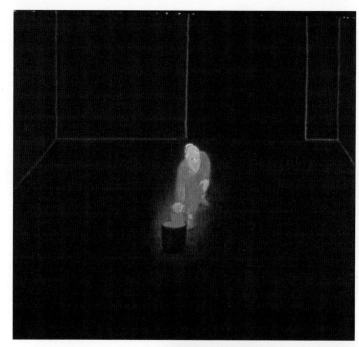

[PLATE 24]
LOVE LETTERS

[PLATE 25] RED MANDONNA

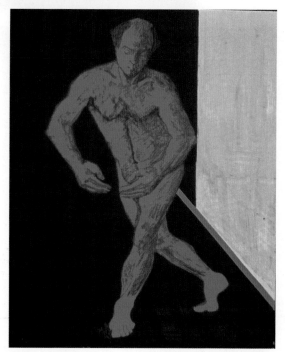

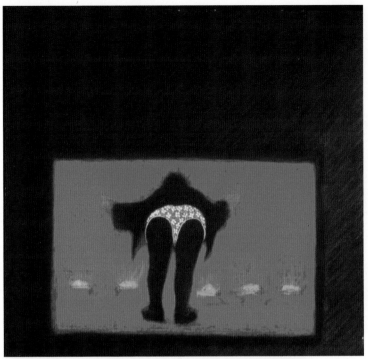

[PLATE 26]
LACE AND LIGHT

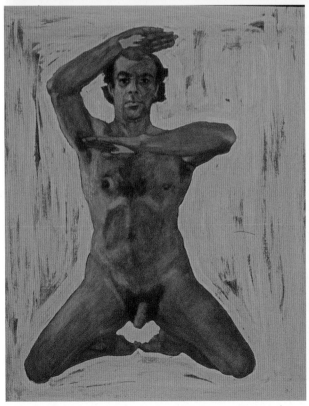

[PLATE 27] GREEN MANDONNA

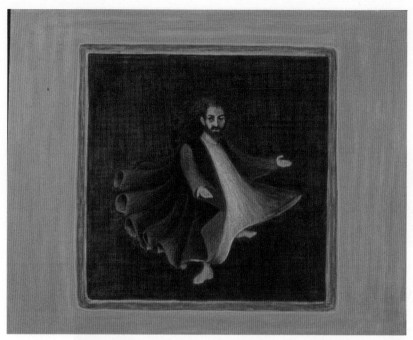

[PLATE 28] THE GYPSY

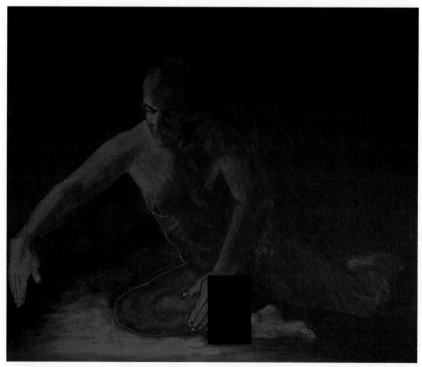

[PLATE 29] ENCODED

CASTING A VESSEL

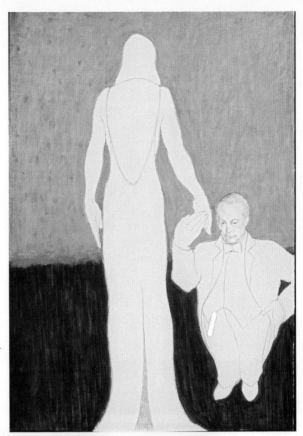

[PLATE 30] CHURCHILL

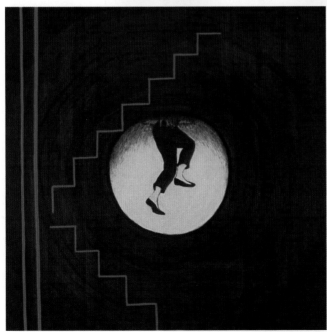

[PLATE 31]
BREAKTHROUGH

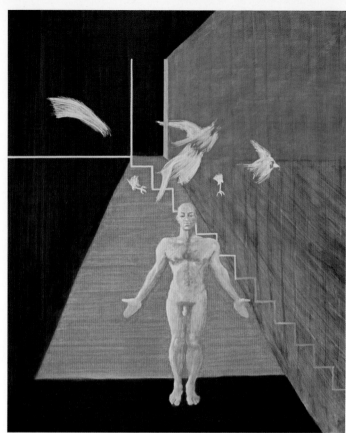

[PLATE 32] BIRTH

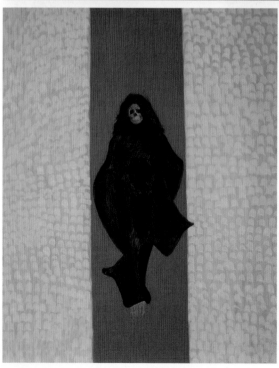

[PLATE 33] FASHIONISTA

CASTING A VESSEL

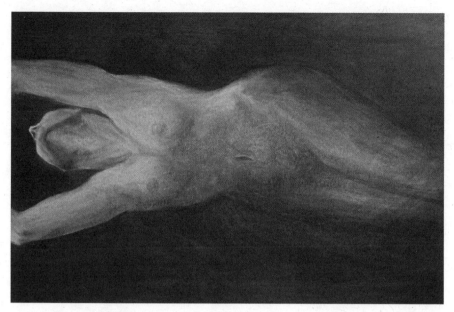

[FIGURE 1] MOORE GESTURE #1

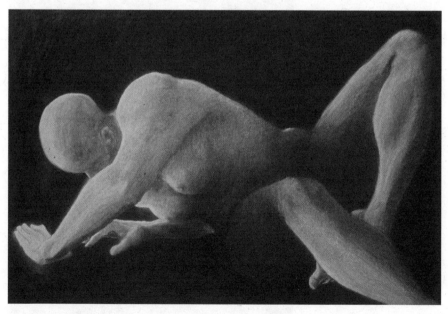

[FIGURE 2] MOORE GESTURE #2

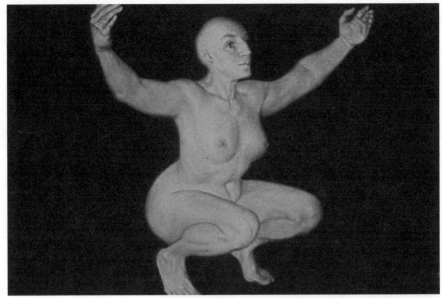

[FIGURE 3] MOORE GESTURE #3

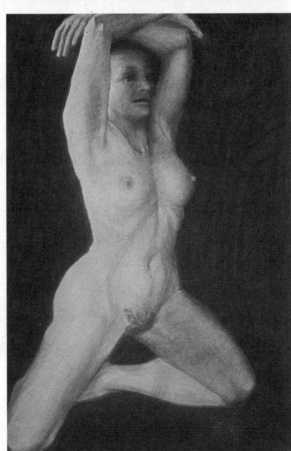

[FIGURE 4] MOORE GESTURE #4

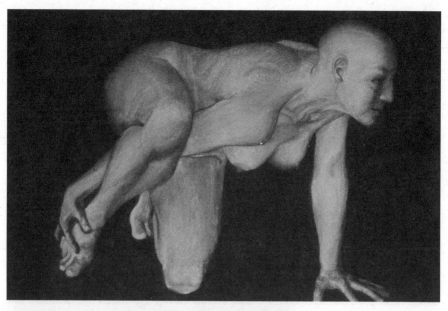

[FIGURE 5] MOORE GESTURE #5

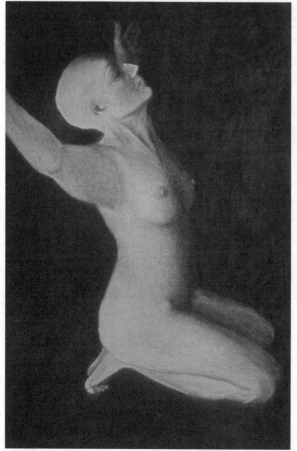

[FIGURE 6] MOORE GESTURE #6

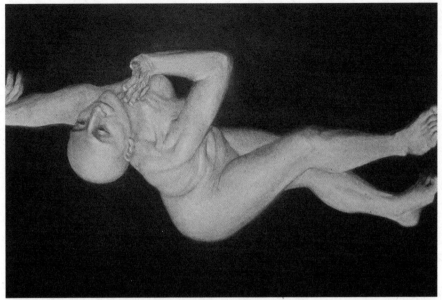

[FIGURE 8] MOORE GESTURE #8

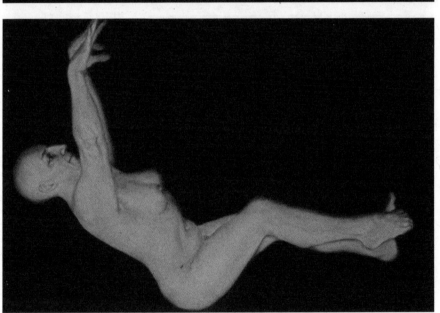

[FIGURE 7] MOORE GESTURE #7

Casting a Vessel, 1997–2005

The *Casting a Vessel* works are based on dreams that occurred in 1998–2005, during the time I was working in analysis on the abuse stories. The paintings in this series were exhibited at the ACA Gallery in Toronto in March 2005. I offer a brief written introduction to the works here, but greater detail concerning what the art helped me to work through is available in chapter 7. The works are reproduced here in the colour section, which follows page 230. See plates 17–33.

In 1997 a dream tells me to paint in egg tempera, a more ecologically friendly medium. To learn the craft of this ancient technique, I needed to stuggle for two years before realizing any art with it. The slowness and care this medium demands proves immensely beneficial to my staying grounded as I worked on the abuse.

Yellow ochre is my favourite colour to the point it has long been the part of my dream language that describes me as an artist. Following the installation of my *Shedding Skins* art at the CAMH, I become anxious, restless, and feel devoid of images to paint. Panicked, I begin work on *Manan Magi #4* (plate 17) using yellow ochre on the background, hoping an image will come to me. The idea for the black vessel outline comes one day—and the next day I know the vessel is meant to hold the three fishers I had sketched in 1986 on the Grand Manan docks in the Bay of Fundy.

I am relieved to have found an image and become absorbed again in the act of painting. The day I finish this work, I do the fateful sitting meditation that will initiate recovery of the story of the three people who abused me in childhood. The three fishermen foretell the abuse recall.

Painted immediately after my 2005 *Casting a Vessel* show, *Fashinista* (plate 33) tells me that my work on the abuse is coming to an end. However, the art and dream processes that fashioned the many deaths of my false selves and rebirths of my new self will remain my chosen venues for growth.

Manan Magi #4, Plate 17, egg tempera on paper, 29 × 30 inches
Through the Grille, Plate 18, acrylic tempera, 61.75 × 23 inches
Wordless, Plate 19, acrylic tempera, 61.75 × 23 inches
Towards an Earth Theology, Plate 20, acrylic tempera, 46.5 × 60 inches
Grilled Fish, Plate 21, egg tempera on board, 20 × 24 inches
The Cardinal, Plate 22, egg tempera on board, 20 × 24 inches
Black Mandonna, Plate 23, egg tempera on board, 20 × 24 inches
Love Letters, Plate 24, egg tempera on board, 16 × 16 inches
Red Mandonna, Plate 25, egg tempera on board, 20 × 24 inches
Lace and Light, Plate 26, egg tempera on board, 16 × 16 inches

Green Mandonna, Plate 27, egg tempera on board, 20 × 24 inches
The Gypsy, Plate 28, egg tempera on board, 20 × 24 inches
Encoded, Plate 29, egg tempera on board, 20 × 24 inches
Churchill, Plate 30, egg tempera, silver point on paper 29 × 39 inches
Breakthrough, Plate 31, egg tempera on board, 16 × 16 inches
Birth, Plate 32, egg tempera on board, 20 × 24 inches
Fashionista, Plate 33, egg tempera on board, 20 × 24 inches

Notes

1　Matthew Arnold, "Stanzas from the Grande Chartruse," in *Arnold Poetical Works*, ed. Chauncey B. Tinker and H.F. Hawley (London: Oxford University Press, 1950), 302.
2　Vita Sackville-West, *The Eagle and the Dove: A Study in Contrasts*, Saint Teresa of Avila [1515–1582], Saint Thérèse de Lisieux [1873–1897] (London: M. Joseph, 1953).
3　Sackville-West, *Eagle and the Dove*.

II Appendix

Clinical Records

Glossary

ROSEMARY

Introduction to Susan's Mental Health Records

In Ontario, the physical clinical record is the property of the health professional or institution where it was prepared. By law, any patient is entitled to a copy of his or her own clinical record. The clinical records for Susan and her uncle Leo Marrin Regan were obtained by the usual means—with a written request and the payment of a nominal fee. The records included here are complete with the exception of a few items—namely, Susan's photograph, the names of hospital staff, and personal information about Susan's siblings.

A glossary at the end of this appendix (p. 286) defines technical terms that are mentioned in the clinical records and later conversations and includes some apparently ordinary words such as *orientation* when these words have a specific technical meaning in mental health practice.

Clinical Records of Leo Marrin Regan

Susan's brother requested the clinical records for their uncle, Leo Marrin Regan, who lived his entire adult life in psychiatric hospitals. The letter from the Kingston Psychiatric Hospital (pp. 241–42) is likely a summary of clinical records for Mr. Regan. This uncle's situation was not known to Susan or her family until 1995, many years after her own hospital admission.

Clinical Records of Susan Schellenberg

Susan requested her own clinical records; her account of receiving the records is included in chapter 5. The nurses' notes, which would have provided information about Susan's activities and status on a daily basis, are unfortunately not available. Dr. Mary Seeman (see chapter 5) pointed out that nursing notes in that period were stored separately and retained for a shorter time than the rest of the clinical record.

Initial Admission Forms

The first pages were likely completed by clerical staff in the admitting department on 2 September 1969, the date of Susan's hospital admission; they provide basic identifying information—name, address, telephone number, and next of kin. Next is a form required by law in circumstances where the person is admitted as an "involuntary" patient, which was the case for Susan's admission. This form was completed by a physician, probably in the emergency department, and outlines the reasons for Susan's involuntary admission. Involuntary status means that the person does not consent freely but is required to come to and remain in hospital because a designated official—usually a physician—believes it necessary because the person suffers from a mental disorder such that there is risk of serious, immediate danger to either him- or herself or to others. Once the necessary legal form is completed, the police have the authority to search for the person and bring him or her to the hospital, and the hospital has the authority to physically prevent the person from leaving until the certificate expires or is lifted by the treating physician. The procedures for certifying a person as an involuntary patient are outlined specifically in law, and are different now from what they were in 1969 when Susan was admitted.

After a person is admitted, he or she is designated a patient. Nursing and medical staff on the hospital ward do further evaluation. In Susan's case, the ward admission record was probably completed by a nurse to provide information about Susan's physical condition, status, and possessions at the time of admission. A medical examination is a routine aspect of admission for psychiatric patients and is intended to ensure that any physical health problems are identified and treated. The physical examination form for Susan was completed by a physician, and provides the doctor's evaluation of her medical health status on admission. Next come laboratory reports on blood and urine tests done just after admission, including a routine test for syphilis (VDRL).

Clinical Notes and Reports

The clinical record is a series of notes made by staff psychiatrists concerning the patient's symptoms, clinical impressions of difficulties, and diagnoses. Information in the notes would have come from interviews with Susan or discussions with nurses or other staff. The social record is based on an interview with Susan's husband. The psychological examination consisted of the psychologist having a series of interviews with Susan and administering several personality tests.

The conference report is based on the conclusions reached in a meeting of all members of the professional team: psychiatrist, nurses, psychologist, social worker, occupational therapist, and any students training in any of these disciplines. At this meeting, all information concerning the patient is reviewed and discussed to determine the final diagnosis, discuss discharge, and make arrangements for follow-up care after the patient is discharged from hospital. The conference report summarizes the conclusions and decisions that were reached from all the interviews, observations, and tests conducted during the patient's time in hospital.

Susan was interviewed during the team conference. Such a patient interview was—and may still be—a routine part of the team conference. Usually the patient is invited into the conference room, introduced to any professional staff he or she has not already met, and asked questions, usually by the psychiatrist. Such interviews are brief, no more than five to ten minutes, and focus on obtaining information that might help to clarify an uncertain diagnosis, determine the current status of patient symptoms, or plan for discharge or treatment changes. It was during the interview with Susan in the team conference that the psychiatrist raised concerns that she might injure her children.

In the final note, we read that Susan was discharged on 26 September 1969 and referred to the public health nurse and to the aftercare clinic for follow-up.

Doctor's Order Form

The doctor's order form consists of the doctor's handwritten directions about practical matters such as medications, permission for the patient to go to various places within the hospital, permission for the patient to leave hospital at certain times, and hospital discharge. The nurses and other staff consult these pages to determine what medication to administer and procedures to follow for each individual patient.

Outpatient Record

The final part of the record consists of the notes from the Lakeshore Psychiatric Hospital Outpatient Services where Susan attended regular appointments after being discharged from the hospital. At these appointments, she met with a psychiatrist who asked about how she was doing and adjusted prescriptions for medication accordingly; a few meetings were with a nurse who would have reported what Susan said and how she appeared to be doing to the psychiatrist in charge of the clinic. The psychiatrist or nurse wrote a brief summary of what occurred and the medication recommended at each follow-up appointment. The physician's orders provide a record of the medication prescribed during this period.

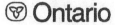

☸ Ontario

Ministry	Ministère	Kingston	Hôpital	Postal Bag 603	Sac postal 603
of	de	Psychiatric	psychiatrique	Kingston ON K7L 4X3	Kingston ON K7L 4X3
Health	la Santé	Hospital	de Kingston	(613) 546-1101	

November 9, 1995

Dear Mr. Regan:

RE: REGAN, Leo

Our records show your uncle as Leo Marrin Regan. He was born January 16, 1895. The Statement of Death is dated February 9, 1960. He lived in Toronto all his life at 509 Sherbourne Street.

His father was born in London, England and had died at age 53. He married Rose Callaghan from Toronto at age 28; Rose was age 24 at the time of their marriage. His father died of Brights' Disease, his mother had diabetes.

At the time of admission, two brothers and two sisters were living, the youngest being 17 years old and the eldest being 26. Three brothers and one sister had died: one boy died of an accident at age 3; one boy died of scarlet fever at age 5; one boy died of pneumonia at 3 weeks; and one sister died with convulsions at five days.

One uncle was said to be somewhat intemperate. One uncle (Jeremiah) had been treated at St. Michael's Hospitals for "nervous trouble".

The patient had been successfully treated for tapeworm eight years prior to admission. He had had scarlet fever, tonsillitis, and appendicitis as a child and convulsions at 3 months.

Leo had a nine month period of depression after his father's death.

He was admitted to hospital October 28, 1915, transferred to Whitby and later transferred to Kingston on July 8, 1931. By 1951 he was a bed-patient and in 1952 he continually lapsed from stupor to sleep. He did not talk or follow instructions. The cause of death is given as

...../2

2748-42 (93/05)

Figure 1a. Summary of Leo Regan's medical and psychiatric history. (Continues next page.)

November 9, 1995   Page 2.

pneumonia due to arteriosclerotic heart disease and catatonic dementia praecox. He was
buried in St. Mary's Cemetary in Kingston. The funeral director was W. Vernon Lindsay.

I trust this is helpful.

Yours truly,

Manager, Clinical Information Services

Figure 1b. *Summary of Leo Regan's medical and psychiatric history (conclusion).*

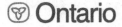

| Ministry of Health | Ministère de la Santé | Queen Street Mental Health Centre | Centre de santé mentale de la rue Queen | 1001 Queen Street West Toronto ON M6J 1H4 | 1001, rue Queen ouest Toronto ON M6J 1H4 |
| | | | | Telephone no./Nº de téléphone | (416) 535–8501 |

Susan Schellenberg

Toronto, Ontario

September 13, 1995

RE: A PHOTOCOPY OF YOUR CLINICAL RECORD

Dear Ms. Schellenberg:

I have photocopied the clinical record as you requested. Please be aware that now that it is in your possession, you are responsible for ensuring its safety. Only you can guarantee that the information contained in the record remains confidential by keeping it safely out of access from other members of the public.

We do charge for photocopies. The first ten pages are free and each additional page is $.25. Please make your cheque for $8.50 payable to the Minister of Finance.

Please remember that you may still complete another Form 28 in the future if you wish to view the file in the Clinical Records Department.

If I can be of further assistance, do not hesitate to contact me.

Yours truly,

Legal Liaison
Clinical Records

2655-42 (93/07)

Figure 2. Covering letter with Susan Schellenberg's clinical records.

1

PROVINCE OF ONTARIO
THE ONTARIO HOSPITAL

Registered No. .... Case Book No. .... 29066 ....

Documentation: .... INVOLUNTARY APPLICATION ....

Name in full: .... SCHELLENBERG, Mrs., Susan Ann ....

Post Office Address or Street Number ....

County .... York .... Municipality .... Islington ....

                                                     City   Town   Village   Township

Probations: Return from Probations:

Date of Admission: .... September 2, 1969

Date of Discharge: _September 26, 1969_

Date of Death: ....

Admitted by Dr .... adm., Clerk ...... at ...... 2045 Hrs. ...... M., Sent ward .... 3 ....

Brought from .... St. Joseph's Emergency ...... by .... Husband Mr. Schellenberg ....

Medical Certificate   { Dr. .... of ....
Made by   { Dr. .... of ....

Maintenance: Pay .... Free .... Per Week ....
                                   Mr.   Schellenberg, husband
Name of Correspondent (relationship): ....

Address: .... home

Telegraph or Telephone Number .... work

Special Remarks: ....

PATIENT'S COPY

Figure 3. Basic data form.

PHYSICIAN'S APPLICATION FOR INVOLUNTARY ADMISSION ✓ 2

Form 1 The Mental Health Act, 1967 Section 8

ONTARIO

Note: This form must be completed in full. In order to be valid, this application must be completed no later than seven days after the examination referred to above. The application is authority to admit only within fourteen days of the date it is completed.

I, the undersigned physician, hereby certify that on the _2_ day of _SEPTEMBER_, 19 _69_

I personally examined _SUSAN A. SCHELLENBERG_
(name of person in full)

ISLINGTON
(home address)

After making due inquiry into all the facts necessary for me to form a satisfactory opinion, I do hereby further certify that he/she suffers from mental disorder of a nature or degree so as to require hospitalization in the interests of his/her own safety or the safety of others.

1. Facts indicating mental disorder observed by myself: (e.g., appearance, conduct, conversation.)

   apathetic. Imitates all movements of husband in detail - feels compelled to do so. Relates events of recent retreat which include visual and auditory hallucinations. Feels that is about to die. At times thinks that is 'The Virgin Mary'. Religious significant to all

2. Other facts, if any, indicating mental disorder communicated to me by others: (State from whom the information was received.) (Husband) recent religious retreat. At church on Aug. 31/69 - went to church of Nativity + took along a painting of the the nativity with her g she presented to the priest. At church, she felt that was asked to be the Mother of Christ. Has not slept for 1 wk. Constantly imitates husband.

3. State reason(s) why no measure short of hospitalization would be appropriate in the case of the above-named person:

   acute schizophrenia - should not be left alone c̄ children and ṟ as out patient at present.

4. State reason(s) why the above-named person is not suitable for admission as an informal patient:

   as above

I hereby apply for the involuntary admission of the above-named person to a psychiatric facility.

Signed this _2_ day of _SEPTEMBER_, 19 _69_

The name and address of the physician must be printed or typed below·

St. Joseph's Hospital
30 THE Queensway

CONFIDENTIAL NOT TO BE DUPLICATED OR USED FOR ANY OTHER PURPOSE WITHOUT FURTHER WRITTEN AUTHORIZATION OF THE PATIENT.

(Signature of physician)

Indicate medication (a) routinely received by the patient:

(b) administered to the patient within the last twenty-four hours

Figure 4. Physician's application for admission.

APPLICATION FOR ADMISSION TO LAKESHORE PSYCHIATRIC HOSPITAL

MALE ____ FEMALE ✓

DOCUMENTATION *Involuntary*

1. O.H.S.C. *91221101*
2. O.M.S.I.P. ____
3. P.S.I. ____
4. Other *Great West Life 20555*

NAME *Schellenberg, Mrs. Susan Ann*

ADDRESS ____ COUNTY *York*

PHONE ____ MARITAL STATUS: S ___ M ✓ SEP ___ D ___ W ___

AGE *34* DATE OF BIRTH *Sept 23-34* PLACE OF BIRTH *Toronto*

CITIZENSHIP *Canadian* ARRIVED IN CANADA ____ IN ONT. *Life*

EDUCATION
LAST GRADE *13 - Took training for nurse* OCCUPATION *housewife* RELIGION *R.C.*

MENTAL SYMPTOMS: *acute schizophrenic state*

PHYSICAL CONDITION: — *has no complaints*

ALLERGIES: — *no* DIABETIC *no.*

PREVIOUS HOSPITAL CARE: *St. Michael's childbirth children — 7, 6, 5-3 yrs. of age.*

REFERRED BY *Dr.* FAMILY DOCTOR *Dr.*

St. Joseph's Hosp. — 1364 Islington Ave. N.

NEXT OF KIN *Mr. — Schellenberg* RELATIONSHIP *husband*

ADDRESS *same as above* PHONE: ____ *work.*

DATE *Sept 2-69* TIME *2145 hrs.* UNIT *3*

SIGNED ____

Figure 5. Application for admission.

FORM 123
25M-67-6123

ONTARIO

PROVINCE OF ONTARIO

Department of Health - Mental Health Branch

Ontario Hospital....*LSPH*...............

WARD ADMISSION RECORD

1. Name of Patient in full: *Shellenberg, mrs. Susan*

2. Date of Admission: *Aug 2/69.*

3. Time of Admission: *2100 hrs.*

4. Temperature, Pulse and Respiration at time of admission: *36 -72 -22*

5. Height *169 cm. 5'6*

6. Weight: *52 Kilos. 114*

7. Color of Eyes: *hazel*

8. Condition of Person on Admission: *clean*
   (General nutrition, cleanliness, vermin, etc.)

9. Skin: *eye operation - no visible scar non apparent*
   (Marks, bruises, scars, tatooing, rash, etc.)

10. Condition of Hair: *brown., clean.*
    (Colour, baldness, vermin, etc.)

11. Condition of Teeth: *good.*
    (Good, bad or artificial. Number and condition of dentures.)

12. Physical Disorders: *non apparent*
    (Deformities, amputations, ruptures, fractures, dislocations, etc.)

13. Condition of Clothing: *clean.*

14. Attitude of Patient on Admission: *co-operative, confused*
    (Co-operative, restive, disturbed, excited, violent, threatening, etc.)

15. Admission Care Given: *Routine*
    (Routine or special care. Tub, shower or bed bath. Treatment given, if any, including sedatives, etc.)

16. Articles Brought with Patient: *See clothing sheet*
    (Suitcase, watch, chain, knives, rings, brooches, money, glasses, etc.)

17. Disposal of Articles Found on Person:

PATIENT'S COPY

....
(Supervisor in Charge)

Figure 6. Ward admission record.

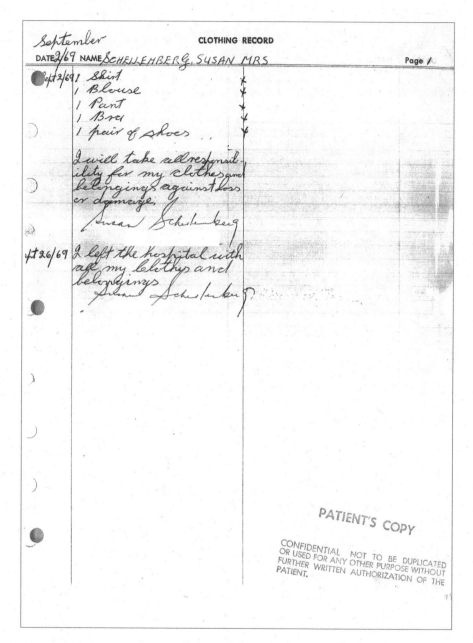

CLOTHING RECORD

September

DATE 2/69 NAME SCHELLENBERG, SUSAN MRS

Page 1

Sept 2/69 1 Shirt ✓
1 Blouse ✓
1 Pant ✓
1 Bra ✓
1 pair of shoes ✓

I will take all responsibility for my clothes and belongings against loss or damage.

Susan Schellenberg

Sept 26/69 I left the hospital with all my clothes and belongings

Susan Schellenberg

PATIENT'S COPY

CONFIDENTIAL NOT TO BE DUPLICATED OR USED FOR ANY OTHER PURPOSE WITHOUT FURTHER WRITTEN AUTHORIZATION OF THE PATIENT.

Figure 7. Clothing record.

EXAMINATION ON ADMISSION

O.H. *S.P.H.*

Case No. *28066*

Hospital Insurance Certificate No. ....

1. Name of patient in full: *Schellenberg Mrs Susan*
   (Surname)   (Given names)

2. Date of admission: *Sept 2-69*

3. Time of admission: *2045 hrs*

4. Accompanied to hospital by: *husband from St Joseph's Emergency*

5. Documentation: *Involuntary*

6. Are the admission papers in order? —

7. Has admission been awarded? *yes*

8. Did the relatives complete the financial arrangements with the business administrator?

9. Mental condition as observed on admission: — *Schizophrenic state
   uncommunicative,*

10. Physical condition (note physical symptoms requiring immediate attention):
    appears satisfactory

11. Assigned to ward: *3*

....
Admitting Physician *Clerk*

Form 105-A

- -

Figure 8. Examination on admission.

DEPARTMENT OF HEALTH FOR ONTARIO
MENTAL HEALTH BRANCH

O. H. ....

PHYSICAL EXAMINATION

Name *SCHELLENBERG, Susan*
(Surname)   (Given names)   Case No. ....

1. Sex *F*   2. Date of birth: *Sept. 23, 1934*

3. Height: *5'6"*   Weight: *112 #* Hair: *auburn* Eyes (colour): *hazel-brown*

4. Circulatory system: *rate 90, regular, no enlargement, BP 130/86 (sit.)*

5. Respiratory system: *low inspiratory wheeze over lt. upper lobe ant. + post.*

6. Digestive system and abdomen: *scaphoid, no organs or masses,*

7. Genito-urinary system: *no C-V tenderness*   *no striae gravidarum para IV*

8. Endocrine system: *thyroid neg.*

9. Nervous system: *drowsy, cranials grossly intact tendon reflexes + +, plantars ↓↓*

10. Skeletal system *neg.*

11. Teeth: *in good repair* Eyes: *react to L+A* Ears: *soft wax lt.* Nose & Throat: *neg.*

Operations: *T+A*   Tumors: *—*   Herniae: *—*   Menses: *finishing menses*

12. Special examinations when indicated or other noteworthy conditions:
Ambulatory Drowsy

13. SUMMARY (of all abnormal findings):

No major physical defects

PATIENT'S COPY

CONFIDENTIAL NOT TO BE DUPLICATED
OR USED FOR ANY OTHER PURPOSE WITHOUT
FURTHER WRITTEN AUTHORIZATION OF THE
PATIENT.

Date *Sept. 3/69*
Form 1 0 5 (25M-67-6148)   ....
                                      signature of examining physician

Figure 9. Physical examination.

PUBLIC HEALTH LABORATORY SERVICE
DEPARTMENT OF HEALTH
SERODIAGNOSIS—STANDARD TEST FOR SYPHILIS

ONTARIO

PATIENT'S NAME _SCHELLENBERG,_____ _Susan_____
SURNAME   FIRST NAME

PATIENT'S ADDRESS_____
STREET

TYPE OF SPECIMEN ____Blood____   CITY OR TOWN _____
DATE COLLECTED _Sept 4/69_

CLINICAL HISTORY:_____
PLEASE CHECK

DR.	**LABORATORY,**	PRENATAL ☐
	LAKESHORE PSYCHIATRIC HOSPITAL	U.S.A VISA ☐ CAN. VISA ☐
	NEW TORONTO, ONTARIO	FOLLOW-UP ☐
		TREATED _____
	_____ONTARIO	PREVIOUS RESULT _____

INSURED BY_____

CERTIFICATE NO._____GROUP NO._____

SURNAME OF SUBSCRIBER_____

YEAR OF BIRTH OF PATIENT_____SEX_____

◄ ALL INSURANCE INFORMATION REQUESTED MUST BE COMPLETED.

FOR LABORATORY USE ONLY

RESULTS	TESTS		REMARKS:
	VDRL	KRP	
NON-REACTIVE	✓		
REACTIVE			
QUANTITATIVE	1:		
UNSATISFACTORY FOR TEST			

Figure 10. Syphilis test result.

Figure 11. Urinalysis test results.

DEPARTMENT OF HEALTH FOR ONTARIO — MENTAL HEALTH DIVISION

LABORATORY REPORTS

Schellenberg Susan

[Surname]   [Given Name]

PAGE

CASE NO. *28066*

PATIENT'S COPY

PASTE 2ND REPORT ON THIS LINE

Name *Schellenberg Susan* Ward *3* Case No. *28066*

Doctor .... Lab. No. ....

| HB. *14.3* GM. | % | HAEMATOCRIT *42.5* % | R.B.C. *4.55* | W.B.C. *5,900* |

SED. RATE *5* MM/HR WESTERGREN

DIFFERENTIAL COUNT	NEUTROPHILES		LYMPHS.	MONOS.	EOSINS.	BASO.	ABNORMAL
	MATURE	YOUNG					
CELLS							

STAINED SMEAR ....

Date *Sept 4/69*   BLOOD (MORPHOLOGY)   Technician (1) (2) (3)

Figure 12. Blood test results.

5. LABORATORY REPORTS:

6. X-RAY REPORT: #1910. Sept.5/69.

No evidence of parenchymatous disease.

7. TUBERCULIN TEST:

..............................1/10cc = 1/20 m.gm.—
..............................1/10cc = 1.0 m.gm.—

8. ADDITIONAL INFORMATION:

CONFIDENTIAL NOT TO BE DUPLICATED OR USED FOR ANY OTHER PURPOSE WITHOUT FURTHER WRITTEN AUTHORIZATION OF THE PATIENT.

9. DIAGNOSTIC IMPRESSION: No evidence of pulmonary tuberculosis.

10. RECOMMENDATIONS: None

PATIENT'S COPY

.M.B.

Figure 13. Tuberculin test result.

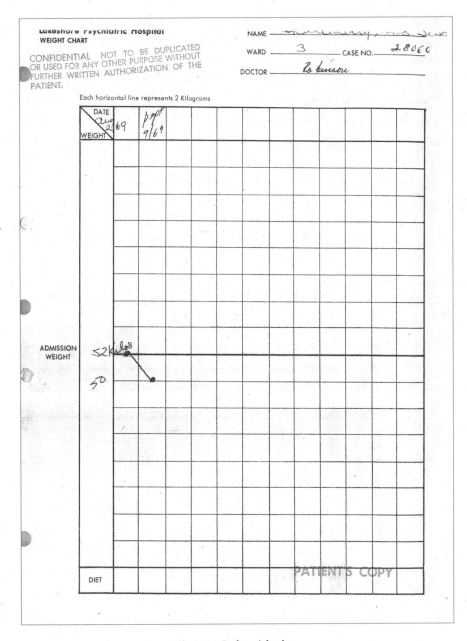

Figure 14. Body weight chart.

DEPARTMENT OF HEALTH FOR ONTARIO
MENTAL HEALTH BRANCH

O.H. L.S.P.H.

PAGE 28066

CLINICAL RECORD

CASE No.

HOSPITAL INSURANCE CERTIFICATE No.

NAME SCHELLENBERG, Susan
(surname) (Christian names)

MENTAL STATUS:
September 10, 1969

Patient is a tall, slender woman, appearing to be stated age of 34 years. She is pleasant and cooperative and enters fully into an interview.

Her most florid psychopathology was seen at admission when she said she heard an inner voice speaking. Then she was pale and tired, and complained of exhaustion. She would blink her eyes from time to time, as though fatigue was overpowering her. The tip of her nose was red. Her voice was pleasant and modulated. She had no thought disorder. However, her response to proverbs is poor, and she makes frequent mistakes in mental arithmetic.

Patient's memory is good. Orientation correct. Intelligence - good average or better. Insight and judgment - fair.

Impression: Paranoid Schizophrenia.

, M.D.

PATIENT'S COPY

CONFIDENTIAL NOT TO BE DUPLICATED OR USED FOR ANY OTHER PURPOSE WITHOUT FURTHER WRITTEN AUTHORIZATION OF THE PATIENT.

Form 127

Figure 15. Clinical record: mental status.

O.H. .... L.S.P.H. ....

CLINICAL RECORD

NAME................ SCHELLENBERG, Susan ....
             (surname)   (Christian names)

ADMISSION NOTE:
September 3, 1969

This 34 year old woman was admitted to this hospital yesterday
on a Physician's Application. Mrs. Schellenberg feels that she is under
God's influence and that her job is to help her husband and children. She
experiences auditory hallucinations consisting of the voice of God which
says such things as "Out of my bones thou shalt be made strong". Mrs.
Schellenberg says that her husband and Gos seem to be the same person.
She says that it was God's will that she marry her husband. This patient
has a thought disorder. Her conversation is vague and loosely associated.
She has not been sleeping for two weeks. She feels exhausted now.

Sept. 5, 1969

This patient said that she slept very poorly the first night in
hospital. Subsequently, she has been sleeping much better and over the
past six days has gradually improved until now when she is almost without
symptoms. Her delusions and hallucinations have disappeared also. She
feels that she was physically and mentally exhausted before coming to
hospital, as a result of having had four children on a yearly basis, and
then going to the religious retreat, ---------------------. She thinks
that after getting rested up in here, she will become totally well again.
She asked now that her medication be reduced.

Sept. 11, 1969

This patient is making steady improvement, and has had her medication
reduced in half. She is being aloud out to do some shopping with her
husband for school clotnes for their children this week. There is virtually
no trace of her acute breakdown which occured about three weeks ago.

Sept. 19, 1969

This patient is considered to have improved greatly, but to be
still in need of hospital care for another week or two. She was disappointed
in learning that she could not be discharged this week-end.

Form 127
100M-6P-1928

Figure 16a. Clinical record: progress report, admission to discharge. (Continues next page.)

O.H. .... L.S.P.H. ....

PAGE 28066

CLINICAL RECORD

CASE No. ....

HOSPITAL INSURANCE

NAME .... SCHELLENBERG, Susan ....

(surname)   (Christian names)

CERTIFICATE No. ....

September 25, 1969

This patient has made a good recovery and will be discharged tomorrow.

DISCHARGE NOTE:
September 26, 1969

Patient was discharged from hospital as of today. Condition was improved.

.... M.D.

Form 127
100M-68-4933

Figure 16b. Clinical record: progress report, admission to discharge (conclusion).

M.H.C. 104-2
15M-68-2809

ONTARIO DEPARTMENT OF HEALTH — MENTAL HEALTH DIVISION

PSYCHOLOGICAL EXAMINATION

Name: SCHELLENBERG, Susan (Mrs.)   Page........1.............   No. 28,066

Born:	Sept. 23, 1934 (aged 35).
Education:	Completed Gr. 13, followed by a 3-year nursing course at St. Michael's Hosp., and then by a one year Public Health nursing course at U. of T. completed at age 22.
Occupation:	After graduation she first worked for 1 year as a nurse in Emergency (St. Mike's), then 1 yr. for the Victorian Order of Nurses, and finally for 1½ years as a public health nurse She quit the latter 6 mos. after her marriage in 1960, (at age 26). In the main housewife since.
Dates Seen:	Sept. 3, (9, 10), 12, 17, 1969.
Referred by:	

BEHAVIOUR:

Mrs. S. was first seen on the ward the day after admission. She sat in a chair and thought and spoke in a very laborious and slow manner, occasionally grimacing and closing her eyes. She then suddenly went into tonic contraction followed by arm movements and generally orgasm-like body tremors. The writer told her to stop it and she immediately did, relaxing. This happened again a little late in the conversation. The writer just watched her. Soon she asked him to stop her. He laid his hand on her arm and said "Stop it". She did, and thanked for it. (She later explained these tremors as her "sharing in Christ's passion", this working through her). At this time she also spoke in her most disclosing fashion (covering up later), and mentioned some of her home conflicts and difficulties - communication with husband, sex, and people being some of the items.

Within a week she was sufficiently improved to do testing. She was cooperative, and apparently anxious and time-conscious. She was eager to talk when given the opportunity - about wanting another child (5th) as she feels she has matured more with every pregnancy; about various community projects (mainly visiting hospitals), and how she considered being here a valuable learning experience.

TESTS ADMINISTERED:

- Intake Survey
- Hartford-Shipley Scale
- M. M. Personality Inventory
- Partial S. C. Test

CONCLUSIONS:

1. Mrs. S. is _estimated_ to presently function in the Average range of intelligence.

2. On personality testing she was sufficiently improved and defensively coping to give a "normal" protocol (on M.M.P.I.). But her ego strength stood low. Otherwise she gave the impression of a deep and slow thinking person who expends

Figure 17a. Psychological examination. (Continues next page.)

M.H.C. 104-2
15M-68-2809

ONTARIO DEPARTMENT OF HEALTH — MENTAL HEALTH DIVISION

PSYCHOLOGICAL EXAMINATION

Name: SCHELLENBERG, Susan (Mrs.)   Page........2...........   No. 28,066

much labour and strenuous effort in giving verbal expression to her thoughts, all accompanied by certain mannerisms (mainly facial).

Drawing on past clinical experience, and considerable probing of her most bizarre thinking, delusions and behaviour whilst actively psychotic, the writer considers her condition at such times to hold a serious element of potential danger, particularly to a family of 4 small children (now ranging age 3 - 7). This revolves around the religious core of her psychosis, and the ascertained fact that at such times she feels totally controlled by other forces (or hypnotized), being a "passive vessel of God's imagination", and thus capable of carrying out anything as directed without being able to exercise any volitional powers.

Clinically, her defensive mechanisms soon become operative again (a great deal of repression and rationalization) and thus largely screening off her former revelations. She seemed to have a great difficulty accepting her breakdown, often stressing how wonderful it was to have it, and how good God was to her thus helping her "to grow and mature". She also blamed much on a run-down condition due to physical ailments at various connected times. Her philosophy of life seems to be rigidly idealistic, with a continuous dictation of "shoulds" active in her mind. She desperately sought for causation of her breakdown in the past and seemed nearly ready to ritually retrace all the events surrounding her religious retreat during which her psychosis emerged.

Mrs. S. attached a large portion of blame to her "undisciplined imagination", and an "inability to listen to the present", being plagued with over-active imagination and absent-mindedness. This she best illustrates with the situation at home when she is cooking, for instance, and becomes completely oblivious of her children trying to contact her as she is off on cloud 9. She also seems obsessed with the idea of more community involvement and this helping her marital situation. (Consider this against her being weak enough in coping with her children as to require the services of a live-in maid, since her 4th pregnancy). "We are not involved enough in community projects and we give money but not ourselves to the needy". The life event with the great impact was "my husband", because - "he has educated, loved, forgiven and stayed with me over all the problems that have lead me to grow up as a woman". Her main interest in life? "Husband, children, art". (The latter seems another obsession in her bid for approval, greatness and recognition. She attends art classes, and seems a pretty good painter). Describing herself? "Growing up". She later explained she meant "just coping". Help thought needed? "Work, discipline, imagination, patience to wait till I can leave hospital". And the last presents quite a challenge to her. She wrote further: "I jump into everything I do and get so involved. The retreat that I made prior to this stay in hospital was too strenuous for me, as I had just gotten over a pericardical infection and was physically incapable of the routine of the retreat". She also wrote: I want to know ---- "God"; Men ---- "can teach women a great deal"; My greatest fear ---- "is that the children will be hurt by or in a car"; My nerves --- "have improved after each pregnancy"; I suffer --- "no loss of dignity when I am loved". This last, she said, meant that though she is sick and here she suffered a loss of dignity because her husband still loves her.

Figure 17b. Psychological examination. (Continues next page.)

M.H.C. 104-2
15M-68-2809

ONTARIO DEPARTMENT OF HEALTH — MENTAL HEALTH DIVISION

PSYCHOLOGICAL EXAMINATION

Name: SCHELLENBERG, Susan (Mrs.) Page.......3........ No. 28,066

In conclusion, this lady has been shy and lacking initiative in her youth. She appears to be, and probably has long been, psychologically fragile. What 'seething caldron of snakes' had become uncovered during her late actively psychotic episode, has now again been lidded, but has not necessarily disappeared. The writer thus feels that with young children in the home her condition warrants careful professional supervision over the near future.

Psychologist.

CONFIDENTIAL NOT TO BE DUPLICATED OR USED FOR ANY OTHER PURPOSE WITHOUT FURTHER WRITTEN AUTHORIZATION OF THE PATIENT.

PATIENT'S COPY

Figure 17c. Psychological examination (conclusion).

SOCIAL RECORD

SCHELLENBERG, Susan

Case Book No. ....

ept. 5, 1969

cial Work.

INITIAL SOCIAL WORK ASSESSMENT:

Informant: Mr.   Schellenberg (husband)

      Islington   (House)
                    (office)
      Vice-President in charge of sales for

    Mr. Schellenberg, a well-set, tall, neat and attractive, clean shaven young man with brown eyes and hair and an honest, open face was seen in an office interview on Sept. 5, 1969. He said that he and his wife are particularly close so he is very concerned about her condition and has been trying to delve into the Retreat she attended to find out just what did happen there.

PRESENTING PROBLEM:

    Early in Aug. patient picked up a virus so was very tired. After their 10 days at a cottage in Muskoka she picked up, however.

    Fri. Aug. 22 - Sat. Aug. 30 patient went on a Retreat in Connection with the R.C. Church. Here apparently she didn't sleep for 7 days and nights, was in a room by herself and was afraid. Four times she thought she was dying, one night went through a complete pregnancy, another night had no feeling in her arms. She heard music and sounds in her ears and hung on to Biblical sayings and poems and certain words that had meaning for her.

    On Friday August 29 they called patient's husband and asked him to take her home; she seemed emotionally drained, looked drawn and her eyes were stary and beady.

    On Sat. patient seemed very tired and lay on the bed with her eyes twitching and flickering till 8 A.M. - her husband couldn't wake her.

    On Sunday, August 31, they (pt. husband and 4 children) went to 10:30 Mass and came home. Soon afterwards he couldn't find her and discovered the car was gone. At 1:10 he got a call from Queensway Hospital saying patient was there and to come down.

    It seems that patient had made a Nativity Scene out of stove pipe wiring and decided to take this picture to the Church of the Nativity. She told her husband later that when she got there she heard music, thought she was the Virgin Mary and floated down the aisle to the Crucifix. This apparently created a stir in the Church and 2 of the people drove her to Queensway Hospital.

    Husband went to the Church of the Nativity to get the car and found patient's scene of the Nativity still in the back seat. At the Hospital, the nurse told him that patient was deeply disturbed emotionally and was schizophrenic and was to see the psychiatrist at 2:30 PM; it was

Figure 18a Social record. (Continues next page.)

SOCIAL RECORD

Cont'd.....

then 2:10. As soon as he saw patient he knew she was in trouble but felt strongly that she would recover better at home with the family so he took her home. She was sitting in a daze and wouldn't go in the house as she thought her husband was the devil speaking. He pulled her into the house and she seemed O.K. At 2:30 patient's mother, 2 aunts and her sister and brother-in-law from Winnipeg arrived and stayed till 5PM. Although patient looked tired and drawn she handled herself well. Patient and her husband talked from 7:30 - 10:30 P.M. and slept less than 2 hours out of the 7 they were in bed, as patient thought she was the Virgin Mary and her husband was God.

Monday, Sept. 1 she decided to go to Mass at 10; she got in the car, backed out of the driveway - was so intense he couldn't stop her - then saw her husband wasn't there, felt God wasn't with her so returned home. She had lunch with her relatives and spent the afternoon and evening with friends but was a little strange - felt someone was laughing at her. At night they slept 3 hours out of 8; again she was wakeful and thought she was the Virgin Mary and got her husband to recite the Rosary.

Tuesday, A.M. was hectic. He took patient and the children to Mass and Communion, then took the children to school. She was "in a bit of a fog". At noon patient said, "There's evil here; there's something going on", and didn't say much else. He made an appointment to see their doctor, Dr. . . . . ; . . . . , at 8 PM. at 5:15 PM patient wouldn't look at her husband, thought something evil would happen and that both were going to die, wouldn't let her husband out of her sight and imitated his every movement. At 6 PM they went for a drive and went to St. Joseph's Hospital Emergency; here Dr. . . saw her at 9:30 PM, spoke to Dr.   and arranged for her admission to this Hospital for that same night, Sept. 2, 1969.

FAMILY SITUATION AND RELATIONSHIPS:

Patient, age 34, married Mr.   Schellenberg, 3 years her senior Dec. 26, 1960; her family didn't look with favour on him as a suitor but she insisted on marrying him because she loved him. They have had no finan cial worries as he is Vice-President in charge of Sales at   . He has many decisions to make and is under pressure at his work; at one time was working 70 hours a week.

He said that he and his wife are very close to each other and have complete trust and confidence in each other. They have their arguments but he always treats her as a lady and they do everything as a family; family unity is very important. He is the head of the family, though; they complement each other.

PATIENT'S COPY

Cont'd.............

Figure 18b. Social record. (Continues next page.)

SOCIAL RECORD

SCHELLENBERG,   Susan   Case Book No....................

Cont'd....

They both wanted to have a large family so she stopped working a
year after marriage. Their children are ((1) a daughter age 7, (2) a son age 6,
(3) a son age 5,(4) a son age 3 :   They agree concerning the discipline of these children. He has always kept a girl - they
get girls on domestic contracts from England and their present girl is
exceptionally good - to help his wife with the children so that she is not
under pressure or over-worked physically.

Patient has a very strong R.C. background. Patient's husband's
father was Protestant and his mother R.C. and the children were christened
R.C.; hisband also took R.C. instruction previous to his marriage.

Patient was described as kind, thoughtful, sensitive, refined,
conscientious and hard working, wanting to help people. She has creative
ability and initiative, is artistic and imaginative, enjoys making rock
gardens and for 3 years has taken painting lessons in the Artists' Work
Shop. She is an excellent mother and cook - has taken cooking courses -
and wants everything done the right way. She feels that we don't do
enought for other people while he feels he should spend more time with his
own family rather than going to help outsiders. He said he himself if
aggressive and strong-willed; he and patient fit together well and complemen
each other. He has a logical, rationalizing mind and is very interested in
sports - football, golf, skiing, swimming, pool - patient goes skiing with
him.

SIGNIFICANT BACKGROUND:

Born Sept. 23, 1934 in Toronto, patient was the 2nd of 4 children.
Father, Joseph Patrick Regan, was of Irish ancestry and was very kind and
generous - always helping people. He was a salesman for John Inglis.
Eleven years ago he had a heart attack and 6 years ago died - was diabetic
and had lost the circulation in the lower part of one leg. Mother, Anne
Ronan, now 58, lives at   One is very aggressive,
determined and strong willed; 3 years ago she had 2 massive strokes and was
in Intensive Care and paralyzed but has come around and even drives a car.
The last 3 or 4 months she has been acting strangely - chuckles inappropriately, stays in the house for 2 days without washing the dishes or
cleaning up, hurts her dearest friends. The parents married late - about
35 - and at first had a hard time financially but father was a super salesman so was able to build up the family fortunes and leave mother comfortably
off. They got along well together; while she was the dominant one, he controlled her and she idolized him.

Patient completed Grade 13 at Loretto Abbey, so led a rather
protected life. She took her R.N. course at St. Michael's Hospital and
specialized in O.R. She found this work hard on her. She was a PHN for
2-3 years and enjoyed it - was conscientious, hard working and aware of
poverty. She stopped working 1 year after her marriage Dec. 26, 1960.

Figure 18c. Social record. (Continues next page.)

SOCIAL RECORD

SCHELLENBERG, ...Susan............   Case Book No. ....:.............

Cont'd.....

PATIENT'S SIBLINGS:

1.

> Note: Text deleted here lists the name, age, place of residence, marital
> status and number of children for each of Susan's siblings; all were

2.
> married and had children:
>> 1. Brother, age 37

3.
>> 2. Susan, age 34
>> 3. Brother, age 30
>> 4. Sister, age 23
> Places of employment and occupation are listed for the men (i.e., the

4.
> two brothers and one broth-in law); all held business positions.

....y ...avo i child.

Patient's husband told something of his own background. His parents
came to Canada from Germany in 1929 or 1930 because of Hitler. His
father, age 68, was a hard working tool and die maker; they were a struggling family. From 1957-1966 parents were in Detroit but are now retired
in St. Catherines. Mr. Schellenberg himself was born in Hamilton but
from age 5-20 was brought up just outside of St. Catherines. He graduated
from Queen's University in Mechanical Engineering. His only sister, 2
years his junior, is happily married, has 4 children, and works as a secretary in St. Catherines.

SUMMARY:

This 34-year-old Roman Catholic mother of 4 children would appear
to have been upset by a week-long R.C. retreat she attended Aug. 22-30.
On Aug. 31 she created a stir in church and was taken to Queensway
Hospital, where a nurse told patient's husband that patient "was deeply
disturbed emotionally and schizophrenic". He insisted on taking her home.
Monday and Tuesday she continued to be disturbed and sleepless, thinking
she was the Virgin Mary and that her husband was alternately God and the
devil and that something evil would happen. Tuesday night husband took
patient to St. Joseph's Emergency where arrangements were made for her
admission to this Hospital for that same night, Sept. 2, 1969.

Patient's childhood and married life would both appear to have been
happy with no overt problems.

PLAN: If and when patient recovers sufficiently to leave Hospital, there
will be no problem concerning her returning home.

PATIENT'S COPY   Social Worker.

31

Figure 18d. Social record (conclusion).

Ontario Department of Health
Mental Health Division   Case No. __28066__

CONFERENCE REPORT

Name   SCHELLENBERG,   Susan
_____
        (Surname)   (Given Names)   O.H. __L.S.P.H.__

Private and Confidential

September 18, 1969

This 34-year-old woman was presented in Conference today, in the presence of the full unit staff, presided over by Dr. ____, She had been admitted on an Involuntary Basis on September 2, 1969. The Physician's Application stated that she was apathetic, imitated all movements of her husband, related recent visual and auditory hallucinations during a religious retreat, feels that she is about to die, and that other times she is the Virgin Mary. It was stated that she had not slept for about a week.

The physical examination on her admission was not remarkable, nor was the chest x-ray. Urinalysis showed a rare white blood cell and red blood cell per high power field. The haemotology was normal.

In the history, it was noted that the patient had been born in 1934, had attained Grade thirteen at Loretto Academy, later trained as a nurse at St. Michael's Hospital, and subsequently had qualified as a Public Health Nurse, owrking in Etobicoke for awhile. It was said that her husband was born in Canada of German descent, and was a university graduate in mechanical engineering with an executive position with the ____ Company.

Recently, the patient had a viral infection in August, which had left her tired. Then on August 22nd, and for eight days following she had entered a religious retreat at ____ under Roman Catholic auspices. It was said that she had no real sleep for about eight nights. On August 31st, after Mass, the husband found his wife at the Queensway Hospital and brought her home. At that time she was sick, and again on September 2nd, he took her to St. Joseph's Hospital from where she was admitted to this Hospital.

The patient met her husband in 1960, and four children have been born to them in a five year period. The patient has a maid at home for the last few years. However, after the second child she had an infectious mononucleosis, and has been occupied at the Artists' Work Shop on an avocational basis.

The mental state indicated a tired young married mother, who frequently blinked her eyes, and told of an inner voice speaking to her. She seemed able to distinguish sharply between good and evil. She spoke of being under the influence of psychological forces that threatened to overwhelm the ego.

In hospital, the patient slept poorly for the first night, but then improved slowly but steadily over the next ten days. Early this week her medication was decreased, and later stopped.

Cont'd............

Figure 19a. Conference report. (Continues next page.)

Case No. 28066

CONFERENCE REPORT

Name SCHELLENBERG, Susan
(Surname)   (Given Names)   O.H. L.S.P.H.

Private and Confidential

Sept. 18, 1969 Cont'd....

In Conference, the patient was cooperative but under visible strain as she answered questions well, although revealing florid psychopathology and weak ego defenses. It was decided that she was suffering from an ACUTE SCHIZOPHRENIC REACTION (295.9), but had had disturbing thinking for sometime. It was felt the prognosis was guarded, especially if she were to undertake another pregnancy, which has been considered by her and her husband.

It was felt that she could be permitted to go out this week-end, as she had on the last week-end, but that medication should be recommenced, and that an explanation should be made to the husband of the serious responsibility she took when she was alone with the children. She was advised to be followed in after-care for some months.

M.D.

Figure 19b. Conference report (conclusion).

28066

FINAL NOTE

NAME: SCHELLENBERG, Susan DATE OF ADMISSION: September 2nd, 1969

DATE OF DISCHARGE: September 26th, 1969

Mrs. Schellenberg has now recovered sufficiently that it is felt she can be discharged to be followed in Aftercare. Since it is felt that should Mrs. Schellenberg's illness recur, there might be some danger to her children, her husband has been advised that she should not be left alone with the children, but should have a housekeeper, who would be there while he is at work. In addition, the Public Health Nurse is being asked to call at Mrs. Schellenberg's home regularly in order to give the patient some emotional support.

The diagnosis is Acute Schizophrenic Reaction.

Treatment has been with medical and nursing supervision, group therapy, supportive psychotherapy and medication. The patient is currently receiving Stelazine 10 mg. b.i.d., Largactil 50 mg. q.h.s. and Cogentin 2 mg. q.h.s.

M.D.

CONFIDENTIAL NOT TO BE DUPLICATED OR USED FOR ANY OTHER PURPOSE WITHOUT FURTHER WRITTEN AUTHORIZATION OF THE PATIENT.

PATIENT'S COPY

Figure 20. Final note.

DEPARTMENT OF HEALTH
MENTAL HEALTH BRANCH

REGISTER No. _____

CASE BK. No. _28066_

REPORT ON PHYSICAL CONDITION ON DISCHARGE OR DEATH

NAME _SHELLENBERG, MRS. SUSAN_   WARD _3_

| Left Hospital _2..1_ | 19 | at | M. | Examined _2..1_ | 19 | at | M. |
| Died | 19 | at | M. | Examined _____ | 19 | at | M. |

CONDITION OF PERSON: (General Nutrition, Cleanliness, Vermin, Etc.) _CLEAN WELL NOURISHED_

Weight _50 Kg._ Pounds

SKIN: (Marks, Bruises, Skin Diseases, Eruption and Locality) _NONE APPARENT_

PHYSICAL DISORDERS: (Deformities, Ruptures, Fractures, Dislocations, Etc.) _NONE APPARENT_

In event of Death describe fully the external appearances of the body at the time of Death:

QUALITY AND CONDITION OF CLOTHING: _CLEAN_

ARTICLES BELONGING TO PATIENT ON DISCHARGE OR DEATH: (See Private Clothing List).

RETURN THIS SLIP TO OFFICE

Date _Sept 26_ 19 _69_   (Signed) _____ Nurse

Form 177
15M-68-1981

PATIENT'S COPY

Figure 21. Report on physical condition on discharge.

LAKESHORE PSYCHIATRIC HOSPITAL   NAME _____

DOCTOR'S ORDER RECORD   CASE NO. _____

DATE ORDERED	ORDER	BY WHOM ORDERED	NURSE'S SIGNATURE
Sept 2/69	Bathroom Privileges		
	Trilafon 10 mgs. I.M. stat		
	Stelazine 10 mgs. in A.M. and then		
	as ordered by staff psychiatrist		
Sept. 4	Stelazine 10 mg. b.d.		
	Largactil 100 mg. h.s. ⎫ 1 week		
	Cogentin 2 mg. h.s. ⎭		
Sept. 8	Group 1		
Sept. 11	Stelazine 10 mg. q.a.m. ⎫		
	Largactil 50 mg. h.s. ⎬ 1 week		
	Cogentin 2 mg. h.s. ⎭		
	May go shopping c̄ husband		
	for school clothes 2 pm – 9 pm today		
Sept 12	Weekend privileges		
Sept 15	Discontinue ⎧ Stelazine		
	⎨ Largactil		
	⎩ Cogentin		
	Ground privileges		
Sept 18	Stelazine 10 mg. b.i.d. ⎫		
	Largactil 50 mg. h.s. ⎬ 2 weeks		
	Cogentin 2 mg. h.s. ⎭		
Sept 19	LOA weekend c̄ husband		
	till Mon. eve		
Sept 25	Discharge tomorrow		
	c̄ meds. Rx		
	Return ____ ____		

Figure 22. Doctor's order record.

LAKESHORE PSYCHIATRIC HOSPITAL

OUTPATIENT SERVICES

Unit After Care Etobicoke   OHIC # : 91221101   Casebook No.: 28066

Surname	Given Names	Date of Birth	First Admission
			Readmission

SCHELLENBERG, Mrs. Susan Ann   23/9/1934

Occupation	Religion	Sex	Marital Status
			S M W Div Sep CL
Housewife	R.C.	Female	Married

Place of birth	Years in Canada		Education
Toronto	Life		Grade 13

Address:	Number	Street	Municipality	County	Phone
1. 127 Lloyd Manor Road			Islington	York	239-7478
2.					
3.					

CONFIDENTIAL NOT TO BE DUPLICATED OR USED FOR ANY OTHER PURPOSE WITHOUT FURTHER WRITTEN AUTHORIZATION OF THE PATIENT.

Responsible relative or friend

Name	Relationship	Address	Phone
1. Mr.	Husband	Same as Above	
2.			

Referring Source   Address

— L.S.P.H.

Family Physician   Address

Professional Staff Coordinator

Presenting problem

Diagnosis

Acute Schizophrenic Reaction

Other Hospitalizations

Date opened	Date closed	Service
September, 26, 1969	Sept 12/72	AFTERCARE ETOBICOKE

June 1972

PATIENT'S COPY

Figure 23. Outpatient services form.

DEPARTMENT OF HEALTH FOR ONTARIO

MENTAL HEALTH BRANCH

O.H. ___L.S.P.H.___

PAGE _____

CASE No. _____

CLINICAL RECORD

HOSPITAL INSURANCE

NAME ___SCHELLENBERG,___ ___Susan___

CERTIFICATE No. _____

(surname)   (Christian names)

AFTER-CARE:
October 10, 1969

    Patient was in for her first after-care appointment this morning accompanied by her husband. Her medication had run out one week earlier th her recall date. She was looking welland feeling well. She had no return of her symptoms. She is looking after her family as before, and in additio attending the Artists' Workshop downtown. Her sleeping and eating habits are good.

    Patient was given a prescription for Stelazine 10 mg. b.i.d., Largactil 50 mg. h.s., and Cogentin 2 mg. h.s. with a return appointment in one month's time, and the prospect of having her medication reduced at the next visit.

                                                  M.D.

November 10, 1969

    Patient and her husband were in for her second after-care appointm She was looking well and feeling well. She has had no return of her sympto She mentioned feeling a little tired at night-time and going to bed early, sleeping soundly until the next morning. It was decided that her medicatio could be reduced by omitting the Stelazine in the evening. Husband offered to keep their present maid until March, which will be a big help in the household. She was given a return appointment for one month in early Decem

                                             , M.D.

December 9, 1969

    Patient was in with her husband for her third aftercare appointme She was looking well and feeling well. She had no symptoms and no complain except for feeling dizzy sometimes when she is stooped over or got up sudde She said that one morning she forgot to take her Stelazine and felt remarka clear for the entire day. As a result, her prescription was renewed with Stelazine ommitted and the Largactil reduced to 25 mg. h.s. Her next appointment is for two months from now.

                                           M.D.

February 2, 1970

    Patient was in with her husband this morning. She was not lookin or feeling quite so well as on her previous visits. She has been out of medication for the last week, and feels that she has not been sleeping so well. However, she has been sleeping deeply enough to have been dreaming, and some of the dreams have been pleasant, although not all of them. She was advised, after some discussion to continue with tranquilizing medicatio namely Stelazine 5 mg. instead of Largactil, for another two months and to come in again in April.

                                          M.D.

Form 127
100M-68-4233

Figure 24a. Clinical records: after-care notes. (Continues next page.)

O.H. LAKESHORE PSYCHIATRIC HOSPITAL

PAGE................

CLINICAL RECORD

CASE No. 28066

HOSPITAL INSURANCE

NAME .... SCHELLENBERG, Mrs. Susan Anne ....
(surname)   (Christian names)

CERTIFICATE No. ....

AFTERCARE
April 7, 1970

Patient was in promptly. About three weeks ago she phoned to say that the medication was making her sluggish, and was advised to discontinue it. She has been getting along well this last winter. She has been going skiing every weekend, usually with the children, but once she and her husba went off for a weekend skiing together. She has not been going to the Artists' workshop, for some time, feeling that it did not help her very

much. She is planning on taking some holidays this summer. She says that she is sleeping about seven hours every night, and waking up about five or six in the morning. Sometimes not being able to fall asleep again.
In general, she looked well this morning, and gave a good account of hersel
She was given a three month interval and a return appointment in July.

M. D.

July 14, 1970

Patient was accompanied by her husband this afternoon.
She was looking rather well, and claimed to be feeling well. Husband gave some examples of her good behaviour over the last few months, and expressed his own gratitude for the supervision and care she received here. She is sleeping well and her household is operating better than it has for many years, as long as the second or third years of their marriage, according to husband. Patient was given an appointment three months from now and will not be taking any medication for that period.

, M. D.

September 22nd, 1970

Husband and wife phoned independently of each other to-day to say that patient had been a little more vague and distant with difficulty in concentrating over the last three or four days. An appointment was given and they came down to be assessed. Patient has been entertaining about every second week-end for the last six months. In addition, she has been looking after two retarded children for the last two or three weeks in the afternoons. Patient had some difficulty concentrating and looked a little more distant and vague. She was given a prescription for Stelazine 5 mg. h.s. with a return appointment in one month.

, M. D.

PATIENT'S COPY

Form 127
100M-68-4233

Figure 24b. Clinical records: after-care notes. (Continues next page.)

CLINICAL RECORD

LAKESHORE PSYCHIATRIC HOSPITAL

Facility

Case Book No. 28068

Ward or Unit 3

Name   SCHELLENBERG, Mrs. Susan Ann

AFTERCARE:
October 20th, 1970

Husband and wife were in to-day. Patient is pregnant again, but
fortunately is looking forward to the child. She has had no symptoms and
no complaints in the last interval. Her prescription was renewed as before
with a return appointment in one month.

., M.D.

November 24, 1970
Husband and wife were in to-day. Patient is getting along
well with her pregnancy, but says she weighs 128 lbs., the most she
has ever weighed. She has no nausea with this pregnancy like the
others. She is going for her check-up with her obstetrician today.
She is sleeping in the afternoons and avoiding extra responsibility
at the present. Her prescription was renewed as before with a return
appointment in two months.

M.D.

January 21, 1971.

Patient was in accompanied by her husband. She is getting along
fairly well and sees her obstetrician regularly, with the next visit
being tomorrow. Her nausea has disappeared. Her prescription was
renewed with a return appointment in two months.

., M.D.

March 18, 1971.

Patient was in accompanied by her husband. She is getting along
fairly well with her pregnancy, and is now about six months advanced. She
has been to her obstetrician recently. She was asked about her need for
medication, and wanted to continue. Her prescription was renewed with a
return appointment in two months.

., M.D.

May 20, 1971.
Patient was looking well and feeling fairly well. She is now
about 2 or 3 weeks from term and she expects to go into the St. Michael's
Hospital for delivery of her baby. Her husband wasn't able to bring her
down this morning so she came by taxi. She is sleeping fairly well and
following a diet given her by her physician. It seems that the four older
children have helped her quite a lot by doing some chores around the house
for her during this last interval. Her prescription was renewed as before
for 2 months.

, M.D. /

Figure 24c. Clinical records: after-care notes. (Continues next page.)

CLINICAL RECORD

LAKESHORE PSYCHIATRIC HOSPITAL......... Case Book No....28065
Facility   Ward or Unit........3

Name SCHELLENBERG,   Mrs. Susan Ann.

AFTERCARE NOTES:

July 20, 1971.

Patient was looking well and feeling well today, as she was in the company of her husband. She had her fifth baby, a boy, about six weeks ago, at St. Michael's Hospital. The baby has been developing very well, and everybody in the family is pleased. Patient's husband is giving his wife as much support and help as he can. At present, the baby is just beginning to discontinue his night feedings. Patient was given a prescription for the same medication as before with a return appointment in two months.

M.D./

September 16, 1971.

This patient tells me that she had a baby in June. Apparently, she had no problems surrounding the baby's birth and has felt quite competent in his care. At the beginning of September, Mrs. Schellenberg had a tubal ligation. There is apparently some strain involved in this as the operation was to have been in the morning and it was delayed until the afternoon. Last week, the patient noted that she was finding her thoughts were racing and that she was having some trouble in sleeping because of the thoughts going through her mind. She is not able to specify any abnormality of her thoughts only that she was under some pressure in thinking. She took 10 mgs., of Stelazine rather than 5 per day for a few days and she says she has felt better since then. I could not detect any psychotic symptoms at present. She looks a little tired but denies any feeling of depression. She says there is no problem in looking after the baby. I suggested to her that she should continue to take 10 mgs., of Stelazine a day for the time being and she has agreed to that. We therefore prescribed Stelazine, 10 mgs., q.h.s. and Cogentin, 2 mgs. q.h.s. The patient has another appointment in one months' time.

-, M.D. /

October 14, 1971.

Patient was smiling and confident today. She was accompanied by her husband. She has a four month old baby at home who is getting along well. She and her husband have had good holidays. The other four children are in school. She is sleeping well and feels that she can go off the 10 mgs. Stelazine to 5 mg If complications develop, she can double up on her medication again. There were nopsychotic symptoms today. Neither was she depressed. Her prescription was made out for Stelazine, 5 mgs., q.h.s., with Cogentin, 2 mgs., q.h.s. for two months.

PATIENT'S COPY   M.D.   /

Figure 24d. Clinical records: after-care notes. (Continues next page.)

CLINICAL RECORD

LAKESHORE PSYCHIATRIC HOSPITAL ....
Facility

Case Book No. 28066

Ward or Unit 3

Name   SCHELLENBERG, Susan

AFTERCARE NOTES
December 21, 1971

Patient was feeling well today. She was accompanied by her four
year old son   She has not been involved in the Christmas rush and has
avoided getting under severe pressure. She thinks she is coming to accept
herself as a chronic patient, but was discouraged from doing this. Her prescrip
was renewed for Stelazine 5 mgm. with Cogentn 2 mgm. h.s. and a return appointm
in three months.

M.D.

March 28, 1972

Patient was feeling well today. She was accompanied by her husband.
Her 5 children are down with chickenpox this week. She has no complaints herself
She did mention there was an odour to her urine, possibly acetone and she mention
that diabetes ran in her family. Her prescription was renewed as before with a
return appointment in three months.

M.D.

June 1 , 1972

This patient was in time for her appointment. She presented no
complaints. There were no thought disorders or perceptual disturbances elicited.
Her mood was within normal limits. She will go on a trip to Japan with her
husband next week. Present medication: Stelazine 5 mg. h.s., Cogentin 2 mg. h.s.
Next appointment in 3 months.

, M.D.

September 12th, 1972.

Patient was in promptly for her appointment. She had run out of pills i
the last week because she has been taking two a night instead of one a night sinc
her husband had a possible heart attack about a week ago, while playing tennis.
He has been in the Toronto General Hospital and although his E.C.G. 's were
negative at first, there are now beginning to show some slight wave changes.
Her youngest son accompanied her and he looked healthy and active. Patient herse
said that she is feeling well without any distress and was becoming more clear
mentally. Her prescription was renewed for Stelazine, 5 mgs., h.s. with Cogentin
2 mgs., h.s. for three months.

M.D.

Figure 24e. Clinical records: after-care notes. (Continues next page.)

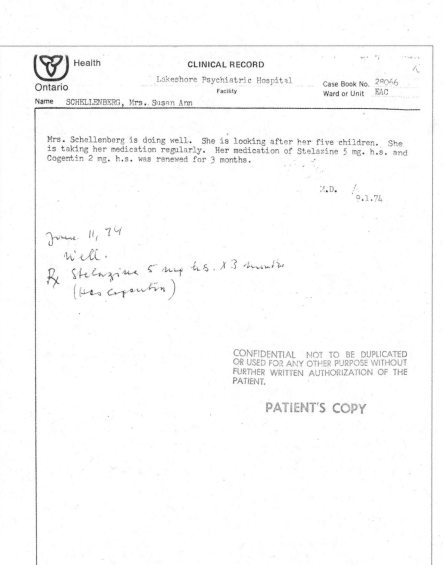

Figure 24f. Clinical records: after-care notes. (Continues next page.)

CLINICAL RECORD

LAKESHORE PSYCHIATRIC HOSPITAL
Facility

Case Book No. ....
Ward or Unit

Name · SCHELLINBERG, Susan (Mrs.)

AFTERCARE NOTES
November 23, 1972

Mrs. Schellinberg was today seen by me and the following medication
was prescribed:

Stelazine 5 mg. h.s.) x 1 month with two repeats to be mailed.
Cogentin 2 mg. h.s. _)

M.D.

February 12, 1973

Mrs. Schillenberg seems very guarded in her conversation and
illicts little information. She says she does take her medication
regularly. Stelazine 5 mgs, h.s. and Cogentin 2 mgs, h.s. - renewed
for three months.

R.N.

April 30, 1973

Mrs. Schellinberg contines to cope satisfactorily. She has five
children under ten years of age and finds the pace rather hectic at times. She
says taking her medication regularly helps her over the rough spots.

Stelazine 5 mg. h.s.)
Cogentin 2 mg. h.s.) renewed x 3 months

R.N.

July 25, 1973

One months medication with two repeats was arranged for Mrs. Schellinberg
today. She is working and apparently doing satisfactory.

Stelazine 5 mg. h.s.
Cogentin 2 mg. h.s.

R.N.

October 9, 1973

Mrs. Schellenberg seems to be keeping a healthy mental attitude. She is
able to cope adequately with her small children and household responsibilities.
Stelazine 5 mg. h.s. and Cogentin 2 mg. was renewed for 3 months.

. R.N.

Figure 24g. Clinical records: after-care notes. (Continues next page.)

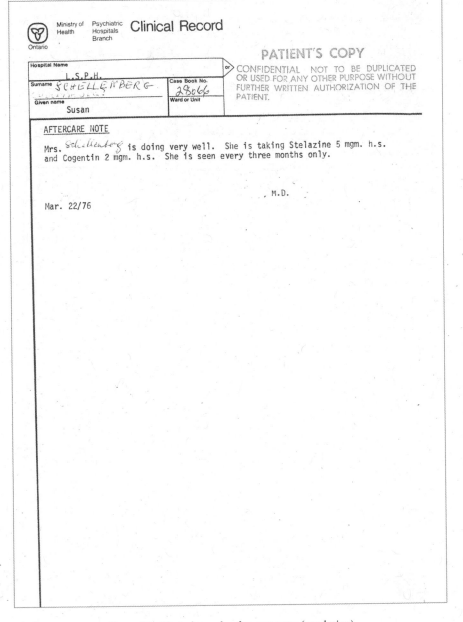

Ministry of Health · Psychiatric Hospitals Branch — **Clinical Record**

Ontario

Hospital Name		
L.S.P.H.		
Surname SCHELLENBERG	Case Book No. 28066	
Given name Susan	Ward or Unit	

AFTERCARE NOTE

Mrs. Schellenberg is doing very well. She is taking Stelazine 5 mgm. h.s. and Cogentin 2 mgm. h.s. She is seen every three months only.

, M.D.

Mar. 22/76

Figure 24h. Clinical records: after-care notes (conclusion).

LAKESHORE PSYCHIATRIC HOSPITAL
TORONTO, ONTARIO

37

PHYSICIAN'S ORDERS

NAME: *Schellenberg Sara*

ADDRESS:

PATIENT ALLERGIC TO

DIAGNOSIS

AGE:

WARD OR UNIT: *23, Sept 34*

CASE BOOK NO.: *28066*

USE BALL POINT PEN ONLY — PRESS FIRMLY   KEY   R — Requisition   D — Discontinued
                                                                CMO — Card Made Out   K — Kardex

DATE	TIME	PHYSICIANS' WRITTEN AND SIGNED ORDERS	R	CMO	D	K
Jan 7, 74		Stelazine 5 mg h.s. + 3 months				
		Cogentin 2 mg OD × 1 month				
		(has still some)				

Figure 25. Physician's order.

LAKESHORE PSYCHIATRIC HOSPITAL
TORONTO, ONTARIO

PHYSICIAN'S ORDERS

38

NAME: _Schellenberg_
Susan

ADDRESS:

AGE: 23, sept 34

WARD OR UNIT: ~~A~~ EP5 offskip

CASE BOOK NO.: 28066

PATIENT ALLERGIC TO

DIAGNOSIS

USE BALL POINT PEN ONLY — PRESS FIRMLY   KEY

R — Requisition   D — Discontinued
CMO — Card Made Out   K — Kardex

DATE	TIME	PHYSICIANS' WRITTEN AND SIGNED ORDERS	R	CMO	D	K
Oct. 9, 74		Stelazine 5 mg h.s. }				
		Cogentin 2 mg h.s. }				
		M ÷ ✗ 3 months				
		please mail				

Figure 26. Physician's order.

LAKESHORE PSYCHIATRIC HOSPITAL
TORONTO, ONTARIO

PHYSICIAN'S ORDERS

39

NAME: Susan Schollenberg

ADDRESS:

AGE: 23/Sept/34 (40)

WARD OR UNIT:

CASE BOOK NO.: E.S. aftercare

PATIENT ALLERGIC TO

DIAGNOSIS

USE BALL POINT PEN ONLY — PRESS FIRMLY   KEY   R – Requisition   D – Discontinued
                                                 CMO – Card Made Out   K – Kardex

DATE	TIME	PHYSICIANS' WRITTEN AND SIGNED ORDERS	R	CMO	D	K
July 2/75		Trifluoperazine 5 mg hs				
		Cogentin 2 mg hs				
		tr. × 1 month				
		Repeat 2×				
Aug 29/75		Same				
		Rx given on private Rx –				
		× 1 mr. Repeat 2×				
		She has medication cost				
		reimbursed				

PATIENT'S COPY   CONFIDENTIAL   NOT TO BE DUPLICATED
OR USED FOR ANY OTHER PURPOSE WITHOUT
FURTHER WRITTEN AUTHORIZATION OF THE
PATIENT.

Figure 27. Physician's order.

LAKESHORE PSYCHIATRIC HOSPITAL
TORONTO, ONTARIO

HO

PHYSICIAN'S ORDERS

NAME: *Schellenberg, Susan*

ADDRESS:

AGE: *23/09/34*

WARD OR UNIT:

CASE BOOK NO.:

PATIENT ALLERGIC TO
DIAGNOSIS

USE BALL POINT PEN ONLY — PRESS FIRMLY   KEY   R — Requisition   D — Discontinued
                                                        CMO — Card Made Out   K — Kardex

DATE	TIME	PHYSICIANS' WRITTEN AND SIGNED ORDERS	R	CMO	D	K
Jan 23/76		*Stelazine 5 mgs.* + *(min)*				
		Cogentin 2 mgs.				
		Repeat 2 x				

Figure 28. Physician's order.

Clinical Records

Figure 29. Outpatient service received.

MINISTRY OF HEALTH REPORT I

PSYCHIATRIC HOSPITAL OUTPATIENT MANAGEMENT

PATIENT SUMMARY OF DIRECT OUTPATIENT SERVICE RECEIVED

FROM JANUARY 1, 1975 TO DECEMBER 31, 1975

FACILITY NEW TORONTO
DATE OF REGISTRATION NOVEMBER 8, 1974
PATIENT NAME SCHEL, SU
CASEBOOK NUMBER 28066

DATE OF CONTACT	TYPE OF SERVICE		LENGTH OF SERVICE (MIN)	CONTACT STAFF	PROGRAM CODE	
07/[illegible]/75	MED. CHEMOTHERAPY	E	12	[illegible]	O-PATIENT	DIAG PHAM
31/[illegible]1/75	MED. CHEMOTHERAPY	E	12	[illegible]	O-PATIENT	DIAG PHAM
06/03/75	MED. CHEMOTHERAPY	E	12	[illegible]	O-PATIENT	DIAG PH
01/04/75	MED. CHEMOTHERAPY	E	12	[illegible]	O-PATIENT	DIAG PHAM
23/04/75	MED. CHEMOTHERAPY	E	12	[illegible]	O-PATIENT	DIAG PHAM
23/05/75	MED. CHEMOTHERAPY	E	4	[illegible]	O-PATIENT	DIAG PH
23/05/75	MED. CHEMOTHERAPY	E	10	[illegible]	O-PATIENT	DIAG PHAM
02/07/75	MED. CHEMOTHERAPY	E	10	[illegible]	O-PATIENT	ETOBICOKE
03/07/75	MED. CHEMOTHERAPY	E	12	[illegible]	O-PATIENT	DIAG PH

NO ACTIVITY FOR 90 DAYS OR MORE

CONFIDENTIAL NOT TO BE DUPLICATED OR USED FOR ANY OTHER PURPOSE WITHOUT FURTHER WRITTEN AUTHORIZATION OF THE PATIENT.

PATIENT'S COPY

3

Figure 30. Outpatient service received.

Glossary

Definitions for this glossary are based on information from *DSM-IV-TR*, *Comprehensive Textbook of Psychiatry/V*, *Dorland's Illustrated Medical Dictionary*, and *Neuropsychological Assessment*.[1] Because an older edition of the DSM would have been in use in 1969, I have indicated terminology, concepts, or practices that are now outdated or not used.

acetone A chemical found in small quantities in normal urine and in larger quantities in the urine of individuals with diabetes. An odour of acetone in the urine can be a sign of a diabetic condition.

acute This term refers to a condition with a short and relatively severe course that requires urgent medical attention.

acute schizophrenic reaction A psychiatric diagnosis used in the past when an individual experienced a sudden, severe emotional disturbance characterized by misinterpretation of and retreat from reality, delusions, hallucinations, ambivalence, inappropriate expression of feelings, and withdrawn, bizarre, or regressive behaviour. The individual diagnosed with this condition was believed to be experiencing symptoms in reaction to environmental conditions, and was viewed as likely to recover. Currently, a person with such symptoms might be diagnosed with a brief psychotic episode, an atypical psychotic episode, or an acute stress reaction. The diagnosis would depend on the nature, duration, and circumstances of patient's difficulties.

aftercare Health services provided to a person after she or he is discharged from hospital as a means of continuing with or monitoring treatment begun during the hospital stay.

ambulatory Patient is able to walk without assistance.

anti-anxiety medication A class of medications used to treat anxiety symptoms.

antipsychotic medication A class of chemically related medications usually prescribed to treat psychotic symptoms such as hallucinations and delusions; medications of this type are also described as major tranquilizers.

arteriosclerotic heart disease Heart disease characterized by thickening and loss of elasticity in the walls of arteries around the heart.

Ativan The trade name for lorazepam, a type of anti-anxiety medication chemically similar to Valium that is prescribed for anxiety or sleep problems.

b.i.d. An abbreviation of the Latin phrase *bis in die*; used as part of prescriptions to indicate that the medication should be taken twice a day.

blood morphology Laboratory tests for the presence of abnormalities in the structure of the blood cells.

BP 130/86 (rt.) This term written after the heading Circulatory System in the physical examination indicates that blood pressure reading was 130/86 on the right arm. This reading was likely considered normal at the time of Susan's hospital admission. The same blood pressure reading would be viewed today as borderline high for a 34-year-old woman (Susan's age at the time of her admission).

brief psychotic episode Under the *DSM-IV* diagnostic system, a brief psychotic episode is a condition where an individual experiences psychotic symptoms such as delusions, hallucinations, or disorganized speech for at least one day and not more than one month, then eventually returns to normal functioning.

Bright's disease A broad descriptive term used in the past for a type of kidney disease characterized by an excess of proteins in the urine and usually due to inflammation of capillaries within the kidneys.

catatonic dementia praecox A psychiatric diagnosis used in the past to describe a condition that would now be roughly comparable to a type of schizophrenia characterized by abnormal movements such as purposeless agitated activity, rigidity, or stupor.

Cogentin The trade name for benztropine mesylate, a medication often prescribed together with antipsychotic medication to reduce the severity of side effects such as tremors, rigidity, drooling, depressed expression, and shuffling gait.

cranials grossly intact, tendon reflexes ++, plantars These phrases written after the heading Nervous System in the physical examination indicate findings from the testing of reflexes in the head, arms, and feet.

C-V tenderness This term written after the heading Genito-urinary System in the physical examination indicates costo-vertebral tenderness, i.e., pain in an area of the back around the kidneys. Such pain could indicate a urinary tract infection.

defensive mechanisms In psychoanalytic theories of personality functioning, the phrase refers to ways of behaving, perceiving, or thinking that are used unconsciously by an individual to regulate feelings. All people use defensive mechanisms; defensive mechanisms are considered to be problematic only when they fail to assist the person in adapting effectively to internal and external realities.

delusion A false belief based on an incorrect inference about external reality that is not consistent with the individual's intelligence and cultural background and cannot be corrected by reasoning.

dissociation The splitting off from one another of ordinarily closely connected behaviour, thoughts, feelings, and sensations. Driving or walking on a familiar route, thinking of something else, and being unable to recall the trip is a common form of mild dissociation. Becoming so absorbed in a movie, book, or other activity that one fails to notice outside sounds or occurrences is another common form of mild dissociation. The sense of watching oneself from outside of one's own body is an example of a greater degree of dissociation.

dissociative states Those states in which complex behaviours take place outside of the awareness of one's predominant consciousness. Trances, blackouts, and identity fragmentation (i.e., multiple personalities) are examples of dissociative states where disruptions have occurred in the ordinarily integrated functions of consciousness, memory, identity, and perception.

DSM-IV An abbreviation for the *Diagnostic and Statistical Manual of Mental Disorders,* Fourth Edition. The *DSM-IV* is a book prepared and published by the American Psychiatric Association, which is a widely used standard reference for the classification and diagnosis of mental disorders.[2]

E.C.G. Electrocardiogram, a graph showing electrical changes in the muscles of the heart during heart beats. Such graphs are often used to investigate possible abnormalities in the functioning of the heart.

ego defences In psychoanalytic theory of personality function, ego defences are ways of behaving, perceiving, and thinking that are used unconsciously by the ego, the part of the personality that mediates between internal wishes and feelings and external reality.

ego strength In psychoanalytic theory, this concept refers to the ego's capacity and effectiveness in carrying out its purpose of assuring the self-preservation of the individual by mediating between internal wishes and feelings and external reality. An individual with great ego strength is able to balance the demands of internal feelings with the requirements of external reality in complex and effective ways. An individual with weak ego strength is unable to maintain an effective balance. An individual with serious emotional difficulties might, for example, become lost in fantasy to the point of disregarding personal care.

flashback Vivid re-experiencing of a highly emotionally charged past event; post-traumatic flashbacks can attain a hallucinatory vividness and involve horrifying memories of past events.

florid psychopathology Emotional disturbances where the individual's symptoms are evident in their most extreme form. For example, a person giving spontaneous, detailed descriptions of conversations with visitors from Mars, seeing visitors from Mars present during an interview with a health professional, and being unable to recognize the unreality of these perceptions would be described as showing florid psychopathology.

haemotology The branch of medicine that treats diseases and conditions of the blood and blood-forming tissues.

hallucinations False sensory perceptions not associated with real external stimuli, e.g., seeing a person in the room when no one is present (visual hallucination) or hearing someone speak when no one is present (auditory hallucination).

Hartford-Shipley Scale A psychological test that measures cognitive functioning and was likely the basis for determining that Susan's intelligence was in the average range. The test may have been used to screen for impairments that could indicate the presence of an organic brain condition. The Hartford-Shipley Scale is now viewed as poorly constructed and of limited use.

h.s. *See* q.h.s.

incoherence of thought or speech Speech that is disorganized and generally not understandable due to thoughts or words running together with no logical or grammatical connection.

insight This term used in the clinical records refers to the patient's ability to understand the true cause and meaning of a situation, particularly the nature of his or her own psychiatric or psychological problems. For example, a patient who sets fires in public buildings and blames his schoolteacher for causing him to do this would be said to have poor insight.

inspiratory wheeze over lt. upper lobe aut. + post These terms written in the physical examination after the heading Respiratory System indicate that when the patient was breathing in, some abnormal sounds could be heard in the back in the area of the upper lobe of the left lung.

intake survey This term in the psychological report probably refers to a questionnaire used at Lakeshore Hospital to gather information about each individual patient's background and psychological difficulties.

involuntary admission Involuntary admission means that the person does not consent freely but is required to come to and remain in hospital because a designated official—usually a physician—believes this necessary (because the person suffers from a mental disorder such that there is risk of serious, immediate danger to either him- or herself or to others). Once the necessary legal form is completed, the police have the authority to search for the person and bring him or her to the hospital, and the hospital has the authority to physically prevent the person from leaving until the date the certificate expires or until the certificate is cancelled by the treating physician.

judgment This term refers to the patient's ability to show good judgment, i.e., to assess a situation correctly and to act appropriately. Clinicians use tests such as asking a patient to tell the meaning of proverbs as a means of testing the patient's ability to reason and form judgments; the actions of the patient in real-life situations are also used by the clinician as a basis for deciding whether a patient shows good or impaired judgment. For example, if a patient believed that it was acceptable to set fires in public buildings, the patient's judgment would be described as poor.

L + A This entry in the physical examination the Eyes heading refers to testing of the eyes to determine the pupils' reactions to light (Light + Accommodation).

Largactil Trade name for chlorpromazine, a type of antipsychotic medication.

LOA This abbreviation in the doctor's order record stands for leave of absence; a doctor's permission (as noted on the order record) is required for a patient to leave the hospital temporarily during hospital treatment without being considered discharged and losing their hospital bed.

loose associations Thinking that is characterized by repeated shifts in ideas from one subject to another in a completely unrelated way; when the problem is severe, speech may become incoherent.

menses Menstruation.

mg Milligrams.

M.M.P.I., M.M. Personality Inventory These terms refer to the Minnesota Multiphasic Personality Inventory, a psychological test of personality functioning and levels of emotional distress. Test interpretation involves comparing the pattern of validity and clinical scale elevations with research findings and relating these elevations and patterns to psychological characteristics and states.

mood disorder A disturbance related to mood, i.e., pervasive and sustained emotion as experienced by the individual. Mood disorders include depression and mania.

neg Abbreviation for negative; in the clinical records, it is written after the heading Skeletal System in the physical examination and indicates that there were no medical findings indicative of pathology.

neuroleptic medication A term used in the past for a class of medications prescribed usually to treat psychotic symptoms such as hallucinations and delusions. This class of medications is currently described as antipsychotics or major tranquilizers.

obsession This term is used in the clinical records to indicate pathological persistence of an irresistible thought or feeling that cannot be eliminated from consciousness by reasoning and is associated with anxiety.

orientation This term refers to the patient's awareness of where he or she is in space and time. Patients with some types of serious problems become seriously disoriented concerning place, time, and person, and may, for example, be unable to recognize that they are in a hospital, unable to state the month or year, unable to state their own names.

outpatient A patient who comes to appointments at a clinic or doctor's office as opposed to an in-patient who stays in hospital. Also used as an adjective to describe health services or clinics where patients come for appointments (as opposed to in-patient services, which are provided to patients staying on a hospital ward).

para IV This term under the Digestive System and Abdomen heading in the physical examination indicates that the patient reported a history of four pregnancies that resulted in the birth of viable offspring (from the Latin *pario*, to bring forth).

paranoid schizophrenia A type of schizophrenia characterized by false beliefs (delusions) concerning persecution, grandeur, control, or the significance of others' behaviour in reference to oneself. For example, an individual suffering from paranoid schizophrenia might experience the radio announcer as repeatedly delivering a special message directed personally to the individual and threatening to poison him or her.

partial S.C. test *See* S.C. test.

perceptual disturbances Abnormalities in perception—that is, in the mental processes that bring sensory information into conscious awareness. Hallucinations are a type of perceptual disturbance.

physician's application The legal form that authorizes the police and hospital staff to require a person to remain in hospital even against their wishes. The form must be completed by an appropriate authority such as a physician or justice of the peace who has seen the person not longer than seven days previously. To complete the form, the authority must document evidence that the person suffers from a mental illness that could result in injury to self or others.

psychodrama A type of psychotherapy characterized by the use of dramatic enactments of emotionally significant material, such as interactions with parents or dreams, to assist the individual in gaining personal insight and resolving emotional difficulties.

psychosis A mental disturbance where the individual is unable to distinguish reality from fantasy. In such a state, an individual is unable to make objective evaluations or reasonable judgments about the world outside him- or herself.

psychotropic medication Medication that has active psychological effects, for example, reduces anxiety or suppresses hallucinations.

q.h.s. Abbreviation for Latin phrase *quaque hora somni*; used as part of prescriptions to indicate that the medication should be taken every evening before sleeping.

rationalization A type of defensive mechanism in which the individual uses rational explanations to justify attitudes, beliefs, or behaviour that might otherwise be unacceptable.

repression A type of defensive mechanism in which an action or feeling is withheld or expelled from consciousness.

Rx Abbreviation for the Latin *recipe* meaning "take;" used in clinical records to mean "prescription" or "treated with."

scaphoid This term under the heading Digestive System and Abdomen in the physical examination indicates a concave abdomen.

schizophrenia Under the *DSM-IV* diagnostic system, schizophrenia is a severe mental disturbance that seriously interferes with an individual's ability to work, care for self, or relate to others for at least six months; individuals diagnosed with schizophrenia have also suffered for at least one month with two or more of the following symptoms: delusions, hallucinations, disorganized speech, grossly disorganized or catatonic behaviour. Dr. Mary Seeman describes further how this diagnosis has changed over the years, and that it is somewhat different now than at the time when Susan was admitted to hospital.

schiziphreniform disorder Under the *DSM-IV* diagnostic system, schiziphreniform disorder is a condition similar to schizophrenia except of shorter duration and less severely incapacitating.

S.C. test The sentence completion test is a psychological test in which the person taking the test is asked to complete a series of incomplete sentences such as "My biggest worry is …" Responses are used to evaluate personality functioning and emotional issues of importance to the patient.

Stelazine Trade name for trifluoperazine, a type of antipsychotic medication.

striae gravidarum This term under the heading Digestive System and Abdomen refers to stretch marks associated with pregnancy.

T+A This entry under the heading Operations refers to tonsils and adenoids. It indicates that Susan reported a history of surgery to remove tonsils and adenoids.

tardive dyskinesia A condition characterized by the development of abnormal movements after taking antipsychotic medication for a period of some months. The movements can include uncontrollable twitches, spasms, and writhing movements and can affect any of the voluntary muscles, including these in eyelids, tongue, larynx, diaphragm, neck, arms, legs, and torso. In some instances, the movements cease when the individual stops taking medication; in other cases, the condition is irreversible, i.e., the movements continue even after the individual stops medication.

thought disorder Disturbance in the form (as opposed to the content) of thought. A person with a thought disorder may, for example, shift repeatedly from one subject to another in a completely unrelated way (loosening of associations), create new words (neologisms) for personal, idiosyncratic reasons, or use illogical constructs.

tonic contraction A muscle contraction that develops slowly and shows a prolonged phase of relaxation. For individuals with mental health difficulties, a tonic contraction can be either voluntary or involuntary and either a nervous manifestation or a drug side effect. The psychologist describes Susan's moving in a manner that involved a tonic contraction, perhaps a lifting of her arm, and seems to regard the movements as an aspect of Susan's difficulties.

trifluoperzine A type of antipsychotic medication, often referred to by its trade name, Stelazine.

Trilafon Trade name for perphenazine, a type of antipsychotic medication.

urinalysis Laboratory tests to determine whether there are any abnormalities in the urine.

VDRL Abbreviation for venereal disease research laboratories. In the clinical records, a check in the box VDRL/Non-Reactive indicates that a blood test for syphilis was negative. At the time of Susan's hospital admission, Ontario law required this test to be performed on all persons admitted to hospital as a means of identifying individuals infected with syphilis. The goal was to prevent the spread of the disease by treating the infected person and identifying any others who might also be infected. The VDRL remains in use.

Notes

1 American Psychiatric Association, *Diagnostic and Statistical Manual of Mental Disorders*, 4th ed., rev. (Washington, DC: American Psychiatric Press, 2000); Harold I. Kaplan, Benjamin J. Sadock (eds.), *Comprehensive Textbook of Psychiatry/V,* 5th ed., Vols. 1–2 (London: Williams and Wilkins, 1989); William Alexander Newland Dorland (ed.), *Dorland's Illustrated Medical Dictionary* (Philadelphia: W.B. Saunders, 1994); and Muriel D. Lezak, *Neuropsychological Assessment*, 2nd ed. (New York: Oxford University Press, 1983).
2 American Psychiatric Association, *Diagnostic and Statistical Manual.*